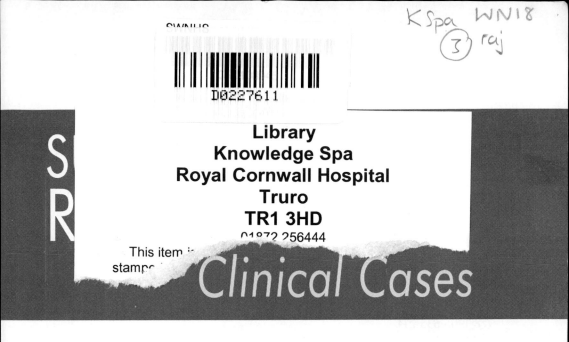

S

R

Clinical Cases

PRABHAKAR RAJIAH MBBS MD FRCR
Diagnostic Radiologist
Cleveland Clinic
USA

BISWARANJAN BANERJEE MBBS FRCS DMRD FRCR
Consultant Diagnostic Radiologist
Tameside General Hospital
UK

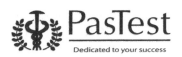

PasTest
Dedicated to your success

© 2008 PASTEST LTD
Egerton Court
Parkgate Estate
Knutsford
Cheshire
WA16 8DX
Telephone: 01565 752000

First Published 2008

ISBN: 1905 635 214
978 1905 635 214

A catalogue record for this book is available from the British Library.
The information contained within this book was obtained by the author from reliable sources. However, while every effort has been made to ensure its accuracy, no responsibility for loss, damage or injury occasioned to any person acting or refraining from action as a result of information contained herein can be accepted by the publishers or author.

PasTest Revision Books and Intensive Courses
PasTest has been established in the field of postgraduate medical education since 1972, providing revision books and intensive study courses for doctors preparing for their professional examinations.
Books and courses are available for the following specialties:

MRCGP, MRCP Parts 1 and 2, MRCPCH Parts 1 and 2, MRCS, MRCOG Parts 1 and 2, DRCOG, DCH, FRCA, Dentistry.

For further details contact:
PasTest, Freepost, Knutsford, Cheshire WA16 7BR
Tel: 01565 752000 Fax: 01565 650264
www.pastest.co.uk enquiries@pastest.co.uk

Cover images: Broken upper arm bone, X-ray
DU CANE MEDICAL IMAGING LTD/SCIENCE PHOTO LIBRARY
Arthritis of the spine, MRI scan
ZEPHYR/SCIENCE PHOTO LIBRARY

Text prepared by Carnegie Book Production, Lancaster
Printed and bound in the UK by Athenaeum Press, Gateshead

CONTENTS

INTRODUCTION

Radiology is a rapidly evolving field with new technological developments emerging every year. It has become an integral component of the diagnostic and therapeutic aspects of every medical speciality and plays a vital role in management of patients. Although the role of plain X-rays in diagnosis is progressively decreasing, they still have their place in the initial stages of patient management. Ultrasound and CT have become the commonly used modalities in diagnosis. MRI is very useful in assessment of musculoskeletal, central nervous and cardiovascular systems.

Radiological pictures are also increasingly used in many postgraduate examinations. Hence it is essential for clinicians and radiologists alike to be well-informed in the appropriate investigation for any clinical case and be aware of the radiological findings in each clinical scenario.

Surgical Radiology: Clinical Cases consists of 200 cases and approximately 360 images. The book is divided into six sections – Gastrointestinal and hepatobiliary radiology, Genitourinary radiology, Musculoskeletal radiology, Neuroradiology, Paediatric radiology and Chest and Cardiovascular radiology. Each case is presented with pertinent history, followed by radiological pictures and 7–10 questions. The second part of each chapter contains the case diagnosis, clinical features, and radiological findings, imaging techniques, diagnostic algorithm, differential diagnosis and management.

The book covers almost the entire gamut of radiological findings in common surgical conditions. The cases include pictures from multiple modalities such as X-rays, ultrasound, Doppler, CT scan, MRI and nuclear medicine, reflecting the current practice. The cases range from the very common to unusual and challenging.

The format of the book, the images and discussion would be ideal not only for surgery and radiology trainees preparing for postgraduate exams, but also for medical students intending to specialise in either of these fields and surgeons and radiologists who wish to update their knowledge on the radiological aspects of common and uncommon surgical conditions.

Dr Prabhakar Rajiah
Dr Biswaranjan Banerjee

1

GASTROINTESTINAL AND HEPATOBILIARY RADIOLOGY

QUESTIONS

Case 1.1

A 67-year-old woman presents with abdominal pain, haematemesis and weight loss. Clinical examination showed a hard mass in the epigastric region.

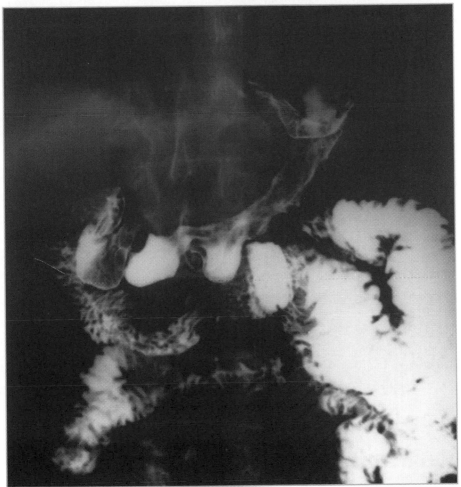

Fig 1.1

1. What do you see on the barium meal?
2. What is the name of this appearance?
3. What is the diagnosis? What causes this appearance?
4. What are the other causes of this appearance?
5. What are the radiological features of this disease?
6. What other investigations are required?
7. What is the treatment?

Answers on pages 63–140

Case 1.2

A 71-year-old man presents with fatigue, abdominal pain and rectal bleeding.

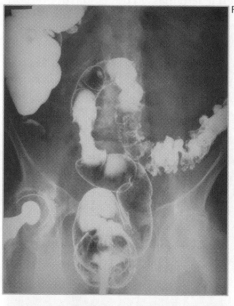
Fig 1.2a

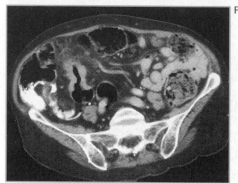
Fig 1.2b

1. What do you see on the barium enema and CT scan?
2. What is the diagnosis?
3. What pre-existing conditions increase the risk of this disease?
4. What investigations are used in early diagnosis of this disease?
5. What are the common locations and type of the lesion?
6. What is the role of radiology in the management of this disease?
7. What is the pathophysiology of this appearance?
8. What is the differential diagnosis and treatment?

Answers on pages 63–140

Case 1.3

A 31-year-old man presents with severe abdominal pain, vomiting, nausea and tenderness. On examination, he is febrile and tachycardic and there is severe rebound tenderness in his abdomen.

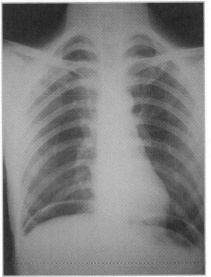
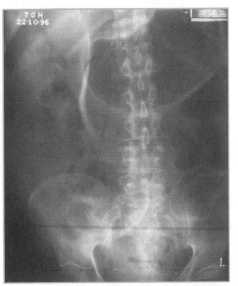

Fig 1.3a   Fig 1.3b

1. What do you observe on the plain X-ray of the chest?
2. What are the findings on the plain X-ray of the abdomen taken in the supine position?
3. What is the diagnosis?
4. What are the radiographic signs of this presentation?
5. What are the causes of this appearance?
6. What other conditions can mimic this abnormality?
7. When can this radiographic abnormality be seen in a patient without any abdominal symptoms?

Answers on pages 63–140

Case 1.4

A 44-year-old woman presented with intermittent right upper quadrant pain, right shoulder pain and vomiting. On examination, there is severe right upper quadrant tenderness.

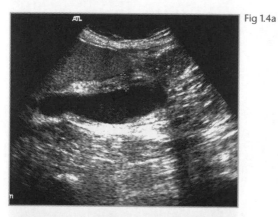

Fig 1.4a

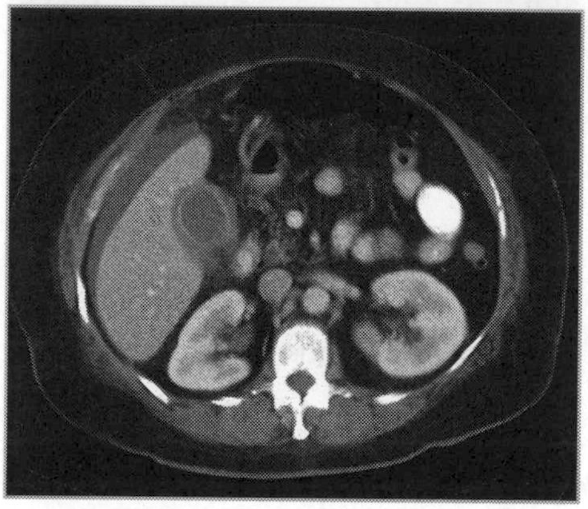

Fig 1.4b

1. What do you observe on ultrasonography and on the CT scan?
2. What is the diagnosis?
3. What are the aetiology and pathophysiology of this disease?
4. What are the radiological features? What other tests can be performed to confirm the diagnosis?
5. What are the complications?
6. What is Mirizzi syndrome?
7. What is the differential diagnosis?
8. What is the role of radiology in the treatment of this disease?

Answers *on pages 63–140*

Case 1.5

A 15-year-old female pedestrian was hit by a truck and presented to the accident and emergency department (A&E) with low BP and upper abdominal pain. On examination, she had tachycardia and tenderness in the left upper quadrant.

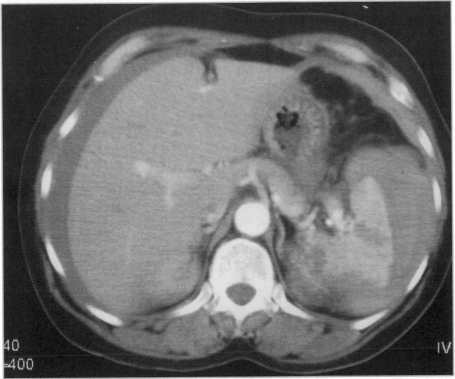

Fig 1.5

1. What do you see on the CT scan of the abdomen?
2. What is the diagnosis?
3. What is the mechanism of injury?
4. What are the clinical features?
5. What are the radiological features and grading?
6. What is the management?
7. What are the indications for surgery and the complications?
8. What are the non-traumatic causes of this disorder?

Answers on pages 63–140

Case 1.6

A 7-year-old girl presents with colicky, right upper quadrant pain, fever and jaundice. On examination, she is febrile and tender in the right upper quadrant. The liver is palpable 1 finger breadth below costal margin.

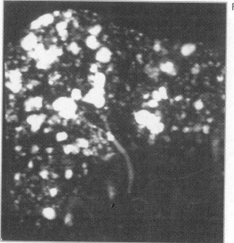
Fig 1.6a

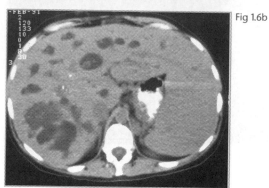
Fig 1.6b

1. What are the findings on MRI of the liver?
2. What are the findings on the CT scan?
3. What is the diagnosis?
4. What is the aetiology?
5. What is the classification of this disease?
6. What are the clinical features?
7. What are the complications?
8. What are the radiological features and differential diagnosis?

Answers *on pages 63–140*

Case 1.7

A 41-year-old man presents with severe haematemesis and jaundice. On examination, he is tachycardic and anaemic.

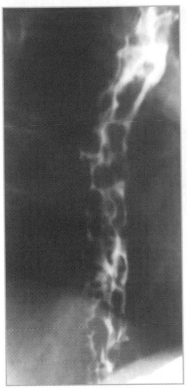

Fig 1.7a

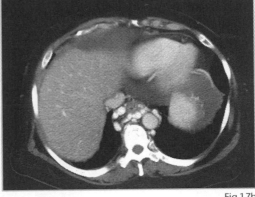

Fig 1.7b

1. What are the findings seen on the barium and CT scans?
2. What is the diagnosis?
3. What are the types of this process and the causes?
4. What is the relevant anatomy?
5. What are the radiological findings?
6. What is the differential diagnosis?
7. What is the treatment?
8. What is the role of radiology in management?

Answers *on pages 63–140*

Case 1.8

A 38-year-old woman presents with abdominal pain, vomiting and distension. On examination, her abdomen is distended and bowel sounds are increased.

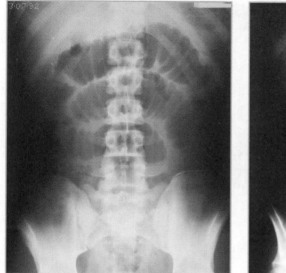

Fig 1.8a

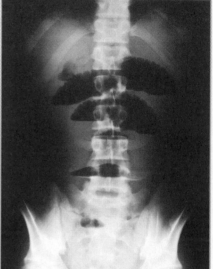

Fig 1.8b

1. What do you see on the plain X-rays of the abdomen?

2. What is the diagnosis?

3. What are the types and causes of this disease process?

4. What are the radiological findings in this disease?

5. What are the variants of this disease?

6. What is the role of the CT scan?

Answers *on pages 63–140*

Case 1.9

A 39-year-old woman presents with right-sided abdominal pain, vomiting, nausea and dyspepsia.

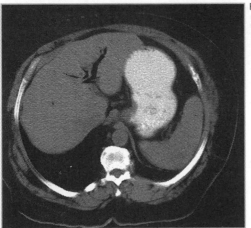

Fig 1.9a

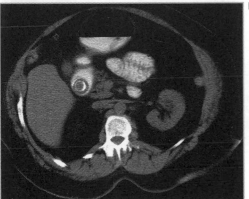

Fig 1.9b

1. What do you observe on these CT scans?
2. What is the diagnosis?
3. What is the aetiopathology?
4. What is the most common site?
5. What are the radiological features?
6. What is Rigler's triad?
7. What are the complications and management?
8. What is the differential diagnosis?

Answers *on pages 63–140*

Case 1.10

A 43-year-old woman presents with vague, dull abdominal pain. Clinical examination is unremarkable. There is no organomegaly.

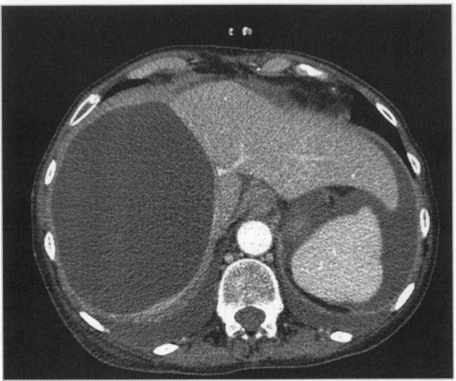

Fig 1.10

1. What do you see on the CT scan?
2. What is the diagnosis?
3. What is the origin of this lesion?
4. What are the imaging features?
5. What is the differential diagnosis?
6. What are the complications?
7. What is the management?

Answers on pages 63–140

Case 1.11

A 47-year-old woman presents with severe epigastric pain. On examination, epigastric tenderness was noted and the patient was tachycardic.

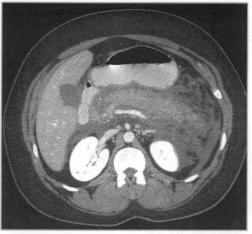

Fig 1.11a

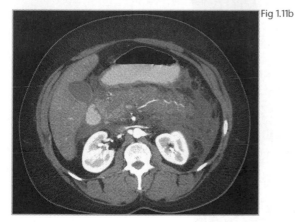

Fig 1.11b

1. What do you see on the first CT scan?
2. What is the diagnosis?
3. What do you see on the follow-up CT scan?
4. What are the clinical features and lab abnormalities in this disease?
5. What are the contributory factors?
6. How is the disease staged?
7. What is the optimal imaging test in evaluation of this disease?
8. How is this patient managed and what are the complications?

Answers on pages 63–140

Case 1.12

A 32-year-old man presented with pain and a lump in the lower abdomen on the left side. Clinical examination revealed a tender lump in the left inguinal region. Bowel sounds were sluggish and his abdomen was distended.

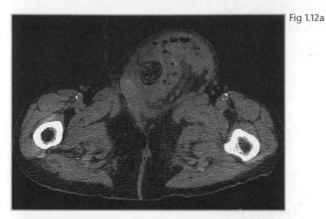

Fig 1.12a

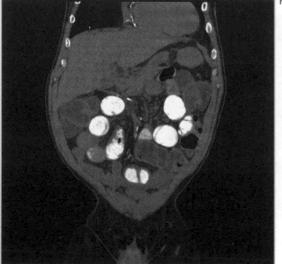

Fig 1.12b

1. What do you see on the CT scans?
2. What is the diagnosis? What complication has developed?
3. What are the common types?
4. What are the clinical features and complications?
5. What are the salient features in imaging?
6. What is the treatment of this condition?

Answers on pages 63–140

Case 1.13

A 55-year-old man presented with dysphagia for solid foods, chest pain and weight loss.

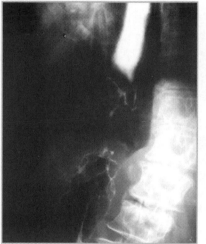

Fig 1.13a

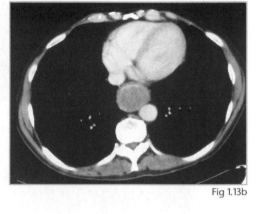

Fig 1.13b

1. What are the findings seen on the barium swallow and the CT scan?
2. What is the diagnosis?
3. What are the histological types?
4. What are the causes and clinical features?
5. What investigations are done routinely and how is the disease staged?
6. What are the important parameters that are assessed on the CT scan?
7. What is the management of a thoracic lesion?
8. What palliative options are available for management?

Answers on pages 63–140

Case 1.14

A 65-year-old man presents with abdominal pain, vomiting and distension. Clinical examination revealed paucity of bowel sounds.

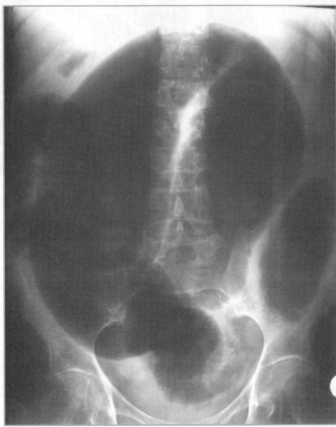

Fig 1.14

1. What do you see on the plain X-ray of the abdomen?
2. What is the diagnosis?
3. What is the aetiology of this condition?
4. What are the predisposing factors?
5. What are the findings on the X-ray?
6. What other investigations can be done?
7. What are the complications?
8. What is the treatment?

Answers *on pages 63–140*

Case 1.15

A 48-year-old woman presents abdominal distension and pain. Clinical examination shows a distended abdomen.

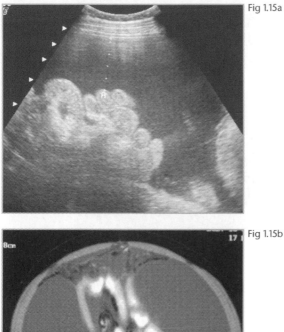

Fig 1.15a

Fig 1.15b

1. What do you see on ultrasonography and on the CT scan?
2. What is the diagnosis?
3. What are the causes?
4. What are the radiological features?
5. How do you differentiate benign and malignant subtypes of this condition?
6. What is the flow of fluid in this condition?
7. What is the earliest site of fluid collection in the abdomen?
8. What are the causes of high-density collection?
9. What is the role of radiology in diagnosis and treatment?

Answers on pages 63–140

Case 1.16

A 32-year-old man presents with abdominal pain and discomfort.

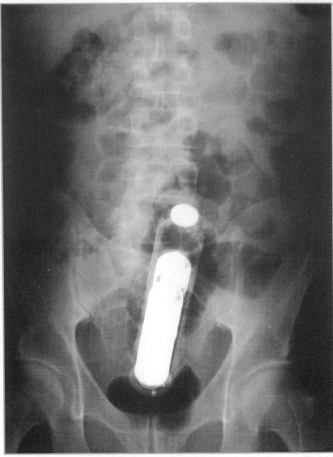

Fig 1.16

1. What is the diagnosis, based on the X-ray?
2. What are the common sites?
3. What are the common objects?
4. What are the reasons?
5. What are the radiological features and the imaging protocol?
6. What are the complications?
7. What is the treatment?

Answers on pages 63–140

Case 1.17

A 19-year-old man presented with chest pain and dyspnoea.

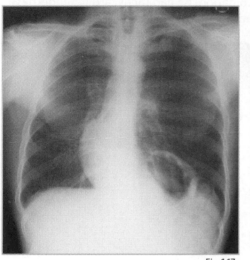

Fig 1.17a

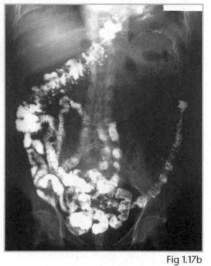

Fig 1.17b

1. What are the findings on the chest X-ray?
2. What are the findings on the barium enema?
3. What is the diagnosis?
4. What is the development of this lesion?
5. What are the clinical features?
6. What are the possible contents of this condition?
7. What is eventration?
8. What is Berquist's triad?

Answers on pages 63–140

Case 1.18

A 27-year-old man was involved in a road traffic accident and presents with right sided abdominal pain. On examination, he had tachycardia, tenderness and guarding in the right upper quadrant of the abdomen.

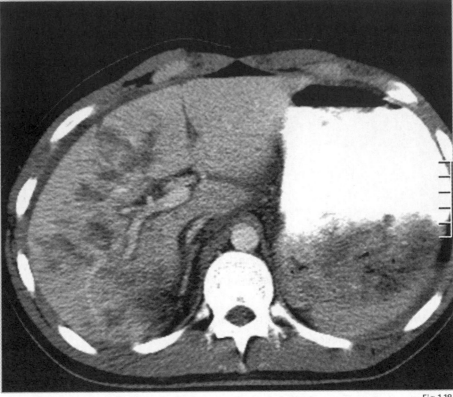

Fig 1.18

1. What do you see on the CT scan of the abdomen?
2. What is the diagnosis?
3. What is the grading of this lesion?
4. What are the common locations?
5. What are the radiological features?
6. What are the complications?
7. What is the treatment?

Answers on pages 63–140

Case 1.19

A 29-year-old woman presents with abdominal pain, tenderness and fever. On examination, there is tenderness in the right upper quadrant.

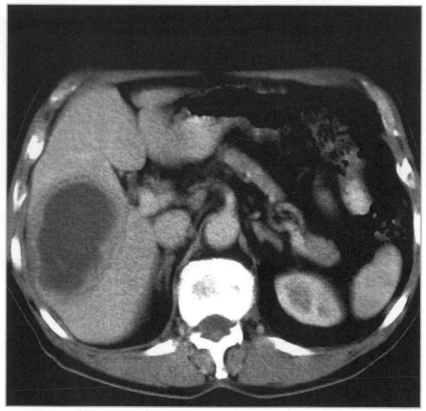

Fig 1.19

1. What do you find on the CT scan?
2. What is the diagnosis?
3. What are the causative organisms?
4. What is the mode of spread?
5. What is the characteristic location?
6. What are the radiological features on ultrasonography, CT and MRI?
7. What is the differential diagnosis?
8. What are the complications?
9. What is the role of radiology in treatment?

Answers on pages 63–140

Case 1.20

A 35-year-old woman presents with jaundice and abdominal pain. On examination, the liver is not enlarged and there is no palpable mass in the upper abdomen.

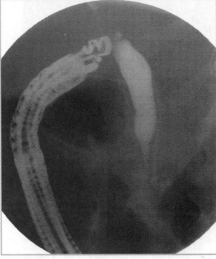

Fig 1.20a

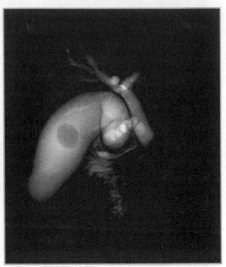

Fig 1.20b

1. What are the findings on the first test?
2. What is the second test? What do you find?
3. What is the diagnosis?
4. What is the differential diagnosis of this condition?
5. What are the principles, advantages and disadvantages of the second test?
6. What diseases can be diagnosed by the second test?
7. What is the role of radiology in treatment?

Answers on pages 63–140

Case 1.21

A 39-year-old woman presents with abdominal pain, vomiting, weight loss and haematemesis. On examination, a mass is felt in the epigastric region.

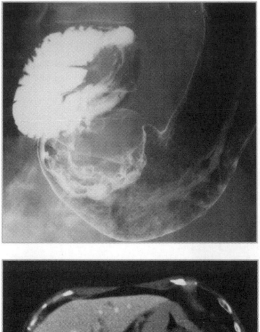

Fig 1.21a

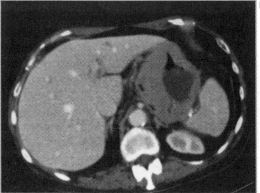

Fig 1.21b

1. What do you see on the barium meal and CT scan of the abdomen?
2. What is the diagnosis?
3. What are the pathological types and patterns of spread?
4. What are the common locations?
5. What are the predisposing factors?
6. What is the pattern of spread?
7. What are the imaging features?
8. What is the differential diagnosis?

Answers on pages 63–140

Case 1.22

A 56-year-old man, with a history of cirrhosis secondary to hepatitis B, presents with right upper quadrant pain and jaundice. The LFT is markedly abnormal. On examination, a non-tender, firm mass was felt in the right upper quadrant.

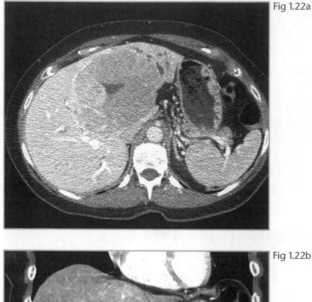

Fig 1.22a

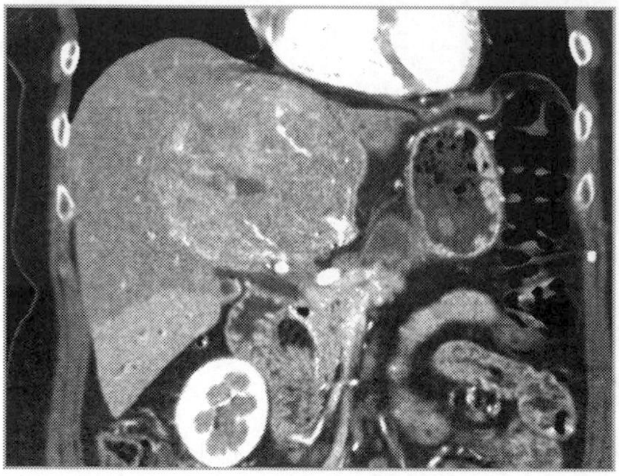

Fig 1.22b

1. What do you see on the CT scan?
2. What is the diagnosis?
3. What are the predisposing factors and clinical features?
4. What are the radiological features?
5. What is the differential diagnosis?
6. What is the management of this condition? What is the role of radiology in management?

Answers *on pages 63–140*

Case 1.23

A 62-year-old man presents with constipation, abdominal pain and distension. On examination, the abdomen is distended and bowel sounds are sluggish.

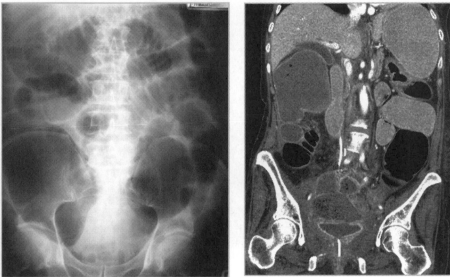

Fig 1.23a   Fig 1.23b

1.   What do you observe on the plain X-ray and CT scan of the abdomen?
2.   What is the diagnosis?
3.   What are the causes of this disease process?
4.   What are the radiological findings in this disease?
5.   What is the role of the CT scan?
6.   What is the role of barium in imaging this disease process?
7.   What is the significance of caecal size?
8.   What are the causes of this disease in children?

Answers on pages 63–140

Case 1.24

A 32-year-old man presents with epigastric pain, fullness and heartburn.

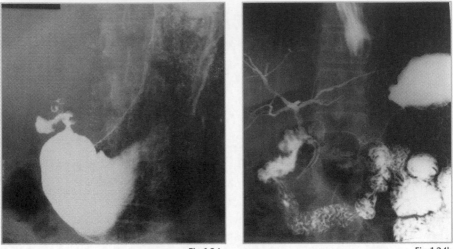

Fig 1.24a   Fig 1.24b

1. What are the findings on the first barium meal picture?
2. What is the diagnosis? What complication has developed in the second picture?
3. What is the aetiology and what are the predisposing factors?
4. What are the characteristic locations?
5. What are the radiological features?
6. What is the differential diagnosis?
7. What are the complications and what is the treatment?

Answers *on pages 63–140*

Case 1.25

A 24-year-old man presents with abdominal pain, back pain and a discharging wound in the perianal region.

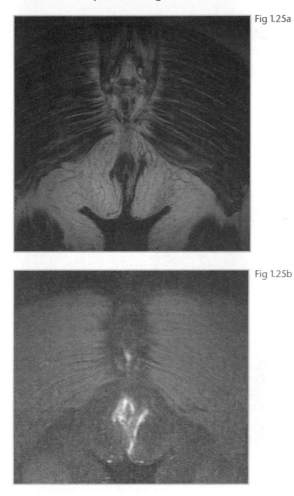

Fig 1.25a

Fig 1.25b

1. What is this investigation and what do you observe?
2. What is the diagnosis?
3. What are the causes of this condition?
4. What is the relevant anatomy of this region?
5. What are the types?
6. What is the role of imaging?
7. What are the important features to be assessed in imaging?

Answers on pages 63–140

Case 1.26

A 39-year-old man presents with severe chest pain after an endoscopic procedure for removal of a foreign body.

Fig 1.26a

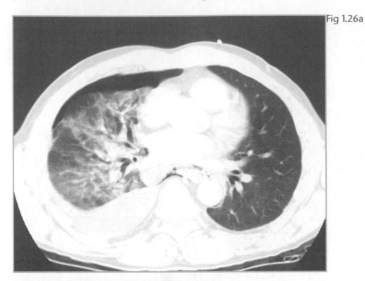

Fig 1.26b

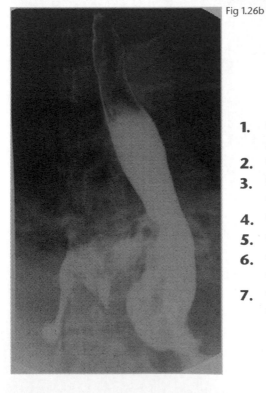

1. What do you observe on the CT scan and contrast swallow?

2. What is the diagnosis?

3. What are the predisposing factors?

4. What is the common location?

5. What are the clinical features?

6. What are the radiological features?

7. What are the complications and treatment?

Answers on pages 63–140

Case 1.27

A 29-year-old immunosuppressed patient develops dysphagia and chest pain. The abdomen was normal.

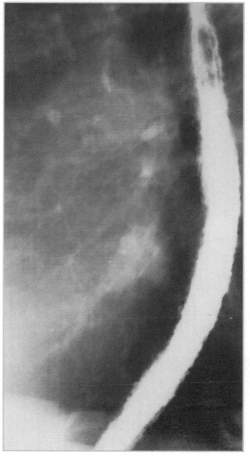

Fig 1.27

1. What do you observe on the barium swallow?
2. What is the diagnosis?
3. What are the predisposing factors?
4. What is the pathophysiology of this disease?
5. What are the radiological features?
6. What are the complications?
7. What is the differential diagnosis?
8. What is the treatment?

Answers on pages 63–140

Case 1.28

A 3-year-old girl presents with right upper quadrant colicky pain, fever and jaundice. On examination, she is febrile, tender on the right upper quadrant, with no palpable mass.

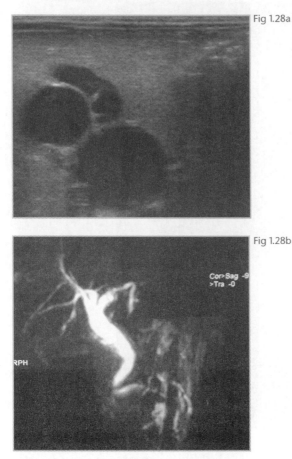

Fig 1.28a

Fig 1.28b

Cor>Sag -9
>Tra -0

RPH

1. What are the findings on ultrasonography of the abdomen?
2. What are the findings on MRI?
3. What is the diagnosis?
4. What are the aetiology and classification of this disease?
5. What are the clinical features and complications?
6. What are the radiological features and differential diagnosis?

Answers on pages 63–140

Case 1.29

A 53-year-old woman presented with colicky right upper quadrant pain. On examination, there is no palpable mass in the abdomen.

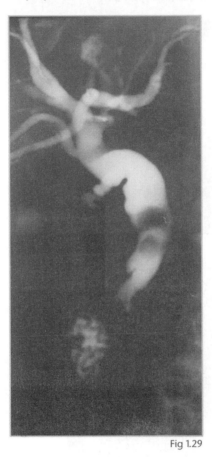

Fig 1.29

1. What do you observe in this investigation?
2. What is the diagnosis?
3. What are the complications of the investigations?
4. What are the clinical features and complications of this condition?
5. What are the common predisposing causes?
6. What are the types based on composition?
7. What are the radiological features?
8. What is the treatment?
9. What is Courvoisier's law?

Answers *on pages 63–140*

Case 1.30

A 12-year-old boy was involved in a road traffic accident and presented with abdominal pain, tenderness and guarding.

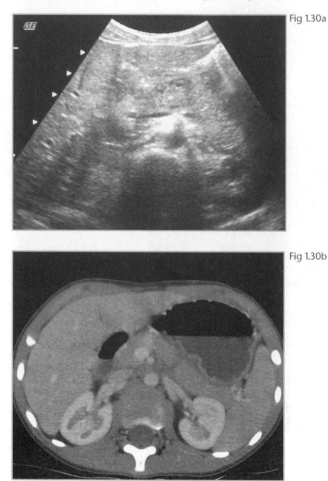

Fig 1.30a

Fig 1.30b

1. What do you see on the ultrasound and CT scans of the abdomen?
2. What is the diagnosis?
3. What is the grading of this lesion?
4. What are the common locations?
5. What are the radiological features?
6. What are the complications?
7. What is the treatment?

Answers on pages 63–140

Case 1.31

A 40-year-old woman presents with abdominal pain, diarrhoea, weight loss and episodes of flushing for several weeks.

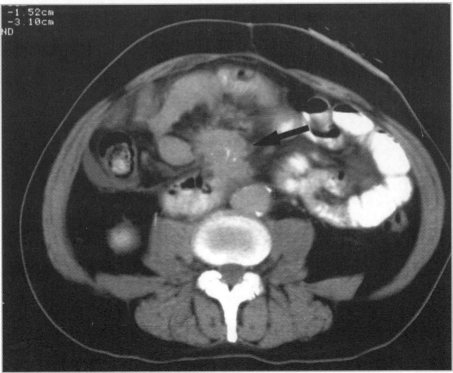

Fig 1.31

1. What are the findings in the CT scan (see arrow)?
2. What is the diagnosis?
3. What are the common sites of this disease process?
4. What are the origin of the disease and the symptoms?
5. What are the radiological features and the characteristic finding?
6. What are the complications?
7. What is the differential diagnosis?
8. What is the treatment?

Answers *on pages 63–140*

Case 1.32

An 11-year-old girl presents with abdominal pain, loss of weight, loose stools with blood and fever. On examination she is febrile. There is tenderness in the right iliac fossa. The bowel sounds were normal.

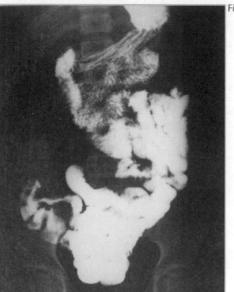

Fig 1.32a

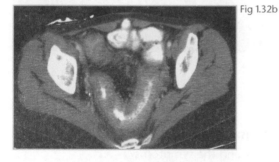

Fig 1.32b

1. What are the findings on the first picture?
2. What do you observe on the CT scan of the abdomen?
3. What is the diagnosis?
4. What are the clinical features?
5. What are the radiological features of this condition?
6. What is the differential diagnosis?
7. What are the complications?
8. What is the treatment?

Answers *on pages 63–140*

Case 1.33

A 37-year-old woman presented with abdominal pain, fever, weight loss and bloody diarrhoea. On examination she has tenderness in the lower abdomen.

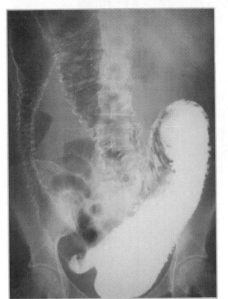
Fig 1.33a

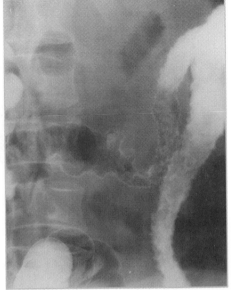
Fig 1.33b

1. What are the findings from the barium enema?
2. What is the diagnosis? What complications do you observe?
3. What are the clinical features?
4. What are the characteristic locations?
5. What are the radiological findings?
6. What are the complications?
7. What is the risk of malignancy?
8. What is the differential diagnosis?
9. What is the treatment?

Answers on pages 63–140

Case 1.34

A 28-year-old man presented with rectal bleeding and anaemia.

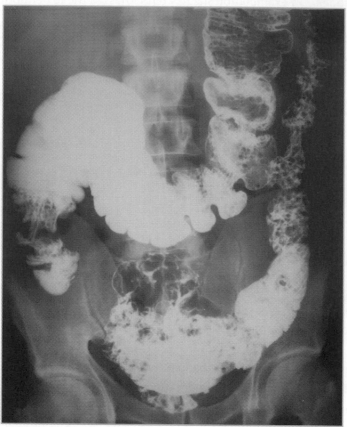

Fig 1.34

1. What are the findings from the barium enema?
2. What is the diagnosis?
3. What syndrome does the patient have?
4. What are the radiological features?
5. What are the histological types of this abnormality?
6. What is the risk of malignancy?
7. What is the management of this condition?
8. What are the other syndromes with similar features?

Answers *on pages 63–140*

Case 1.35

A 63-year-old man presents with rectal bleeding and anaemia. Clinical examination shows no abdominal mass, but a hard mass was felt on per rectum examination.

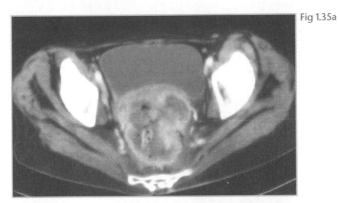

Fig 1.35a

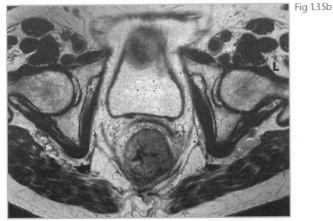

Fig 1.35b

1. What are the findings seen on the CT and MR scans?
2. What is the diagnosis?
3. What are the histological types and the predisposing factors?
4. What are the diagnostic tests used?
5. What are the radiological features and complications?
6. What are the important parameters that are assessed by CT and MRI?
7. What is the radiological differential diagnosis?
8. What is the role of radiology in treatment?

Answers *on pages 63–140*

Case 1.36

A 57-year-old woman presents with chest pain, heartburn, dysphagia and vomiting.

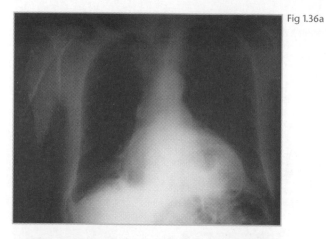

Fig 1.36a

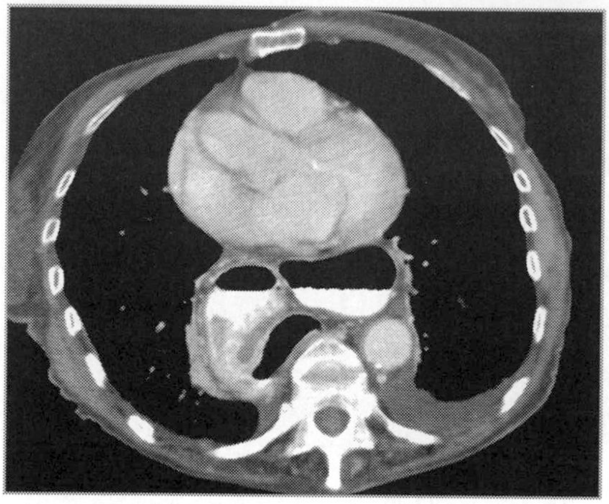

Fig 1.36b

1. What do you observe on the plain X-ray and CT scan?
2. What is the diagnosis?
3. What are the types?
4. What are the radiological features?
5. What is Saint's triad?
6. What are the complications?
7. What is the differential diagnosis?
8. What is the treatment?

Answers *on pages 63–140*

Case 1.37

A 37-year-old woman presents with dysphagia, coughing and vomiting.

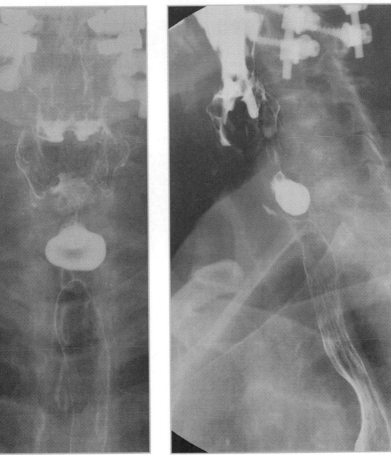

Fig 1.37a

Fig 1.37b

1. What do you see on the barium swallow?
2. What is the diagnosis?
3. What is the pathophysiology of this disease?
4. What are the clinical features?
5. What are the radiological findings?
6. What are the variants of this disease?
7. What is the treatment?
8. What are the complications and associations?

Answers *on pages 63–140*

Case 1.38

A 35-year-old woman presents with dysphagia for liquids and chest pain.

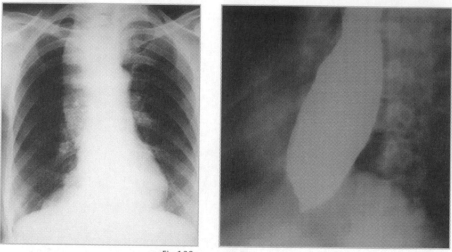

Fig 1.38a   Fig 1.38b

1. What do you see on the chest X-ray and barium swallow?
2. What is the diagnosis?
3. What is the pathophysiology of this disease?
4. What are the radiological findings?
5. What is Hurst's phenomenon?
6. What are the variants of this disease?
7. What is the differential diagnosis?
8. What are the treatment and complications of this disease?

Answers on pages 63–140

Case 1.39

A 54-year-old woman presents with dysphagia, heartburn, regurgitation and coughs. The first picture was taken during swallowing of barium and the second picture after completion of drinking of barium.

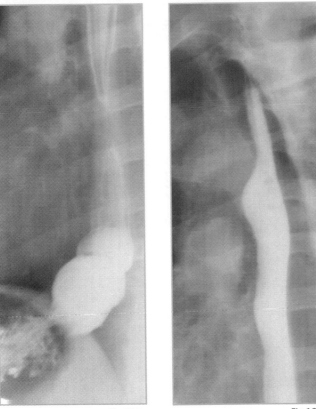

Fig 1.39a   Fig 1.39b

1. What do you see on this investigation?
2. What is the diagnosis?
3. What is the mechanism of development of this condition?
4. What radiological tests are useful for diagnosis?
5. What other tests are useful in diagnosis?
6. What are the radiological findings?
7. What are the complications?
8. What is the treatment of this disease?

Answers on pages 63–140

Case 1.40

A 13-year-old girl presents with flank pain, nausea and vomiting, and weight loss. On examination there is no palpable mass or tenderness in the abdomen.

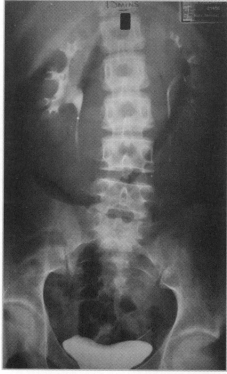

Fig 1.40a

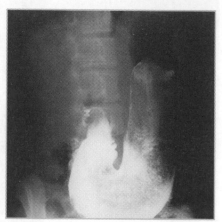

Fig 1.40b

1. What are the findings on the intravenous urogram (IVU)?
2. What do you observe from the barium meal?
3. What is the diagnosis?
4. What are the predisposing factors of this condition?
5. What are the various subtypes and clinical features?
6. What are the radiological findings and complications?
7. What is the treatment?

Answers on pages 63–140

Case 1.41

A 52-year-old man presents with severe epigastric pain, abdominal distension and retching. On examination, there is severe tenderness in the epigastric region, with no palpable mass.

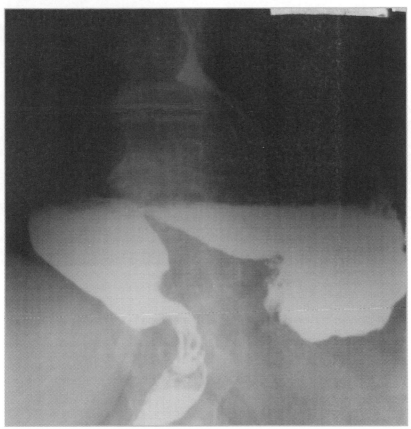

Fig 1.41

1. What are the findings from this barium meal?
2. What is the diagnosis?
3. What causes this condition?
4. What are the types?
5. What are the radiological features?
6. What is Borchardt's triad?
7. What are the complications and associations?
8. What is the differential diagnosis?

Answers on pages 63–140

Case 1.42

A 50-year-old man presents with severe, right-sided, colicky abdominal pain, constipation and vomiting. On examination, there is diffuse tenderness in the abdomen and bowel sounds are diminished.

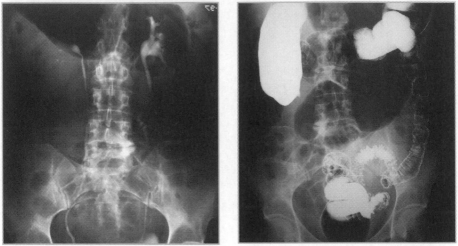

Fig 1.42a   Fig 1.42b

1. What do you see on the IVU and barium enema?
2. What is the diagnosis?
3. What condition is always associated with this?
4. What are the predisposing factors?
5. What are the types?
6. What are the radiological findings?
7. What are the complications?
8. What is the treatment?

Answers *on pages 63–140*

Case 1.43

A 36-year-old woman presents with jaundice, fever and abdominal pain.

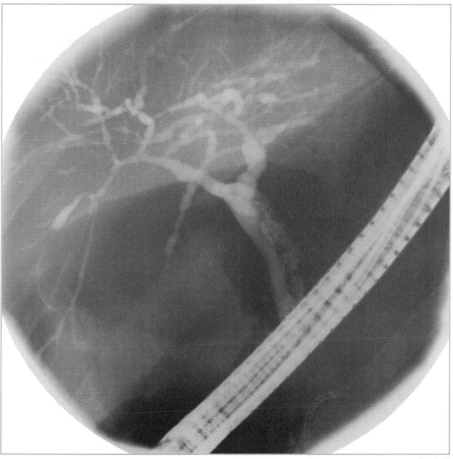

Fig 1.43

1. What do you observe with this test?
2. What is the diagnosis?
3. What is the most important disease associated with this condition?
4. What is the most common location?
5. What are the radiological findings?
6. What are the major complications?
7. What is the differential diagnosis?

Answers on pages 63–140

Case 1.44

A 43-year-old woman presents with abdominal pain, diarrhoea and weight loss. On examination, there is mild tenderness in the epigastric region and a cystic mass is palpated.

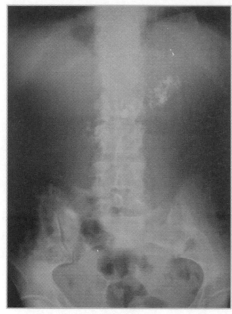

Fig 1.44a

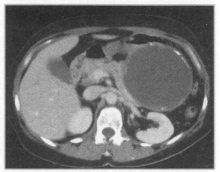

Fig 1.44b

1. What do you see on the X-ray and the CT scan of the abdomen?
2. What is the diagnosis?
3. What is the classification of this disease?
4. What are the causes?
5. What are the imaging features?
6. What are the complications?
7. What is the most important diagnostic dilemma?
8. What is the role of radiology in treatment?

Answers on pages 63–140

Case 1.45

A 28-year-old man presents with severe pain in the lower abdomen, nausea and vomiting. On physical examination there is rebound tenderness in the right lower quadrant. His WBC count is raised. Radiological tests were ordered.

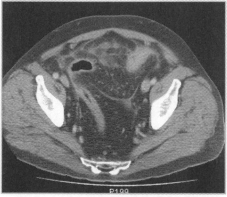
Fig 1.45a

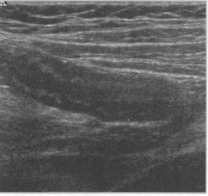
Fig 1.45b

1. What do you see on the CT scan?
2. What do you see on the ultrasound of the right lower quadrant of abdomen?
3. What is the diagnosis?
4. What is the pathophysiology?
5. What are the clinical features?
6. What are the radiological features?
7. What are the complications?
8. What is the clinical course and treatment of this disease?

Answers on pages 63–140

Case 1.46

A 47-year-old male presents with lower abdominal pain and history of intermittent lump in the left groin. On examination, there is no palpable mass, but increased cough impulse is noted in the left groin.

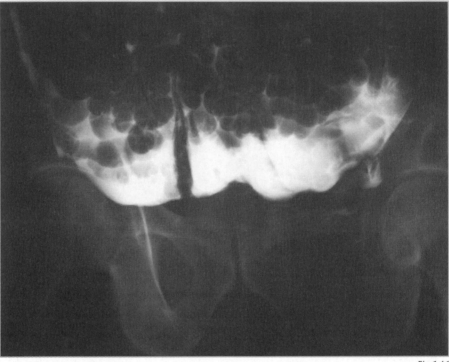

Fig 1.46

1. What is this investigation?
2. How is it performed?
3. What is the relevant anatomy?
4. What do you find on this examination?
5. What are the indications?
6. What are the complications of this procedure?

Answers on pages 63–140

Case 1.47

A 37-year-old man presents with right lower quadrant pain. On examination, there is swelling and tenderness in the right lower quadrant. The WBC count is 14 000/ml .

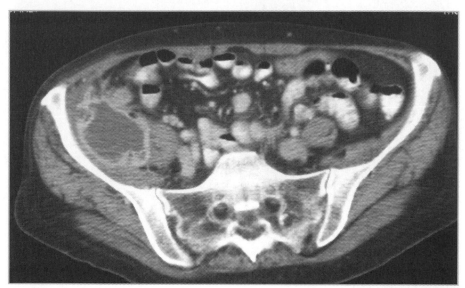

Fig 1.47

1. What do you see on the CT scan?
2. What is the diagnosis?
3. What is the pathophysiology?
4. What are the radiological features?
5. What is the differential diagnosis?
6. What is the treatment?

Answers on pages 63–140

Case 1.48

A 38-year-old woman presents with swelling in the right inguinal region. On examination the swelling is soft and fluctuant.

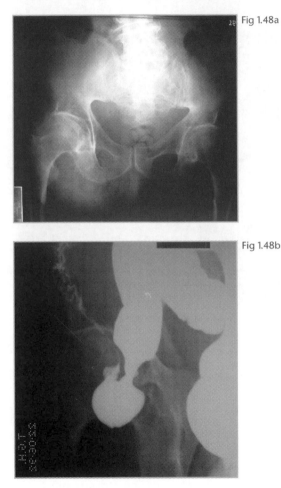

Fig 1.48a

Fig 1.48b

1. What do you see on the X-ray?
2. What do you see on the contrast study?
3. What is the diagnosis?
4. What is the anatomical location of this lesion?
5. What are the clinical features?
6. What are the salient features in imaging?
7. What are the complications?
8. What is the treatment?

Answers *on pages 63–140*

Case 1.49

A 55-year-old man presented with left lower quadrant pain and tenderness.

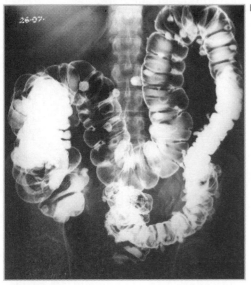

Fig 1.49a

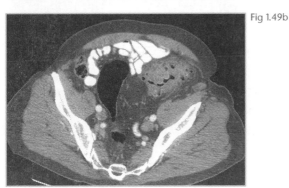

Fig 1.49b

1. What do you see on the barium enema, which was done 1 year earlier?
2. What are the findings on the CT scan?
3. What is the diagnosis?
4. What are the predisposing factors?
5. How does this disease develop?
6. What are the complications?
7. What are the radiological features?
8. What is the treatment?
9. What is the most important differential diagnosis?

Answers on pages 63–140

Case 1.50

A 61-year-old man presents with jaundice and abdominal pain. On examination a tender mass is felt in the right upper quadrant.

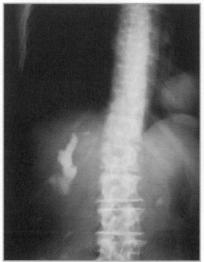

Fig 1.50a

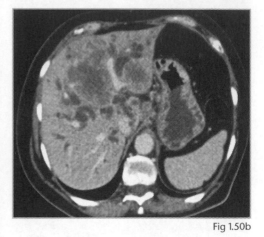

Fig 1.50b

1. What do you see on the cholangiogram and the CT scan?
2. What is the diagnosis?
3. What are the other types of this disease?
4. What are the common locations?
5. What are the radiological features?
6. What is the differential diagnosis?
7. What is the treatment?
8. What are the radiological procedures that are useful in these patients?

Answers on pages 63–140

Case 1.51

A 52-year-old woman presented with jaundice, abdominal pain and weight loss.

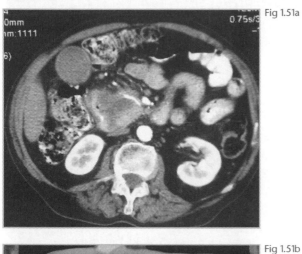

Fig 1.51a

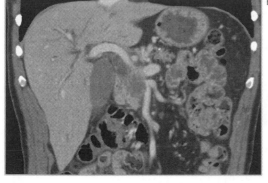

Fig 1.51b

1. What do you see on the abdominal CT scan?
2. What is the diagnosis?
3. What is the pathology?
4. What are the predisposing factors?
5. What is the pattern of spread?
6. What are the imaging features?
7. What are the most important features to be assessed by CT?
8. What is the differential diagnosis?

Answers *on pages 63–140*

Case 1.52

A 37-year-old woman presents with abdominal pain and altered LFTs.

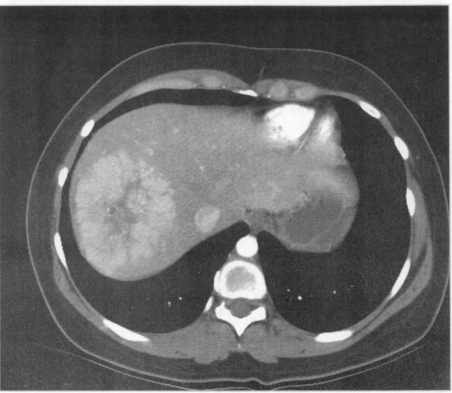

Fig 1.52

1. What are the findings on the abdominal CT scan?
2. What is the diagnosis?
3. What are the predisposing factors and associations?
4. What is the relationship between oral contraceptives and this disease?
5. What is the pathognomonic feature in pathology and radiology?
6. What are the findings on CT and MRI?
7. What are the complications?
8. What is the differential diagnosis?

Answers *on pages 63–140*

Case 1.53

A 20-year-old man presents with right-sided chest pain and tachypnoea. On examination there are reduced breath sounds in the right base.

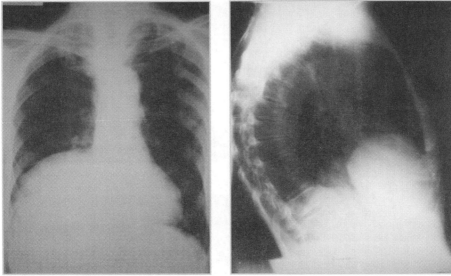

Fig 1.53a   Fig 1.53b

1. What are the findings on the X-ray?
2. What is the diagnosis?
3. What is the development of this lesion?
4. What are the clinical features?
5. What are the organs involved in this lesion?
6. What are the radiological features?
7. What is the differential diagnosis?

Answers on pages 63–140

Case 1.54

A 37-year-old woman presents with vague abdominal pain. Clinical examination is unremarkable.

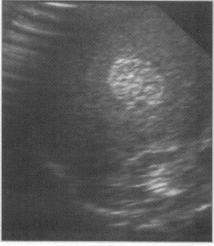

Fig 1.54a

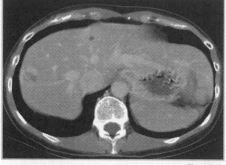

Fig 1.54b

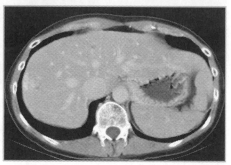

Fig 1.54c

1. What do you see on ultrasonography?
2. What do you observe on the CT scan?
3. What is the diagnosis?
4. What is the pathology?
5. What is Kasabach–Merritt syndrome?
6. What are the imaging features?
7. What is the differential diagnosis?
8. What are the complications
9. How will you confirm the diagnosis and what is the treatment?

Answers *on pages 63–140*

Case 1.55

A 54-year-old woman presents with weight loss and abdominal distension.

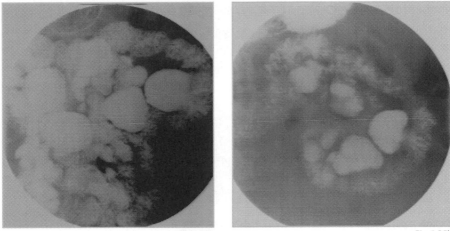

Fig 1.55a   Fig 1.55b

1. What do you find on the barium study?
2. What is the diagnosis?
3. What is the most common location of this disease?
4. What are the radiological features?
5. What are the clinical features and complications?

Answers on pages 63–140

Case 1.56

A 37-year-old woman presents with vague abdominal pain. Clinical examination is unremarkable.

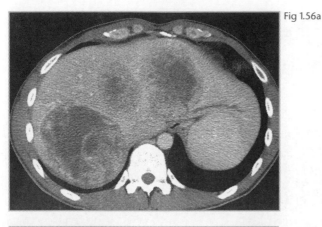

Fig 1.56a

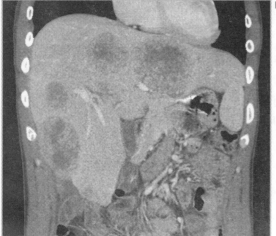

Fig 1.56b

1. What do you observe on the CT scan?
2. What is the diagnosis?
3. What are the primary lesions that give this appearance?
4. What are the imaging features?
5. Which of these lesions exhibit calcification?
6. What is the differential diagnosis?
7. What is the treatment?
8. What is the role of radiology in management?

Answers on pages 63–140

Case 1.57

A 73-year-old man presents with sudden onset of severe abdominal pain and abdominal distension. Clinical examination shows decreased bowel sounds. The patient is hypotensive, tachycardic and acidotic

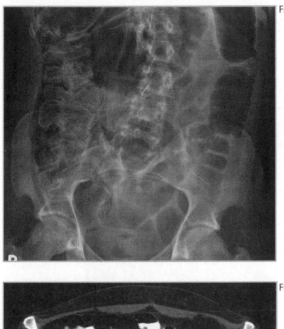
Fig 1.57a

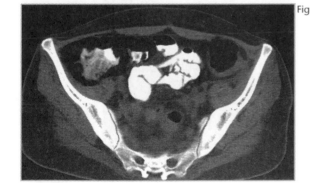
Fig 1.57b

1. What are the findings on the X-ray and the CT scan?
2. What is the diagnosis?
3. What are the other causes of this appearance? What chest conditions produce this appearance?
4. What are the radiological features and differential diagnosis?
5. What are the causes and features of bowel ischaemia?

Answers *on pages 63–140*

Case 1.58

A 5-year-old boy presents with difficulty swallowing, an itching sensation in the throat and drooling. On examination his oropharynx appears normal. There is no evidence of enlargement of tonsils and cervical lymph nodes. There is no tachypnoea or features of respiratory distress.

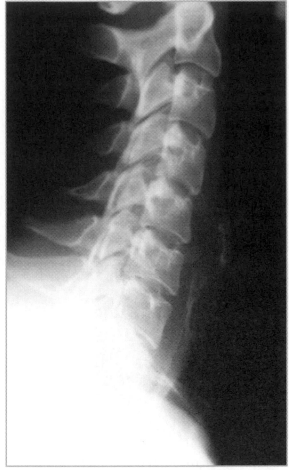

Fig 1.58

1. What do you observe on the lateral X-ray of the neck?
2. What is the diagnosis?
3. What are the predisposing factors and common locations?
4. What are the radiological features?
5. How is this condition managed and what are the complications?

Answers on pages 63–140

Case 1.59

A 57 year old male underwent appendectomy and was in ICU. On the fourth post operative day, he developed fever and abdominal pain. Clinical examination revealed abdominal tenderness, more severe on the left side. His WBC count was 21,000/ml.

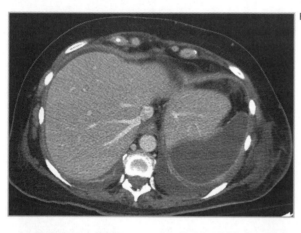

Fig 1.59a

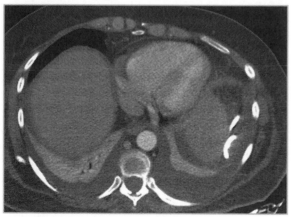

Fig 1.59b

1. What are the findings on the first CT scan?
2. What is the diagnosis?
3. What has been done on the second CT scan?
4. What is the pathophysiology?
5. What are the radiological features?
6. What is the treatment?
7. What is the role of radiology in treatment?

Answers on pages 63–140

Case 1.1: Answers

1. The barium meal shows a severely contracted stomach, with irregular walls. Even on delayed images (not shown here), the appearance persisted.

2. This appearance is called linitis plastica.

3. Scirrhous gastric carcinoma. Linitis plastica is usually caused by diffuse infiltration of the stomach submucosa by a scirrhous tumour.

4. Gastric cancer is the most common cause of the linitis plastica appearance. The other causes of this radiological appearance are: chronic gastric ulcer with severe spasm, corrosive ingestion, radiation, lymphoma, pseudolymphoma, metastasis, tuberculosis (TB), Crohn's disease, syphilis, histoplasmosis, actinomycosis, toxoplasmosis, hepatic chemoembolisation, sarcoidosis, amyloidosis, eosinophilic gastritis and polyarteritis nodosa.

5. The characteristic appearance in barium is a leather-bottle stomach, which is a diffusely narrowed stomach with wall thickening, and no change in configuration with peristalsis. The morphological types of gastric carcinoma are ulcerative, polypoid, scirrhous, superficial spreading and multicentric.

6. Endoscopy with biopsy is done to confirm the diagnosis. A CT scan is useful for assessing local spread to adjacent organs, vascular invasion, lymphadenopathy, liver metastasis and distal metastasis.

7. Treatment options are surgery and chemotherapy. The selection of the surgical procedure depends on the location of the tumour, the growth pattern seen on biopsy specimens and the expected location of the lymph node metastases. For proximal third gastric cancer, an extended gastrectomy, including the distal oesophagus, is performed. Middle third cancer requires total gastrectomy. Distal third gastric cancers undergo total gastrectomy if the biopsy shows 'diffuse-type' carcinoma and subtotal gastrectomy if the biopsy reveals 'intestinal-type' adenocarcinoma.

Case 1.2: Answers

1. The barium enema shows concentric narrowing of the sigmoid colon, with overhanging edges, the characteristic apple-core lesion. The second investigation is a CT scan; this shows concentric thickening of the wall of the sigmoid colon, which is narrowing the lumen.

2. Carcinoma of the distal sigmoid colon.

3. 93% of colorectal carcinomas arise from pre-existing adenoma. Predisposing factors are – a past history of adenoma/carcinoma, dysplasia, family history, inflammatory bowel disease (Ulcerative colitis, Crohn's disease), history of endometrial/ovarian/breast carcinoma, irradiation, ureterosigmoidstomy and polyposis syndromes.

4. Double contrast barium enema is used for screening patients who present with altered bowel habits or rectal bleeding. Double contrast enema has a sensitivity of up to 97% for detection of polyps > 1 cm. Polyps which are > 2 cm, broad, sessile with irregular margins are suspicious for malignancy. Virtual colonoscopy is equally effective in diagnosing early polyps, especially in older patients who cannot be put through the rigorous barium enema. Air is insufflated in the colon and CT scan images are acquired in the prone and supine position. The computer reconstructs the images and an image similar to colonoscopy is obtained. In most centres, colonoscopy is routinely used for colonic bleeding, but caecum is not visualised in some cases and 10% of small polyps are missed.

5. The most common location is the rectosigmoid region. Other locations are the descending colon (10%), transverse colon (12%), ascending colon (8%) and caecum (8%). Colonic cancers can be fungating polypoid, annular, tubular and ulcerating. Calcification is seen in mucinous carcinoma. Histologically they can be adenocarcinomas, mucinous carcinomas, or squamous or adenosquamous carcinomas. Left-sided lesions are annular and present early with obstruction, but right-sided lesions are polypoidal and present late with chronic anaemia

6. Barium enema is used to diagnose these lesions and for finding synchronous lesions in other segments of colon. CT is used for staging the tumour, which can be seen as a polypoidal mass or thickened bowel wall. It also detects local invasion, which is seen as pericolonic soft tissue stranding or mass. Spread to lymph nodes, liver, lungs and bones can be assessed.

7. Apple-core appearance is produced by an annular ulcerating carcinoma, resulting from tumour growing along the lymphatic channels that parallel the circular muscle fibres of the inner layer of muscularis propria. The tumour is seen as annular constriction with overhanging edges.

8. Lymphoma is another tumour which can produce apple core appearance. Less common causes are diverticulitis, chronic Crohn's disease/ulcerative colitis, ischemic colitis, infections (LGV, TB, amoeboma) and benign tumours (villous adenoma). In carcinoma of the pelvic colon, the left half of colon and rectum are resected along with mesocolon and paracolic lymph nodes. Follow up treatment depends on histology and Duke's classification.

Case 1.3: Answers

1. The chest X-ray shows air under the diaphragmatic domes.

2. Supine abdominal X-ray shows clear visualization of the outer and inner lining of the bowel wall as a result of presence of air outside the bowel wall and the normal intraluminal gas (Rigler's sign). The outline of falciform ligament is also visible.

3. Pneumoperitoneum caused by hollow viscus perforation.

4. X-ray findings – In an erect film, air collects under the diaphragm. In supine views, diagnosis may depend on subtle findings.

    A. **Rigler sign** – air on both sides of bowel (indicates > 1000ml of gas)

    B. **Foot ball sign** – large pneumoperitoneum outlining entire abdomen

    C. **Telltale triangle sign** – air between 3 loops of bowel

    D. **Inverted V sign** – outlining of both lateral umbilical ligaments

    E. **Outlining** of medial umbilical ligaments, falciform ligament

    F. **Urachus sign** – outlining middle umbilical ligament

    G. **Doges cap sign** – Triangular collection in Morrisons pouch

    H. **Falciform ligament sign** – Linear lucency in the right upper quadrant.

I. **Ligamentum teres sign** – vertical, slit/oval area between 10-12 ribs

J. **Ligamentum teres notch** – V shaped inverted, under liver

K. **Cupola sign** – gas below central tendon of diaphragm.

L. **Visualization** of diaphragmatic muscle slips.

---

5. Causes of pneumoperitoneum:

(a) Trauma: blunt/penetrating

(b) Iatrogenic: postoperative (absorbed in 1–24 days, air after 3 days is suspicious), laparoscopy, endoscopy, enema tip injury, needle biopsy, peritoneal catheter placement, peritoneal dialysis, paracentesis, misplaced thoracocentesis tube, intussusception reduction, chemoembolisation of liver tumours

(c) Gastrointestinal tract diseases: hollow viscus perforation, perforated appendix/sigmoid diverticulitis/Meckel's diverticulitis, foreign body, inflammatory bowel disease, toxic megacolon, obstruction, tumours, imperforate anus, necrotising enterocolitis, spontaneous perforation of stomach, Hirschsprung's disease and meconium ileus

(d) Ruptured pneumatosis intestinalis

(e) Idiopathic perforation in preterm infants

(f) Extension from chest (pneumomediastinum, bronchopleural fistula)

(g) Gas-forming peritonitis

(h) Introduction through female genital tract (tubal patency tests, pelvic examination, intercourse, douching, knee–chest movements).

---

6. False positive – gas filled structures such as diverticulum, Chiladiti syndrome (hepatic flexure interpsosition between liver and diaphragm), diaphragmatic hernia, abscess, subdiaphragmatic fat, omental fat between liver and diaphragm, basal atelectasis, irregular diaphragm and pneumothorax. **False negative** – Erect X-ray should be taken 5 minutes after keeping the patient in erect position, to give time for free gas to rise up under diaphragm. Lateral decubitus films are more sensitive and can be used for confirmation. Ultrasound is useful in skilful hands to identify air.

---

7. Sealed silent perforation (diabetes, elderly, severely ill, steroids), postoperative, dialysis, jejunal diverticulosis, ruptured pneumatosis intestinalis/stercoral ulcer, post embolisation and extension from pneumomediastinum.

Gastrointestinal Answers

Case 1.4: Answers

1. Ultrasound shows a thick, oedematous wall of the gallbladder, which has some deris within its lumen. The CT scan shows a thick, enhancing wall. There is also some free fluid around the liver. No gallstone is seen.

2. Acute acalculus cholecystitis.

3. Acute cholecystitis is acute inflammation of the gall bladder, mostly caused by a calculus obstructing the cystic duct. 10% are acalculus, which may result from obstruction of cystic duct by mucous or sludge or infection of bile. It is common in patients with major trauma, burns or recovering from surgery.

4. Ultrasound is the most useful imaging modality used in diagnosis. Normal gall bladder measures < 5cm and the normal wall thickness is 3–5mm. In ultrasound, stones are identified in the gall bladder or common bile duct. The wall of gall bladder is thickened, measuring > 5mm. The wall has a stratified appearance with a middle layer of oedema and echogenic layers on either side of it. The gall bladder is distended and measures > 5cm. Sonographic Murphy sign is positive (tenderness in the right upper quadrant on palpation). CT scan shows distended gall bladder, thick wall, stranding of pericholecystic fat and pericholecystic fluid. Further confirmation can be obtained with HIDA (hydroxyl iminodiacetic) scan, which is a scintigraphic investigation. It gives functional information about gall bladder and cystic duct patency. When the gall bladder is not visualised even after 4 hours, it is indicative of acute cholecystitis with obstruction of cystic duct due to oedema.

5. Gangrene (shaggy, irregular wall, pseudomembrane inside gall bladder, echogenic necrotic mucosa inside), perforation (gall stone escaping the gall bladder into peritoneal cavity, collection adjacent to gall bladder, irregular wall and defect in gall bladder, free air), empyema (distended gall bladder, echogenic internal echoes), abscess, gall stone ileus (stone migrating into bowel and causing obstruction – gall stone in bowel, dilated bowel loops gas in bile ducts) and Bouveret syndrome (stone eroding into duodenum, with duodenal obstruction).

6. Mirizzi syndrome is dilatation of intrahepatic ducts due to obstruction of common hepatic duct caused by pressed by an impacted stone within the cystic duct or neck of gall bladder, overlying the common hepatic duct.

7. Thickening of the gall bladder is non specific and can be seen in chronic cholcecystitis, carcinoma, variants of cholecystitis, hypoalbuminemaia, renal failure, hepatitis, right heart failure, ascites, hepatic venous or lymphatic obstruction, cirrhosis and graft versus host disease.

8. Ultrasound guided percutaneous drainage can be done if there are pericholecystic abscess or empyema.

Case 1.5: Answers

1. The CT scan shows completely irregular and disrupted architecture of the spleen, with hypodense areas indicating laceration and perisplenic collection, suggestive of haematoma. There is free fluid around the liver as well, which is probably a haemoperitoneum.

2. Splenic rupture secondary to trauma.

3. Blunt abdominal trauma is the most common cause of splenic rupture. The spleen is the most common organ in the abdomen to be involved in blunt trauma. It is often associated with other visceral or bowel injuries, rib fractures, left renal injury and diaphragm injuries. Of those with left rib fractures 20% have splenic injuries; 25% of those with left renal injury have splenic injury.

4. Left upper quadrant pain/tenderness, shoulder pain, abdominal distension and circulatory collapse are features of splenic injury.

5. CT is the procedure of choice for the diagnosis of splenic injuries. Splenic injuries can be haematomas, lacerations, vascular injuries or perisplenic hematoma. **Hematoma** – a round hypodense inhomogenous region with or without hyperdense clot. **Subcapsular hematoma** – a crescenteric region of hypodensity along the splenic margin. **Contusion** – mottled enhancement; **laceration** − linear, hypodense parenchymal defect connecting the opposing visceral surfaces; **fracture** − hypodense haematoma with separation of splenic fragments, a laceration extending across two capsular surfaces; **shattered spleen** − multiple lacerations; **perisplenic hematoma** − a sentinel clot adjacent to spleen. **Active extravastation** − of high density contrast indicates vascular injury/pseudoaneurysm. **Haemoperitoneum** − indicates splenic capsular disruption. There are many grading systems for splenic injury. **Grade I** − tear < 1cm, subcapsular < 25%; **II** − tear 1−3cm, subcapsular 25−50%, parenchymal − < 5cm; **III** − tear > 3cm, trabecular vessels involved, subcapsular > 50%, parenchymal > 10cm; **IV** − segmental/hilar vessels with devascularisation; **V** − shattered spleen or total devascularisation. Ultrasound can detect free fluid and large injuries, but less sensitive than CT scan.

6. Differential diagnoses of splenic injury include patchy enhancement in arterial phase of CT scan, normal lobulations, unopacified jejunum mimicking spleen and ascites/bile leak mimicking haemoperitoneum. Management is conservative in haemodynamically stable patients. Surgical resection is indicated for haemodynamically unstable patients and higher grades of injury. Splenic embolisation is an alternative. Complications are scar, fibrosis, pseudocyst, pseudoaneurysm and delayed rupture

7. Haemodynamically unstable patient, higher grades of injury, presence of haemoperitoneum, associated injuries and comorbid factors are all taken into consideration when surgery is planned. Bleeding, injury to adjacent structures, infection, thrombocytosis and splenosis are some of the complications of splenectomy. Immunisation against capsulated organisms such as *Haemophilus* spp., pneumococci and meningococci are indicated because a normal spleen phagocytoses capsulated organisms.

8. Infections, congestive splenomegaly, infiltrative disorders and tumours are other causes of non-traumatic splenic rupture.

Case 1.6: Answers

1. MRI (T2-weighted sequence) shows multiple cystic lesions, which are bright (hyperintense) as a result of their fluid content. Common hepatic and bile ducts are normal.

2. The CT scan shows multiple hypodense (less dense than adjacent liver) lesions in the liver. Some of these cysts have small dense nodules within them. Liver and spleen are marginally enlarged.

3. Caroli's disease.

4. Choledochal cysts are congenital anomalies with cystic dilatation of the biliary tree. Caroli's disease is segmental saccular dilatation of intrahepatic bile ducts, which is probably secondary to perinatal hepatic artery occlusion or hypoplasia of fibromuscular wall components.

5. The LaTodani classification of choledochal cysts:

Type I (80-90%): saccular or fusiform dilatations of the common bile duct:

     − IA: saccular, entire extrahepatic bile duct or most of it

     − IB: saccular, limited segment of the bile duct

     − IC: fusiform, most or all of the extrahepatic bile duct

Type II: diverticulum arising from the common bile duct

Type III: choledochocele arising from the intraduodenal portion of the common bile duct

Type IVA: multiple dilatations of the intra- and extrahepatic bile ducts

Type IVB: multiple dilatations involving only the extrahepatic bile ducts

Type V (Caroli's disease): consists of multiple dilatations limited to the intrahepatic bile ducts.

6. Caroli's disease is seen in childhood or older age groups. It presents with recurrent cramps, fever, jaundice and cirrhosis, with portal hypertension in late cases. It is associated with renal tubular ectasia, medullary sponge kidney, a choledochal cyst and congenital hepatic fibrosis.

7. Complications include bile stasis with cholelithiasis, cholangitis, liver abscess, septicaemia and cholangiocarcinomas. In patients without hepatic fibrosis, the frequency and severity of cholangitis determine the prognosis. In those with hepatic fibrosis, cholangitis and portal hypertension are the complications.

8. Ultrasonography shows multiple cystic structures, which are dilated biliary radicles converging towards porta hepatis. These are more prominent in the superior aspect of the liver. Portal branches protrude into the cysts. Extrahepatic ductal dilatation is seen only if there is another cause such as a stone. Doppler ultrasonography is used for evaluating the liver and portal hypertension. CT has the characteristic central dot sign, where the portal radicles are completely surrounded by dilated bile ducts. Sludge or calculi are seen in dilated ducts. Magnetic resonance cholangiopancreatography (MRCP) can be done and it shows segmental saccular dilatation of bile ducts. Hepatobiliary nuclear scans can demonstrate communication between cysts and bile ducts. Ultrasound-guided aspiration of cysts will confirm the presence of bile and the diagnosis of cholangitis. A common differential diagnosis is polycystic liver disease, which is usually associated with multiple renal cysts.

Case 1.7: Answers

1. The barium swallow shows longitudinal, tortuous filling defects in the lower oesophagus. The CT scan shows enhancing, dilated, plexiform, vascular structures surrounding the distal oesophagus, which appears thickened.

2. Oesophageal varices.

3. Oesophageal varices are plexus formed by dilated subepithelial veins, submucosal veins and venae comitantes of vagus nerves outside muscularis. There are two types. Uphill varices carry collateral blood from the portal vein via the azygos vein to the superior vena cava (SVC). Downhill varices carry blood from the SVC via the azygos into the inferior vena cava (IVC)/portal vein and are seen in the upper oesophagus. Uphill varices are the most common and caused by cirrhosis, splenic vein thrombosis, obstruction of hepatic veins/IVC and marked splenomegaly. Downhill varices are caused by obstruction of the SVC distal to entry of the azygos vein as a result of lung cancer, lymphoma, goitre, mediastinal tumours and mediastinal fibrosis.

4. The anterior branch of the oesophageal vein drains into the left gastric vein. The posterior branch drains into the azygos and hemiazygos veins.

5. Barium swallow is often used in diagnosis. Varices are seen as thickened folds, with tortuous, radiolucent, filling defects. It might be missed in conventional barium swallow. Thin barium is used and images are acquired with a Valsalva manoeuvre/deep inspiration or left anterior oblique projection with the patient in a recumbent position. Occasionally varices are incidentally discovered on a CT scan done for cirrhosis. The oesophageal wall is thickened and there are bilateral vascular structures surrounding the oesophagus, which show serpiginous contrast enhancement.

6. The common differential diagnoses are varicoid carcinoma of the oesophagus (fixed appearance, no variation with Valsalva manoeuvre) and candidiasis (irregular ulcerations).

7. Bleeding oesophageal varices are treated with resuscitation, oesophageal tube (Sengstaken Blakemore) placement, drugs (IV vasopressin), endoscopic sclerotherapy or variceal banding. Surgical procedures are portosystemic shunt, oesophageal devascularisation or liver transplantation in advanced liver disease.

8. Radiology can be used in the management of severe bleeding. X-ray is used to confirm the position of oesophageal tube. Percutaneous transheptic embolisation of gastro-oesophageal varices is done by catheterisation of gastric collaterals that supply blood to the varices through the transhepatic route. An TIPSS (transjugular intrahepatic portosystemic shunt) is used if the medical and endoscopic treatment fail. In this procedure, a stent is placed between the portal and hepatic veins, which releases the portal hypertension.

Case 1.8: Answers

1. The first plain X-ray (supine) shows dilated loops of small bowel in the central part of the abdomen. Complete mucosal folds are seen within the bowel lumen. The second X-ray (erect) shows fluid levels within dilated bowel loops.

2. Small bowel obstruction.

3. Small bowel obstruction can be **Dynamic or adynamic**. In dynamic form, peristalsis works against a mechanical obstruction. In adynamic form, peristalsis is either completely absent (paralytic ileus) or feeble for propulsion of intestinal contents. Adhesions, hernia, tumours, volvulus, intussusceptions and gall stone ileus are the common causes of mechanical obstruction in adults. Classification based on disease process. **Congenital** – Atresia, duplication, stenosis, midgut voluvus, Meckel's diverticulum; **Extrinsic** – Adhesions, hernia, volvulus, extrinsic neoplasm; **Luminal** – foreign bodies, meconium ileus, intussusception, intrinsic tumour; **Intramural** – Tumours, inflammatory, ischemia radiation, haemorrhage, strictures. Common causes of adynamic ileus are post operative ileus and ileus due to peritonitis, hypokalemia or acute conditions such as pyelonephritis, pancreatitis, appendicitis and pneumonia.

4. X-rays are the mainstay in the diagnosis. In a normal abdomen, there might be gas in three to four variably shaped loops < 2.5cm in diameter. In obstruction, there are dilated loops of small bowel. Jejunal loops have frequent and high valvulae conniventes. Ileum has sparse or absent valvulae conniventes. Small bowel loops are centrally placed and show valvulae conniventes. Large bowel loops are in the periphery and show haustrations. Erect films show distended small bowel loops (> 3cm) with air–fluid levels. There is little or no gas in the distal small bowel. A stepladder appearance is seen in lower obstruction. A string-of-beads appearance is seen with air entrapped in the volvulae in obstruction. Occasionally the bowel loops are completely filled with fluid and there is no gas in the abdomen. The point of obstruction is identified if there is sudden transition from a dilated to a non-dilated loop. Water-soluble contrast can be orally administered and follow-up films are done after 3 and 24h. In complete small bowel obstruction, there is no passage of contrast after 3–24h. In low-grade small bowel obstruction there is some flow of contrast distal to the obstruction with visualisation of folds. In high-grade obstruction, there is delay in arrival of contrast, which is diluted and hence the folds are not clearly seen. In adynamic ileus, dilated small and large bowel loops are seen, but the small bowel distension decreases on serial films. There is delayed but free passage of contrast material.

5. In **closed loop obstruction**, two points along course of single bowel loop are obstructed at a single site, caused by adhesion of incarcerated hernia. The bowel loop is fixed. There is a U or C shaped bowel loop, with coffee bean sign (gas tilled loop) or a fluid filled loop. Beak sign and whirl sign indicate point of obstruction in CT scan.

Strangulated obstruction is due to impaired circulation at the site of obstruction. In addition to features of closed loop obstruction, there is vascular compromise, with no enhancement of bowel wall or delayed prolonged enhancement, mesenteric haziness due to oedema, congested mesenteric vasculature, localised mesenteric fluid/haemorrhage and gas in intestinal wall/portal vein.

6. A CT scan is used for diagnosis of obstruction (dilated, loops > 2.5cm; small bowel faeces sign — gas bubbles mixed with particulate matter proximal to obstruction), detecting the level of obstruction and cause of obstruction.

Case 1.9: Answers

1. The first CT scan shows gas in the biliary tree (pneumobilia). The second CT scan shows a dense opacity within the lumen of the duodenum. There is stagnation of oral contrast in a moderately distended stomach.

2. Bouveret syndrome. This is gastric outlet obstruction caused by impaction of gallstones in the gastric pylorus or the first part of the duodenum. The gallstone has eroded through the GB or CBD wall into duodenum, allowing air from the duodenum to enter the bile ducts.

3. Gallstone ileus is small bowel obstruction caused by gallstones. It accounts for 25% of intestinal obstruction in patients aged > 60 years. Predisposing factors are gallbladder disease, gallbladder carcinoma or peptic ulcer disease. It occurs in 15% of those with biliary enteric fistula. Clinical features are intermittent, colicky, right-sided pain, nausea, vomiting, abdominal distension and constipation. It is seen in the fifth and sixth decades.

4. The most common site of lodgement of the calculus is the terminal ileum. Other sites are the proximal or distal ileum, pylorus, sigmoid and duodenum (2–3%).

5. Abdominal X-ray and ultrasonography are useful in diagnosis. X-rays show dilated bowel loops, which are fluid filled or with air—fluid levels. There is gas in the biliary tree, secondary to erosion of the gallstone into the bowel and the resulting fistula. The gallstone is visualised (in

25%), in a loop of bowel, proximal to which dilated bowel loops are seen (> 3cm). Ultrasonography shows displaced gallstones and pneumobilia. A barium study will show a cholecystoduodenal, choledochoduodenal, cholecystocolic, choledochocolic or cholecystogastric fistula. In Bouveret syndrome, the stomach is dilated as a result of gastric outlet obstruction. Diagnosis may be difficult when the stone is of the same density as the oral contrast. Oral contrast can also be seen entering the gallbladder as a result of the fistulous communication.

6. Rigler's triad is diagnostic of small bowel ileus. It is the combination of dilated, obstructed, small bowel loops, pneumobilia and a calcified gallstone in the small bowel.

7. Recurrence, obstruction, perforation and ischaemia are the complications. Endoscopy is done and the stone is removed with mechanical, electrohydraulic or laser lithotripsy. Surgery is often not desirable because patients are poor surgical candidates secondary to concomitant illnesses and advanced age. If surgery is performed, enterolithotomy alone may be adequate treatment in elderly people, and subsequent cholecystectomy may not be required.

8. Other causes of small bowel obstruction such as adhesions, hernia, volvulus and tumours can be confused with gallstone ileus, but they don't have gas in the biliary tree.

Case 1.10: Answers

1. The CT scan shows a large, well-defined, fluid-filled, hypodense lesion in the right lobe of the liver. The lesion does not have any internal debris or air and does not show any contrast enhancement of its wall.

2. Simple cyst of the liver.

3. Hepatic cysts usually refer to non-parasitic cysts of the liver, and are believed to be of congenital origin as a result of defective development of aberrant intrahepatic bile ducts or a bile duct hamartoma that fails to develop normal connections with the biliary tree and contains thin serous fluid. They are lined by cuboidal epithelium with thin fibrous stroma. They are seen in 2.5% of the population and more common in women. They are usually solitary, but may be multiple.

4. Simple liver cysts are frequently seen on imaging. Ultrasonography shows a simple cyst as a well-defined anechoic lesion, with posterior acoustic enhancement (bright opacity behind the dark cyst) and no internal contents. The CT scan shows a homogeneous hypodense cyst, with well-defined margins and a regular wall with no solid component or wall enhancement. On MRI the cyst is hypointense (dark) in T1 and hyperintense (bright) in T2.

5. Differential diagnoses of liver cysts:

   Congenital: simple cyst, bile duct hamartoma, Caroli's disease

   Infection: hydatid, abscess

   Traumatic Iatrogenic: haematoma, biloma, seroma

   Syndromes: polycystic kidney disease, polycystic liver disease, tuberous sclerosis

   Tumours: cystic metastasis (sarcoma, colorectal, ovary, carcinoid), biliary cystadenomas, cystadenocarcinomas, cavernous haemangioma, undifferentiated sarcoma, ovarian cancer metastasis

   Miscellaneous: pseudocyst, haematoma, biloma, seroma.

6. Infection and haemorrhage are complications.

7. Simple hepatic cysts do not require any treatment. They are often incidental findings on imaging and asymptomatic. Large cysts producing symptoms may be aspirated under ultrasound or CT guidance. Sclerosants (ethanol/sodium tetradecylsulphate) can be injected to collapse the cyst and prevent reaccumulation as a result of continuous fluid secretion.

Case 1.11: Answers

1. The initial CT scan shows an enlarged pancreas, which shows normal contrast enhancement, except for a small area of non-enhancement in the head. There is fluid around the pancreas, which extends anterior to both kidneys, especially on the left side.

2. Acute pancreatitis.

3. On the second CT scan, the entire gland is dark and shows very little enhancement, implying development of pancreatic necrosis.

4. Epigastric or right upper quadrant pain/tenderness, nausea, vomiting, fever, hypotension, tachycardia, tachypnoea, jaundice and decreased bowel sounds are the clinical features. Raised serum amylase (> 5 times of normal level are diagnostic) and lipase are the common abnormalities seen in acute pancreatitis. Combined estimation of lipase and amylase is more accurate. Triglyceridemia can cause spurious lowering of amylase and lipase in pancreatitis. Other abnormalities include raised white blood cell (WBC) count, altered liver function tests (LFTs) and abnormal electrolytes (especially hypocalcaemia).

5. Alcohol abuse and biliary stones are the most common causes of acute pancreatitis. Other causes include medications, hyperlipidaemia, trauma, carcinoma, pancreas divisum, cardiopulmonary bypass, infections and peptic ulcer disease.

6. Pancreatitis is graded and staged using Ranson's criteria, APACHE II and CT severity index. CT grading of pancreatitis (scores given in parentheses):

    Grade A: the pancreas appears normal (0)

    Grade B: pancreas is enlarged and oedematous (1)

    Grade C: inflammation extends to peripancreatic tissue (2)

    Grade D: one fluid collection, without abscess (3)

    Grade E: multiple fluid collections or pancreatic abscess (4).

    Grades of necrosis < **30% – 2; 30–50%** – 4; > **50% –** 6. The combined score of CT grading and necrosis is calculated and the severity depends on the score. The CT scan is done in non-contrast, arterial and venous phases. Areas of necrosis do not enhance in the arterial phase and this is an important prognostic indicator.

7. Usually acute pancreatitis is a clinical diagnosis. CT scan is used when the diagnosis is indeterminate or for evaluation of severity and complications. Ultrasonography is done for assessment of gallstones.

8. Nil by mouth, nasogastric intubation, parenteral nutrition, analgesics, antibiotics, electrolyte and fluid replacment are required for management of the acute stage. Collections are drained under CT guidance. Pancreatic phlegmon, necrosis, abscess, pseudocyst and pseudoaneurysms,

haemorrhagic pancreatitis, pancreatic ascites, biliary obstruction and thoracopancreatic fistula are the local complications. Fat necrosis, hypocalcaemia, acute respiratory distress syndrome (ARDS), pleural effusion, consolidation, acute circulatory failure and acute renal failure are the systemic complications.

Case 1.12: Answers

1. The first CT scan shows a large mass in the left inguinal region. There are tortuous loops of bowel within this mass. The second scan shows dilated loops of small bowel in the abdomen.

2. Incarcerated left inguinal hernia with small bowel obstruction.

3. Inguinal hernias can be direct or indirect. Indirect inguinal hernia occurs through the deep inguinal ring, which is lateral to the inferior epigastric artery and superior to the inguinal ligament and extend for a variable distance into the inguinal canal. It can pass through the canal, emerge via the superficial ring and extend into the scrotum. Contents may be small bowel loops, mobile colon segments (caecum, sigmoid, appendix), mesenteric fat or urinary bladder. Direct hernia occurs through the inferior aspect of Hesselbach's triangle, and lies medial to the inferior epigastric artery.

4. Patients with inguinal hernia present with dull aching pain and lump, made worse with exercise or straining. On examination, a soft or firm lump, which is more prominent with provocative manouevres is seen. Cough impulse is noted. In inguinal hernia, the neck of the sac is situated above and medial to the ligament. Complications are incarceration, obstruction and strangulation. When the hernia is strangulated, there is pain, tenderness, swelling and redness with toxic features. Obstruction presents with nausea, vomiting, constipation and distension. Obesity, heavy lifting, coughing, straining, ascites, peritoneal dialysis, VP shunt, COPD, family history are predisposing factors.

5. In ultrasound, indirect inguinal hernia is seen lateral to the inferior epigastric artery. Direct inguinal hernia arises medial to the inferior epigastric artery in the Hesselbach's triangle. Ultrasound differentiates a groin swelling from abscess, lymph node or aneurysm. In CT scan, the sac is situated medial to the pubic tubercle. Complications such as

obstruction and strangulation can be diagnosed. Contrast herniography is useful in diagnosis of early incomplete and post operative small hernias, which are clinically indeterminate.

6. Elective repair is herniotomy or herniorrhaphy. The steps of hernia repair are – (i) reduction of contents and excision of hernia sac; (ii) repair of transversalis fascia and internal ring; (iii) reinforcement of posterior wall; (iv) repair of external oblique, creating smaller external ring. Emergent surgery is required for complications. Resection of bowel may be necessary for bowel infarction. Truss may be used in patients, with reducible hernias, who are not fit for surgery. Conventional repair may aggravate respiratory symptoms in those with large hernias and chronic respiratory disease. Limited procedure such as widening mouth of the hernia, to avoid obstruction may be sufficient.

Case 1.13: Answers

1. The barium swallow shows hold up of barium in the oesophagus due to an irregular stricture in the distal part of the oesophagus. The CT scan shows a concentric soft-tissue mass in the distal oesophagus, with enlargement of the oesophageal outline.

2. Oesophageal carcinoma.

3. Squamous carcinoma is seen in the mid-third of the oesophagus and adenocarcinoma is seen in the distal third.

4. Predisposing factors for squamous cell carcinoma are smoking, alcohol, Plummer–Vinson syndrome, achalasia, caustic strictures, chronic hot liquid ingestion, nitrosamines, poor oral hygiene and tylosis palmaris. Adenocarcinoma is caused by metaplastic degeneration of columnar epithelium (Barrett's) in distal oesophagus due to chronic inflammation caused by gastro-oesphageal reflux. Dysphagia for solids initially but later for solids and liquids, pain, weight loss and haematemesis, hoarseness and respiratory symptoms are the symptoms of oesophageal cancer.

5. Routine blood tests, endoscopy, endoscopic ultrasound, bronchoscopy in the mid-third of the oesophagus, CT of the thorax and upper abdomen, and a bone scan are investigations used for diagnosis and staging. Tumour staging is better done with endoscopic ultrasound:

Tis – carcinoma *in situ*

T1 – invasion of lamina propria/submucosa

T2 – muscularis propria

T3 – adventitia

T4 – adjacent organs

N1 – regional lymph nodes

M1 – distal metastasis, coeliac lymph nodes in lower oesophageal tumours, non-regional nodes in mid-oesophageal tumour and cervical nodes in upper oesophageal tumour. In distal oesophageal tumours, laparscopy may be helpful in detecting extension of tumour below the phrenicoesophageal ligament.

6. Oesophageal cancer is seen as a thickening of the oesophageal wall with narrowing of the lumen. This appearance is non-specific and can be seen in benign conditions as well. Extension outside the oesophagus, invasion of adjacent structures such as trachea, bronchi, aorta and mediastinum, regional lymphadenopathy in the thorax and abdomen, and liver and pulmonary metastases are assessed by the CT scan. Barium swallow is often the initial test used in diagnosis. The tumour is seen as an irregular stricture and shouldering is seen proximally or distally, which differentiates it from benign oesophageal strictures.

7. Transhiatal or transthoracic oesophagectomy with gastric pull-through is done to manage resectable oesophageal tumours. Other options are the Ivor Lewis procedure (laparotomy and posterolateral right thoracotomy), the McKeown procedure (anterolateral right thoracotomy, laparotomy and cervical anastomosis) and the left thoracoabdominal approach. Bypass surgery provides an alternative food passageway when the oesophagus is completely obstructed by cancer.

8. Expandable metallic stents can be inserted under fluoroscopic guidance through the diseased stenotic segment. Radiation, laser ablation and photodynamic therapy are other palliative options.

Case 1.14: Answers

1. The X-ray shows a huge distended loop of sigmoid colon, arising from the pelvis and extending to the left upper quadrant under the dome of the diaphragm (coffee bean appearance). There is no haustra in the dilated colon and the walls appear thickened.

2. Sigmoid volvulus.

3. Sigmoid volvulus is the most common volvulus in the gastrointestinal tract. It is caused by unusual narrow attachment of the root of a long sigmoid mesocolon to posterior abdominal wall, resulting in the close proximity of the two limbs of the sigmoid colon, making it vulnerable to twisting. The loop can be rotated any degree, although 360° is the most common type.

4. Overloading of pelvic colon and adhesive band of pelvic colon are contributory factors. It is common in elderly, neurological and psychiatric patients. Chronic constipation, high roughage diet and lead poisoning are predisposing factors.

5. An X-ray is enough for the diagnosis of sigmoid volvulus. A distended sigmoid colon is seen (inverted 'U' shape), with the limbs of the sigmoid loop directed toward the pelvis and the apex extending to the dome of the diaphragm.

    Coffee-bean **sign** – distinct midline crease, caused by gas in the sigmoid colon, surrounding thickened oedematous walls. The colonic haustra are lost, walls are thickened and there might be air–fluid levels. If the loop is full of fluid, it might be seen as a soft-tissue density lesion. In the supine film, a dilated sigmoid reaching the level of transverse colon (**northern exposure sign**) is a reliable sign of volvulus.

6. A barium or CT scan can be done, but is not necessary. Barium swallow shows a '**bird of prey**' sign, which is the tapered hook-like end of the barium column at the site of twisting. A CT scan shows the '**whirl sign**' which is caused by twisted mesentery formed by afferent and effect loops.

7. Obstruction, ischaemia and perforation are the complications.

8. In patients without ischaemia or perforation, sigmoidoscopic decompression of the rectum can be attempted. Sigmoidopexy is done for those with recurrent volvulus and complications. Resection of bowel may be necessary when there is a suspicion of impending gangrene.

Case 1.15: Answers

1. Ultrasonography of the abdomen shows a clear fluid collection in the peritoneal cavity, with centrally floating bowel loops. The CT scan shows fluid collection in the peritoneal cavity on either side of centrally floating bowel loops.

2. Ascites.

3. Ascites is an abnormal accumulation of intraperitoneal fluid. Common causes of ascites are related to:

Portal hypertension – Cirrhosis, hepatic outflow obstruction, congestive cardiac failure, constrictive pericarditis, Budd Chiari syndrome.

Malignancy – Intraperitoneal primary tumor or peritoneal metastasis

Renal – chronic renal failure, nephrotic syndrome.

Inflammatory/Infective – Peritonitis, pancreatitis, TB, Fitz Hugh Curtis syndrome, filariasis

Endocrine – Myxoedema, Meig's syndrome, ovarian stimulation syndrome.

Miscellaneous –Trauma

4. On the X-ray, the abdomen is distended, with bulging flanks and centrally placed bowel loops. The peritoneal flank stripe is thickened. The space between the properitoneal fat and gut is > 3mm, with medial displacement both of the lateral liver margin (Hellmer's sign) and of the ascending and descending colon. A white-out appearance of the abdomen is seen.

Radiological changes are seen only when the fluid measures > 500 ml. Ultrasonography is very sensitive and can detect 5–10 ml fluid. On ultrasonography a transudate is seen as a clear collection and an exudate has internal echoes or internal septations. On a CT scan, even small quantities of fluid are detected. The density of the collection can indicate the nature.

5. Occasionally it might be possible to differentiate benign and malignant ascites. Benign fluid collection is usually clear, but occasionally shows septations or loculations; the bowel loops are free floating and the gallbladder wall appears thick. Benign ascites is seen primarily in the greater sac and not in the lesser sac. Malignant ascites is highly echogenic with internal contents and loculations, the bowel loops are fixed and the gallbladder wall is not thickened. Associated masses indicate malignancy. Malignant ascites is seen equally in greater and lesser sacs. Presence of coarse internal echoes indicates blood and fine internal echoes are caused by chyle. Multiple septa indicate TB or pseudomyxoma peritonei.

6. Fluid from supramesocolic compartment extends along the shelves on the mesenteric side of the small bowel loops and drops into the inframesoclic compartment and then into the pelvis. From the pelvis, the fluid flows along the paracolic gutters. The fluid in the right paracolic gutter extends all the way to the right subhepatic spaces, but, on the left, is limited by the phrenicocolic ligament.

7. In a supine patient, the earliest site of fluid collection is Morrison's pouch (hepatorenal). The most dependent part of the pelvis is the pouch of Douglas.

8. High-density ascites indicates haemoperitoneum, infection or malignancy. Trauma, TB and ovarian/appendiceal tumour (pseudomyxoma) are also causes of high-density ascites.

9. Fluid is aspirated under ultrasound guidance for diagnostic and therapeutic purposes. Ultrasound guidance enables aspiration from even small collections, and helps avoid vascular structures, bowel loops and bladder. Therapeutic paracentesis is performed in refractory or tense ascites. Albumin 5 g should be supplemented for each litre aspirated > 5 l. TIPSS is useful in refractory ascites.

Case 1.16: Answers

1. A sexual aid in the rectum, a rectal foreign body.

2. Foreign bodies are common in the orifices. They might be inserted into the rectum or vagina, urethra, ear, nose or throat. Rectal foreign bodies are directly inserted or very rarely swallowed and reach the rectum after gastrointestinal tract transit.

3. Swallowed foreign bodies in the rectum could be toothpicks, popcorn, bones or sunflower seeds. Inserted foreign bodies are sex toys, batteries, glass bottles, light bulbs and cans. Clinical presentation is with pain or a request to remove the foreign body.

4. Objects could be inserted for sexual gratification. Children do it out of curiosity. It is seen in psychiatric patients who have an altered perception, orientation and understanding. Pseudotherapeutic procedures done by non-traditional medical practitioners are another cause. Drug traffickers might insert contraband substances into the rectum to escape detection.

5. Radio-opaque foreign bodies are usually seen on plain films. Anteroposterior (AP) and lateral views are required. A chest X-ray in the upright position is done to exclude perforation. The most important information is whether the foreign body is high or low lying in relation to the rectosigmoid junction. Low-lying foreign bodies are palpable and removed by endoscopy. High-lying objects are difficult to visualise and remove.

6. Bowel wall injury, bleeding, perforation, ischaemia and sepsis are the complications.

7. Low-lying foreign bodies that are smooth, non-friable and non-breakable can be removed with forceps under proctoscopy in the Emergency Department. Foreign bodies at higher levels can be removed by flexible endoscopy. Laparotomy is required for laceration, perforation, infection, high-lying objects, glass objects, friable or breakable objects, sharp or non-smooth objects and dangerous objects.

Case 1.17: Answers

1. The X-ray of the chest shows an abnormal, lucent structure in the inferior aspect of the left hemithorax, which is causing mild displacement of the heart to the right side.

2. The barium enema shows contrast opacified large and some small bowel loops. The distal transverse colon and splenic flexure are seen herniating into the left side of the chest.

3. Bochdalek's type of diaphragmatic hernia.

4. The diaphragm has a ventral component, which is formed by septum transversum over 3–5 weeks and gradually extends posteriorly to envelop the oesophagus and great vessels. This fuses with the foregut mesentery to form the posteromedial aspects of the diaphragm by week 8. Lateral margins develop from the thoracic wall. Posterolaterally, the pleuroperitoneal canal fuses the last. Bochdalek's hernia is formed as a result of failure in fusion of the cephalic or pleuroperitoneal fold, resulting in an open pleuroperitoneal canal.

5. Bochdalek's hernia is more common on the left side. The right side is involved in 15% and it is bilateral in 5%. It manifests in the neonatal period or earlier, because it is a large hernia and produces symptoms. It constitutes about 90% of diaphragmatic hernias. Occasionally it presents later in life and can be detected as an asymptomatic, incidental finding.

6. On the left side, omental fat, bowel, spleen, left lobe of liver, kidney and pancreas can herniate. On the right side, liver, gallbladder, small bowel and kidney can herniate. The X-ray shows bowel loops inside the chest cavity Mediastinal shift is seen to the opposite side, when the hernia is large. When the stomach/bowel herniates into thorax, corresponding lucencies are not seen in the stomach. Complications of diaphragmatic hernia are pulmonary hypoplasia and persistent fetal circulation.

7. Eventration results from a congenitally hypoplastic, thin diaphragm, causing upward displacement of abdominal contents. This is located in an anteromedial location on the right side and involves the entire dome on the left side.

8. Berquist's triad is seen in traumatic diaphragmatic hernia and consists of rib fractures, fracture of the spine/pelvis and traumatic rupture of the diaphragm. It is seen in blunt or penetrating trauma. Usually they are < 1cm, and produce the collar sign, which is a waist-like constriction at the site of entry of bowel loops.

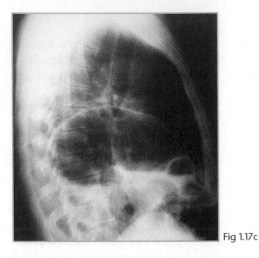

Lateral chest X-ray in same patient.

Fig 1.17c

Case 1.18: Answers

1. The CT scan of the abdomen shows multiple hypodense, linear areas in the right lobe of the liver. There is no biliary dilatation. There is hypodensity surrounding the contrast-enhanced portal veins. There is mild free fluid around the liver.

2. Hepatic injury with laceration.

3. Liver trauma is divided into six categories:

   (a) subcapsular haematoma < 20%, tear, < 1 cm

   (b) haematoma 10–50%, tear 1–3 cm deep, < 10 cm long

   (c) haematoma > 50%, ruptured haematoma, > 10 cm, tear > 10 cm long

   (d) laceration/disruption of 25–75% of a lobe, one to three segments in one lobe

   (e) disruption > 75% of one lobe, more than three segments in one lobe, juxtahepatic venous injury

   (f) hepatic avulsion.

4. The right lobe is more commonly involved. Left lobe injury is associated with injury to the duodenum, colon and pancreas. Most of the lesions are perivascular, paralleling right and middle hepatic arteries and posterior branches of the right portal vein.

5. Contrast-enhanced CT is the imaging modality of choice for hepatic trauma. Subcapsular haematomas are seen as a crescenteric, hyperdense, hypodense or isodense collection compressing the liver parenchyma. Lacerations are seen as irregular linear areas of hypodensity. A characteristic feature of liver trauma is periportal hypodensity, which is probably a result of haemorrhage, bile and dilated periportal lymphatics caused by elevated central venous pressure or injury to the lymphatics. Liver devascularisation and infarcts are seen as hypodense wedge-shaped areas in the periphery of the liver. Active bleeding is seen as a hyperdense area and active contrast extravasation can be detected. Haemoperitoneum is seen as a high-density fluid collection in the abdomen. Intrahepatic or subcapsular gas can be seen as a result of necrosis. Ultrasonography is also a good diagnostic tool, except small, subtle injuries and actively bleeding vascular injuries.

6. The complications are haemobilia, arteriovenous (AV) fistula, pseudoaneurysm, biloma, infection and delayed rupture.

7. Most cases of blunt liver traumas are managed conservatively when the patient is haemodynamically stable. Active bleeding requires transcatheter embolisation or surgery. Bile collection in liver or peritoneum requires percutaneous drainage under imaging guidance. Surgery is indicated in cases of ongoing blood loss and signs of general peritonitis.

Case 1.19: Answers

1. The CT scan shows a large hypodense lesion in the right lobe, which shows a thick rim of enhancement in the periphery. There is no biliary dilatation.

2. Liver abscess.

3. Liver abscess could be pyogenic or amoebic. *Escherichia coli*, aerobic streptococci, *Staphylococcus aureus* and anaerobic bacteria cause pyogenic liver abscess. Amoebic abscess is caused by *Entamoeba histolytica*.

4. The infection can be by ascending cholangitis (obstructive biliary disease), portal phlebitis (appendicitis, colitis, diverticulitis), infarction (sickle cell disease, embolism), direct spread from adjacent infections (cholecystitis, peptic ulcer, subphrenic abscess), trauma (rupture, wounds, biopsy, surgery), indwelling catheters or cryptogenic (45%).

5. Amoebic abscess is common in the posterosuperior segment of the right lobe. Pyogenic abscess is usually solitary and in the right lobe. There is preferential distribution of blood flow in the liver. The blood that flows from the superior mesenteric vein is distributed to the right lobe and splenic vein to the left lobe. Amoebic abscess usually spreads from primary infection in the ileocaecal junction. Hence it is common in the right lobe.

6. Ultrasonography shows a hypoechoic lesion with well-defined rim and internal debris or septations. A CT scan shows a hypodense, loculated cavity with a thick wall, which enhances. Gas can be seen within the cavity. A cluster of abscesses indicates biliary spread. MRI shows low signal in T1 and high signal in T2 with rim enhancement. Multiple abscesses are seen in 10% (usually biliary rather than haematogenous spread).

7. Differential diagnoses include hepatic cysts, haematoma, hydatid cyst, polycystic kidney disease, cystic metastasis (gastric, ovarian), necrotic hepatoma, large haemangioma and biliary cystadenoma. The most important feature that differentiates abesses from the others is the presence of rim in enhancement in contrast enhanced CT. Presence of gas is also helpful.

8. Complications are septicaemia, rupture into the subphrenic space/ peritoneal cavity/pleural cavity/pericardium, empyema and biliary obstruction. Amoebic abscess can rupture into the colon, right adrenal gland or bile ducts.

9. Liver abscesses are treated with antibiotics. Large abscesses are drained percutaneously under imaging guidance and broad spectrum antibiotic cover.

Case 1.20: Answers

1. The first test is ERCP (endoscopic retrograde cholangiopancreatography). There is a smooth, tight narrowing of the distal common bile duct, with proximal dilatation.

2. The second test is MRCP, which is a non-invasive modality for examining the biliary system. This shows a smooth, tight narrowing of the distal common bile duct. A gall stone is also noted.

3. Benign biliary stricture.

4. Differential diagnoses of benign strictures are postoperative (90%), trauma, sclerosing cholangitis, recurrent pyogenic cholangitis, acute/chronic pancreatitis, erosion by calculus, pseudocyst, perforated duodenal ulcer, abscess, papillary stenosis, radiation, hepatic artery chemoembolisation, chemotherapy infusion, AIDS and choledochal cyst. Malignant strictures are seen in pancreatic carcinoma, ampullary carcinoma, cholangiocarcinoma, metastases and lymph node compression.

5. MRCP is a type of MRI that exquisitely demonstrates the biliary tree. The following are the advantages over ERCP: it is non-invasive, involves no radiation, anaesthesia is not required, it is not operator dependent and it is cheaper. The sequences are all heavily T2 weighted, which shows all fluid-containing structures as high signal intensity. Multiple coronal oblique images of the pancreaticobiliary system are obtained. Initially thick coronal images are taken. Subsequently thin collimation images are taken in the coronal plane. Three-dimensional images of the biliary tract are acquired in radial planes. Dynamic imaging of the lower biliary system can be done for evaluation of whether a focal area of narrowing opens. High-resolution images are acquired for characterisation of subtle lesions. It is used when ERCP is contraindicated or not possible or failed, and when there is biliary enteric anastomosis. The disadvantages are: subtle lesions are missed as a result of the non-distended state, intrahepatic ducts and peripheral pancreatic duct cannot be seen because of low spatial resolution, and it delays treatment because it is a duplication of imaging.

6. MRCP is useful in evaluation of choledocholithiasis, intrahepatic ductal pathologies, chronic pancreatitis, malignant or benign obstruction, strictures, pseudocysts, biliary cystadenomas, congenital abnormalities and after biliary surgeries/reconstructions.

7. Percutaneous or ERCP biliary drainage with an endoprosthesis or metallic stents is used to relieve biliary obstruction under image control.

Case 1.21: Answers

1. The barium meal shows an irregular mass in the gastric antrum. The CT scan shows circumferential thickening of the stomach wall.

2. Gastric carcinoma.

3. Gastric carcinoma is the third most common gastrointestinal malignancy after colorectal and pancreatic cancer; 95% are adenocarcinomas and 5% squamous and adenosquamous carcinomas. The tumours can be polypoidal fungating, ulcerating, infiltrating/scirrhous, superficial spreading or advanced bulky cancer.

4. The most common location is the antrum and pylorus. Six per cent are seen in the lesser curvature and 10% involve the greater curvature. The oesophagogastric junction is involved in 30%.

5. Smoking, smoked and pickled food, nitrites, nitrates, *Helicobacter pylori* gastritis, chronic atrophic gastritis, pernicious anaemia, gastrojejunostomy, partial gastrectomy, and adenomatous and villous polyps are predisposing factors.

6. The tumour spreads locally along the peritoneal ligaments (along **gastrocolic ligament** to transverse colon and pancreas, along **gastrohepatic and hepatoduodenal ligament**s to liver), lymph nodes (draining the site of tumor which then pass to celiac and superior mesenteric group of nodes), haematogenously (liver, lung, bones), peritoneal seeding (in peritoneum, ovaries, rectal wall). Ovaries may be the only site of transperitoneal spread (Krunkenberg's tumour). Involvement of left supraclavicular node is Troisier's sign.

7. A barium meal is used for diagnosing early stage disease. A double-contrast barium study is obtained. Early cancer can be of the following types:

Type I: protruded > 5mm

Type II: superficial < 5mm

Type IIa: slightly elevated

Type IIb: flat

Type IIc: slightly depressed

Type III: excavated/ulcerated.

In the advanced stages, the tumour is seen as a filling defect, polypoidal mass, thickened folds, ulceration or diffuse infiltration along the wall (linitis plastica). A CT scan is used for local staging. There is irregular thickening of the gastric wall, with surrounding soft-tissue stranding (normal wall thickness < 5mm). Nodules can be seen on the serosal surface. Spread to the oesophagus and duodenum, adjacent lymph nodes and peritoneal seeding are noted. Distant metastasis can be evaluated.

8. Differential diagnoses of gastric filling defects are intrinsic lesions such as polyposis, leiomyoma, TB, lymphoma, Crohn's disease, sarcoidosis, sarcoma, metastasis, ectopic pancreas and haematoma or extrinsic impression by lymph nodes, or pancreatic, liver, splenic or renal mass. Lymphoma is the most common tumour that can be confused in a CT scan. In lymphoma, there is more extensive and homogeneous wall thickening, but there is a lesser perigastric component. Enlarged lymph nodes are seen, even below the level of renal veins (adenocarcinoma nodes – not seen below the renal vein).

Case 1.22: Answers

1. There is large, round mass with central areas of necrosis in the left lobe of the liver. There are several abnormal distorted vascular channels within the mass. The left portal vein is not visualized.

2. Hepatocellular carcinoma (HCC).

3. Alcohol, hepatitis B, hepatitis C, haemochromatosis, aflatoxin, biliary cirrhosis, androgenic steroids, oral contraceptives, thorotrast and porphyria cutanea tarda are predisposing factors. It is more common in the Far East, Asia and sub-Saharan Africa. Pruritus, jaundice, splenomegaly, variceal bleeding, cachexia, hepatic encephalopathy, right upper quadrant pain, ascites and other signs of liver failure are features of hepatoma. Laboratory findings include elevated α-fetoprotein; other lab findings are expected in a cirrhotic liver.

4. Hepatoma can be focal, multifocal or diffuse. A CT scan in an arterial and portal phase is usually adequate to establish the diagnosis, which is confirmed by ultrasound- or CT-guided biopsy. MRI and contrast ultrasonography are also useful. Ultrasonography shows an expansive tumour. A hypoechoic rim at the periphery of the tumour is a result of a fibrous capsule or compressed parenchyma. Ill-defined margins are seen in more invasive tumours. On a CT scan, HCC is seen as a hypodense mass, with a hypodense rim of capsule. The tumour is bright if there is superimposed haemorrhage. Large tumours are heterogeneous, as a result of areas of haemorrhage or necrosis. The characteristic appearance is seen after contrast enhancement. As the tumour is supplied by the hepatic artery, it is very bright and enhances in the arterial phase, but the contrast rapidly washes out and the tumour is seen as a hypodense mass in the portal phase. Invasion of the portal vein and other structures can be seen. MRI also shows similar features. The lesion is dark on a non-contrast scan and shows early arterial enhancement with quick washout in the portal venous images. Angiography shows vascular tumour, with hypertrophied neovasculature. Cirrhotic patients undergo yearly ultrasonography and α-fetoprotein for screening development of HCC.

5. **Metastasis** is multifocal and does not enhance in the arterial phase, except the vascular metastasis such as renal carcinoma, thyroid carcinoma, phaeochromocytoma, neuroendocrine tumours and sarcomas. **Haemangiomas** are the most common benign tumours in liver and might be difficult to differentiate from hepatomas when they are large. They usually show a different pattern of enhancement, which is nodular and slow filling in delayed phases. They show positive uptake in Technetium labelled RBC Scintigraphy and have very high signal in heavily T2 weighted images. **Adenomas** and **focal nodular hyperplasia** are also vascular tumours, but they do not show rapid washout and are isodense on the delayed scans. Scar is seen in **focal nodular hyperplasia** and **fibrolamellar carcinoma**.

6. Surgery is the treatment of choice. Only 5% are cured with surgery. Radiology is useful in palliative treatment of HCC. Hepatic artery chemoembolisation, percutaneous alcohol ablation, radiofrequency ablation and microwave/laser ablation are carried out under image control. In hepatic artery chemoembolisation, Lipiodol (iodised poppy seed oil) is used along with chemotherapeutic agents, such as doxorubicin (Adriamycin) and embolic material such as gelfoam. The Lipiodol is selectively taken up by the tumour and cleared very slowly and hence the chemotherapeutic agent is selectively delivered to the tumour, without toxic side effects.

Case 1.23: Answers

1. Supine X-rays of the abdomen, shows dilated loops of small and large bowel, with abrupt cut off at the level of the sigmoid colon. There is no gas in the rectum. CT scan shows dilated small and large bowel loops, up to the level of a soft tissue in the sigmoid colon.

2. Large bowel obstruction, caused by a tumour in the sigmoid colon.

3. Causes of large bowel obstruction:

    Luminal: faecal impaction, gallstone, intussusception

    Mural: tumours, inflammation (ulcerative colitis, Crohn's disease), infection (TB, amoebiasis, actinomycosis, schistosomiasis), radiation, ischaemia, trauma, haematoma

    Extrinsic: adhesions, volvulus, hernia, extrinsic tumours such as metastasis, endometriosis.

4. The plain film shows dilated loops of large bowel. The caecum is dilated. If the ileocaecal valve is competent, the small bowel loops are normal. If it is incompetent, gas escapes into the small bowel and there is dilatation of small bowel loops as well. Gas–fluid levels distal to the hepatic flexure usually indicate obstruction unless there is diarrhoea, or after an enema (dilated bowel loops with fluid levels).

5. The CT scan is useful for finding the cause of the obstruction. Usually large bowel obstruction results from a tumour. A CT scan can help in evaluating the cause of obstruction and assessing extraluminal structures and spread.

6. Use of barium is avoided in emergency situations, for fear of leakage into the peritoneal cavity which results in peritonitis and peritoneal toilet may be difficult during laparatomy. Retained barium in colon makes colonoscopy difficult to perform. Hence, if there is doubt about obstruction, a water-soluble contrast enema can be done to localise the site of the obstruction.

7. The critical diameter of the caecum is 10–12 cm. In large bowel obstruction, usually the caecum is the most dilated portion. A caecum > 12 cm indicates impending perforation.

8. The causes of large bowel obstruction in children are meconium plug syndrome, colonic atresia, imperforate anus, Hirschsprung's disease and small left colon syndrome.

Case 1.24: Answers

1. The barium meal shows deformed and irregular duodenal cap. On the second film, barium is noted within the biliary system.

2. Duodenal ulcer, with choledochoduodenal fistula.

3. Normal duodenum is protected from damage by gastric acid and the proteolytic enzyme pepsin by a mucous layer, bicarbonate secretion and prostaglandins. Duodenal ulcer results from an acid imbalance that might be caused by high acid production or inadequate protective factors. Predisposing factors are NSAIDs (inhibition of COX1, which decreases protective prostaglandins), steroids, *Helicobacter pyloric* infection (increased gastric acid production by cytokines, immunological response against duodenal mucosa secondary to bacterial colonization in gastric metaplasia induced by high acid, proteases, urease), smoking, alcohol, caffeine, Zollinger-Ellison syndrome, mastocytosis, chemotherapy, radiation and cocaine use.

4. 95% of all duodenal ulcers are seen in the bulbar region and are more common in the anterior wall. 5% are seen in post bulbar region with the majority in the medal wall above papilla. Ulcers in the post bulbar region especially beyond the ampulla and in the jejunum are suspicious of Zollinger Ellison-Syndrome due to gastrinomas.

5. Barium meal is sparingly used nowadays since the diagnosis is made by endoscopy. In early stages, a round or oval ulcer is seen in the duodenal bulb. Kissing ulcers are seen as ulcers opposite to each other in the anterior and posterior wall. Giant ulcers are large and measure >2cm. Most of the ulcers present with deformity of the duodenal bulb. The deformity can be a cloverleaf deformity or an hourglass stenosis.

6. Differential diagnosis for duodenal narrowing and deformity are – tuberculosis strongyloidiasis, Crohn's disease, sprue, malignancy, pancreatitis, pancreatic carcinoma and trauma.

7. Complications are obstruction, perforation (anterior wall), bleeding (posterior wall) and penetration with sealed perforation. Duodenal ulcer is the commonest cause of bowel perforation. Pneumoperitoneum is seen on a plain x ray. CT scan of the abdomen can be used to confirm and find the location of perforation. Leak of air and contrast can be demonstrated from the site of duodenal ulcer. Fistula can develop to the bile duct. Treatment depends on the etiology and presentation. *H. pylori* induced ulcers receive eradication therapy regimen. For NSAID ulcers, the drugs are discontinued and proton pump inhibitors are used. Bleeding ulcers are treated with endoscopic therapy (cautery/epinephrine/argon plasma coagulation). H2 receptor antagonists and proton pump inhibitors are also used. Failure of endoscopic therapy for bleeding, recurrent bleeding and perforation are indications for urgent surgery. Vagotomy with pyloroplasty or antrectomy is done in patients who are refractory/intolerant/no compliant to medical management."

Case 1.25: Answers

1. This is MRI of the perianal region. These are coronal T1 and STIR sequences. The latter suppresses the fat and displays fluid-filled structures as bright areas. A linear high signal lesion is seen extending from above the level of the internal sphincter to the skin surface on the left side.

2. Fistula *in ano.*

3. The causes are: Crohn's disease, infection, surgery, iatrogenic, radiation, malignancy, trauma, ischaemia, foreign body and idiopathic. It is more common in men.

4. The anal canal has an external sphincter of skeletal muscle attached to the anococcygeal ligament, perineal body and urogenital diaphragm, merging proximally with the puborectalis muscle, which in turn merges with levator ani. The internal sphincter is the distal termination of the circular muscle of the gut. The longitudinal muscle is between the external and internal sphincters and has no sphincter function. The intersphincteric plane is found between the longitudinal muscle and the external sphincter. Ischiorectal fossa is lateral to the sphincter complex. The mucosa lining the anal canal is divided by the dentate line (pectinate line), which is 2 cm from the anal verge. Above this line the mucosa is columnar, made of longitudinal anal columns of Morgagni, the distal aspects of which are linked to each other with anal valves; these have pockets called crypts of Morgagni or anal sinuses, into which the anal glands empty. The cryptoglandular hypothesis is that the fistulae originate as infection in anal glands. Two-thirds of these glands are in the intersphincteric space, where infection begins and manifests acutely as abscess and chronically as fistula.

5. Fistulae connect two epithelial surfaces. There is an internal enteric opening in the anal canal at the level of the dentate line, which is usually the 6 o'clock position. The fistula reaches perianal skin by a variety of routes.

Parks classification: intersphincteric (along intersphincteric space without penetrating external sphincter – 45%); **trans-sphincteric** (crosses external sphincter and reaches ischioanal fossa – 30%); **suprasphincteric** (spreads upward in the intersphincteric space arching over puborectalis and crossing the levator plate – 20%); **extrasphincteric** (no intersphincteric infection, enters rectum or anorectal junction directly – 5%).

Diverticular disease, rectal Crohn's disease and carcinoma are causes. Secondary tracts are extensions from the primary tract and can be intersphincteric, ischioanal or supralevator. Ischioanal fossa is the most common site. Extensions in the horizontal plane are called horseshoe if there is ramification on each side of the internal opening.

6. The majority of anal fistulae have simple tracks that are easily identified during surgery. In 5–15%, the tracks are complicated with secondary extensions outside the anal sphincter, horseshoe fistulae, and ischiorectal and supralevator abscesses. Failure to recognise these secondary extensions will result in surgical failure. MRI enables assessment of all these features.

7. The following features should be assessed by imaging for a through evaluation of an anorectal fistula:

    (a) **primary track**: superficial, intersphincteric, suprasphincteric, trans-sphincteric, extrasphincteric, sinus

    (b) **abscess**: intersphincteric, ischiorectal, supralevator.

    (c) **horseshoeing**: intersphincteric, infralevator, supralevator

    (d) **internal opening**: location

    (e) **external opening**: location.

Case 1.26: Answers

1. The CT scan shows air in the posterior mediastinum (just anterior to the vertebra) and right-sided hydropneumothorax. Contrast swallows show leakage of contrast into the mediastinum, from the lower oesophagus.

2. Oesophageal rupture.

3. Oesophageal rupture is seen commonly after iatrogenic injury (endoscopy, stricture dilatation, bougie, surgery, intubation), spontaneous rupture (Boerhaave's syndrome – rupture of distal oesophagus after an episode of vomiting) and chest trauma.

4. The common locations of rupture are cervical and upper thoracic oesophagus. The left posterolateral wall of the distal oesophagus, just superior to the gastro-oesophageal junction, is another common location of rupture.

5. Chest pain, dyspnoea, dysphagia, odynophagia, sepsis and hypotension are clinical features.

6. Plain X-ray findings in oesophageal rupture are extensive pneumomediastinum, subcutaneous emphysema, left pleural effusion and left lower lobe atelectasis. Extrapleural air in lower mediastinum between parietal pleura and diaphragm is called V sign of Naclerio. Mediastinal widening indicates development of mediastinitis. The diagnosis and site of rupture is confirmed with a contrast swallow, which shows the leak in 90% of patients. If the leak is not demonstrated in a contrast swallow and

the clinical suspicion is high, a CT scan should be carried out immediately after the contrast swallow, which demonstrates even a small leak. CT scan shows mediastinal air, haematoma, oesophagal wall thickening, contrast leak, pleural effusion and lung changes secondary to aspiration.

7. Complications of oesophageal rupture are mediastinitis, mediastinal abscess and SVC obstruction. Severe cardiorespiratory disturbance can be seen in the acute stage. Small tears are managed conservatively. If the tear is large and recognised early, surgical repair is carried out.

Case 1.27: Answers

1. Barium swallow shows a shaggy outline of the oesophagus with multiple, small, superficial ulcerations along its entire length, giving it an irregular contour.

2. Candida oesophagitis.

3. Candia oesophagitis is seen in immunosuppressed individuals such as those with HIV, leukaemia, chronic disease, diabetes, immunosuppressive therapy in renal/hepatic/pancreatic/cardiac transplantation, steroids, chemotherapy, radiotherapy or antibiotics. It is also seen in patients with sluggish oesophageal motility such as scleroderma, achalasia, strictures and after surgeries such as fundoplication.

4. *Candida albicans* is an opportunistic fungal infection. It has creamy-white plaques covering friable erythematous mucosa. Clinically there is dysphagia, odynophagia, chest pain and oral thrush. It is commonly seen in the upper half of the oesophagus. Oesophageal candidiasis is an indicator of HIV.

5. Barium swallow shows a cobblestone appearance in the early stages due to mucosal nodularity. Longitudinal plaques are also seen. The characteristic appearance is a shaggy ouline of the oesophagus, which has an irregular serrated contour caused by a combination of ulcers, plaques, erosions, pseudomembranes and haemorrhage. The lumen is narrowed in the later stages and there are tertiary peristaltic contractions. Strictures are rare. Intramural diverticulosis may be seen. Double-contrast swallow is the most sensitive investigation.

6. Complications are stricture, systemic candidiasis and gastric bezoar.

7. Differential diagnoses: reflux oesophagitis, superficial spreading carcinoma, varices, artefacts, herpes oesophagitis, glycogen acanthoses, caustic ingestion, Barrett's oesophagus, pseudodiverticulosis and papillomatosis.

8. Treatment is with antifungal medications such as ketoconazole or fluconazole.

Case 1.28: Answers

1. Ultrasonography shows a dark hypoechoic, tubular structure at the porta hepatic, lying medial to a distended gall bladder. This is a prominent common bile duct.

2. MRI shows fusiform dilatation of the common bile duct. There is no dilatation of the intrahepatic biliary radicles.

3. Choledochal cyst, type IA.

4. Choledochal cysts are congenital anomalies with cystic dilatation of the biliary tree. The following is the LaTodani classification of choledochal cysts:

   Type I (80–90%): saccular or fusiform dilatations of the common bile duct

   - **IA**: saccular, entire extrahepatic bile duct or most of it
   - **IB**: saccular, limited segment of the bile duct
   - **IC**: fusiform, most or all of the extrahepatic bile duct

   Type II: diverticulum arising from the common bile duct

   Type III: choledochocele arising from the intraduodenal portion of the common bile duct

   Type IVA: multiple dilatations of the intra- and extrahepatic bile ducts

   Type IVB: multiple dilatations involving only the extrahepatic bile ducts

   Type V (Caroli's disease): consists of multiple dilatations limited to the intrahepatic bile ducts.

5. Choledochal cyst is seen in childhood or older age groups. It presents with recurrent abdominal cramps, fever, jaundice, cirrhosis with portal hypertension in late case(s). Complications include bile stasis with cholelithiasis, cholangitis, liver abscess, septicaemia and cholangiocarcinomas.

6. Ultrasonography shows cystic dilatation of the bile duct. The location depends on the type of choledochal cyst. Demonstration of communication with the biliary tree is essential for making a diagnosis. Doppler ultrasonography is used to evaluate the liver and portal hypertension. A CT scan shows a dilated duct, and coronal and sagittal reconstructions show continuation with the bile duct. Sludge or calculi are seen in dilated ducts. MRCP can be done and shows dilatation of bile ducts. Hepatobiliary nuclear scans can demonstrate communication between the cysts and bile ducts. Ultrasound-guided aspiration of cysts will confirm the presence of bile and the diagnosis of cholangitis. Differential diagnoses include other causes of liver cysts such as simple liver cyst, abscess, hydatid cyst and cystic tumours.

Case 1.29: Answers

1. This investigation is ERCP. It shows multiple filling defects in the distal portion of the common bile duct. The proximal common bile duct and intrahepatic biliary radicles are dilated.

2. Choledocholithiasis.

3. Complications of ERCP are acute pancreatitis, acute cholangitis, bleeding and perforation. MRCP (magnetic resonance cholangiopancreaticography) is an alternative, non-invasive technique now available to demonstrate the biliary tree.

4. Clinical features of choledocholithiasis are colicky right upper quadrant pain, nausea, vomiting and dyspepsia. Complications of gallstones are acute cholecystitis, perforation, abscesses and gallstone ileus. Complications of common bile duct stones are jaundice, acute cholangitis and acute pancreatitis. Gall stones have a recognised association with gall bladder and bile duct carcinomas.

5. Biliary stasis, infection, haemolysis and enteral resection are the common predisposing factors in the formation of a gallstone.

6. Cholesterol stone, mixed stone and pigment (calcium bilirubinate) are the two types of gallstones.

7. In cholangiography (percutaneous or ERCP), stones are seen as filling defects within the contrast-opacified bile ducts. Common bile duct stones are seen on ultrasonography as bright opacities with distal dark acoustic shadowing. Proximal ducts are dilated. Stones are better seen if there is common bile duct dilatation. On CT the stone is seen with a target sign (intraluminal mass with crescenteric ring). On MRI and MRCP, the stone is seen as a dark object within the bright bile in the biliary ducts. Air bubbles can be confused for stones on ERCP or MRCP, but they always collect in the non-dependent portion of the system.

8. Laparoscopic cholecystectomy is the procedure of choice for symptomatic gallstones in surgically fit patients. Ursodeoxycholic acid is used to dissolve pure cholesterol stones. Extracorporeal shock wave lithotripsy (ESWL) is not as effective as in renal stones

9. **Courvoisier's law**: in the presence of jaundice, an enlarged gallbladder is unlikely to result from gallstones; rather, carcinoma of the pancreas or the lower biliary tree is more likely. This can be explained by the observation that the gallbladder with stones is usually chronically fibrosed and, so, incapable of enlargement.

Case 1.30: Answers

1. Ultrasonography of the abdomen shows a linear, vertical discontinuity in the pancreatic body. There is disruption of the pancreatic duct. The CT scan shows a vertical split in the body of the pancreas.

2. Pancreatic laceration. Pancreatic injuries are uncommon (0.4/100 000 of trauma). Injury may follow blunt or penetrating trauma. Most blunt injuries are caused by direct contact with the steering wheel or secondary to seat belt injury or handlebar injury in cyclists/motorcyclists.

3. Classification of pancreatic trauma:

I: simple superficial contusion, minimal parenchymal damage without ductal injury (most common).

II: deep laceration/perforation/transection of body/tail; pancreatic duct may be damaged

III: severe crushing, perforation/transection of the pancreatic head, with or without duct injury, but intact duodenum

IV: combined pancreaticoduodenal injuries:

(a) with mild pancreatic injury

(b) with severe pancreatic injury and duct disruption.

4. The most common location of pancreatic trauma is the junction of the body and tail. Transection is more common to the left of the superior mesenteric vessels and occurs when there is compression over the spine. Injuries to the right of midline cause serious crushing injuries to the pancreas and duodenum.

5. Ultrasonography and CT are used for diagnosis of pancreatic trauma. With CT, contusion is seen as an area of focal hypodensity in the pancreas. Acute haematoma is seen as a high-density area. Laceration is seen as a focal area of linear disruption in the pancreas. Fluid collection can be seen around the superior mesenteric artery, transverse mesocolon and lesser sac, and between the pancreas and splenic vein. There is thickening of the pararenal fascia. Other features are pancreatic enlargement, fluid separating the splenic vein and pancreas, high-density fat around the pancreas and intra-/extraperitoneal fluid. ERCP is useful for assessing ductal injuries. MRCP is a non-invasive modality for assessing the pancreatic duct.

6. Pancreatitis, pseudocyst formation, pseudoaneurysm, portal vein thrombosis, abscess and fistula are the complications Many patients have delayed presentations with recurrent pancreatitis and pseudocysts. A patient with a post-traumatic pseudocyst should be considered to have a tear of the duct unless proved otherwise.

7. Grade I injuries do not require surgery, unless there are serious associated injuries to other organs. Grade II injuries require only drainage, if the main duct is intact. For distal ductal injury, distal pancreatic resection and drainage of pancreatic bed with or without splenectomy is done. Surgery for grade III injuries depends on the ductal injury status. Grade IV injuries always require surgery, which is usually pancreaticoduodenectomy.

Case 1.31: Answers

1. The CT scan shows a spiculated mass with specks of calcification, located in the mesentery close to a small bowel loop. There are linear fibrotic bands extending from the mass into the mesentery and some fixity to a loop of bowel.

2. Carcinoid tumour of the small bowel and extension into the mesentery.

3. Carcinoid tumour is the most common primary tumour of the small bowel. In the bowel, the most common location is the small bowel, of which the ileum is involved in 90%. Other locations are the jejunum, duodenum, stomach, appendix, colon, rectum, pancreas, liver and biliary tract. A third of these tumours are in the small bowel, with metastases. A third of these tumours are multiple.

4. Carcinoid tumours arise from Kulchitsky's cells in the crypts of Leiberkühn. They may be asymptomatic or present with pain, obstruction, weight loss, palpable mass, perforation or gastrointestinal haemorrhage. Carcinoid syndrome is seen in 7%, characterised by episodic diarrhoea, obstruction, bleeding, malabsorption, flushing of skin and right heart failure from endocardial fibroelastosis, leading to tricuspid regurgitation and pulmonary valve stenosis, wheezing and fever. Carcinoid syndrome is regarded as a sign of malignancy. It is usually seen in tumours with metastasis or primary pulmonary or ovarian carcinoids. There is increased excretion of 5-HIAA in the urine.

5. Plain X-ray findings include soft-tissue mass, calcification and obstruction, none of which are specific. Barium may show kinking (characteristic finding) and separation of bowel loops. The most specific technique is somatostatin receptor scintigraphy. Ultrasound is poor in detecting the primary, but useful in hepatic metastasis. Angiogram shows a sunburst appearance. On the CT scan, there is a focal mesenteric mass with spiculated margins and radiating stellate strands along the neurovascular bundles, indicating a marked desmoplastic reaction, which is the characteristic finding. Calcification is seen. There is retraction and shortening of the mesentery with thickened small bowel loops. Necrotic lymph nodes and vascular liver metastasis can be seen. An angiogram shows a sunburst appearance. CT enteroclysis is a new technique that obviates the need for a barium study. In this technique, a negative oral contrast is administered to distend the lumen and thin-slice CT images are obtained and reconstructed in multiple planes.

6. Complications are obstruction, perforation, haemorrhage, right heart failure and carcinoid syndrome.

7. Differential diagnoses: desmoid tumours (in Gardner syndrome), small bowel adenocarcinoma, lymphoma, retractile mesenteritis, metastasis, and pancreatic/gastric/colonic carcinoma.

8. Carcinoid syndrome is managed by medication with somatostatin analogues (ocreotide) which alleviates symptoms by reduction of hormonally active tumour bulk. Primary tumour is resected if detected early or when it causes obstruction.

Case 1.32: Answers

1. The first study is a small bowel study with barium. A long segment of the terminal ileum is narrowed with small ulcerations. The caecum appears normal.

2. The CT scan shows diffuse circumferential wall thickening of a loop of ileum, in the pelvis. In addition, there is increased density of fat in the adjacent mesentery and retroperitoneum, with creeping fat sign.

3. Crohn's disease of the small bowel.

4. Crohn's disease is a chronic inflammatory disease of the bowel with discontinuous, asymmetrical involvement of the gastrointestinal tract. Pathologically Crohn's disease is characterised by transmural involvement and granulomas. Clinical features include diarrhoea, rectal bleeding, abdominal pain (crampy or steady right lower quadrant/periumbilical, relieved by defecation), weight loss, anaemia and joint pain. Children might have growth failure and delayed puberty. Physical findings may reveal right lower quadrant tenderness, mass, perianal fistulae, skin changes (erythema nodosum/pyoderma gangrenosum), uveitis and peripheral arthritis.

5. A barium meal shows involvement of the terminal ileum in the form of thickened and nodular folds, aphthous ulcers, cobblestone mucosa or medial caecal defect. There is ridigity of small bowel loops with

wide separation. Postinflammatory polyps, mucosal granularity and pseudodiverticula can be seen. A CT scan shows homogeneous thickened walls or a double-halo configuration (lumen surrounded by oedematous hypodense mucosa and soft-tissue density muscularis and serosa). There are skip lesions of asymmetrical bowel wall thickening. A characteristic feature on CT is the creeping fat sign, where there is massive proliferation of mesenteric fat separating the bowel loops. Dilated bowel loops, sinus, fistula, adenopathy and abscesses are other features.

6. Radiological differential diagnoses are: TB (involvement of caecum, pulmonary TB), infection with *Yersinia* spp. (resolution in 3–4 months), radiation enteritis, lymphoma (no spasm, nodular/aneurysmal), actinomycosis, and carcinoid and eosinophilic gastroenteritis.

7. Complications are fistula, sinus, abscess, perforation, toxic megacolon, hydronephrosis and small bowel adenocarcinoma. Fatty liver, liver abscess, gallstones, cholecystitis, sclerosing cholangitis, urolithiasis, hydronephrosis, amyloidosis, cystitis, clubbing, seronegative spondyloarthropathy, erosive arthritis, avascular necrosis, osteomyelitis, septic arthritis and abscesses are other complications.

8. Treatment consists of 5-aminosalicylic acid (5-ASA) preparations, antibiotics such as metronidazole, corticosteroids, immunosuppressants (methotrexate, 6-mercaptopurine, azathioprine, antibodies to tumour necrosis factor [TNF] α). Surgery is performed when medical therapy fails and complications develop.

Case 1.33: Answers

1. Barium enema shows absence of haustrations in the colon. There are multiple small ulcers, scattered throughout the colon, but more prominent in the descending colon, which is also rigid and non distensible. There are mucosal islands noted in the transverse colon. The transverse colon is grossly distended near the hepatic flexure. In the second picture, there is an irregular, ulcerative mass in the transverse colon, close to the splenic flexure.

2. Ulcerative colitis. Complications seen here are toxic megacolon and carcinoma.

3. Ulcerative colitis is an idiopathic inflammatory bowel disease, with symmetrical continuous involvement of the colon. It presents with bloody diarrhoea, fever and cramps. Extracolonic features are iritis, pyoderma gangrenosum, erythema nodosum, pericholangitis, sclerosing cholangitis, chronic active hepatitis, rheumatoid arthritis, spondylitis and thrombotic complications.

4. Usually, ulcerative colitis begins in the rectum and spreads proximally and symmetrically. Rectosigmoid is involved in 95% of cases. When the colitis extends proximal to the splenic flexure it is called universal colitis, and when it extends to the terminal ileum it is termed as backwash ileitis.

5. The findings on the barium enema depend on the stage. In the acute stage there is fine mucosal granularity and tiny superficial ulcers. Collar-button ulcers, double tracking and thumbprinting are other findings. Pseudopolyps are seen as a result of scattered areas of oedematous mucosa and re-epithelialised granulation tissue within an area of denuded mucosa. The presacral space is widened as a result of inflammation. Rectal folds are obliterated. In later stages, the haustra are lost. Inflammatory polyps are seen and the colon is short and rigid. The term 'burnt-out colon' is used when there is distensible colon with no haustral markings and no mucosal pattern. Postinflammatory polyps are small sessile or filiform polyps.

6. Complications are toxic megacolon (most common cause of death, transverse colon > 55cm), strictures, obstruction and perforation, fistula formation, scelerosing cholangitis, arthritis including sacroileitis, nephrolithiasis and colonic carcinoma.

7. There is a 5% risk of malignancy in patients with ulcerative colitis. Risk starts after 10 years and is 0.5% per year for colitis. It is higher if the onset is at age < 15 years, if there is pancolitis or when it is in the rectosigmoid. The lesion is usually annular or polypoid.

8. Differential diagnoses:

   Familial polyposis: haustrations are seen; no inflammation in polyps

   Cathartic colon: more extensive changes are seen in the right colon

   Crohn's disease is the most important clinical differential diagnosis, and is more common in a small bowel with deep ulcers, thick ileocaecal valve, eccentric location and transmural skip lesion. Megacolon is uncommon, but fistulae may be seen. There is a slightly increased risk of carcinoma.

In ulcerative colitis, the colon is involved and the rectum always involved. There are shallow ulcers with loss of haustrations and a gaping ileocaecal valve. There is symmetrical involvement with no skip lesions. Megacolon is common and there is a high risk of carcinoma.

9. Treatment is with 5-ASA derivatives, steroids and immunosuppressants. Surgery is done when complications develop.

Case 1.34: Answers

1. The barium enema shows the entire colon studded with multiple small polyps. This is more prominently seen in the left colon, because the transverse colon and ascending colon are filled with barium. There is no mass.

2. Colonic polyposis.

3. Familial adenomatous polyposis (FAP). FAP is an autosomal dominant disease with 80% penetrance, characterised by tubular/villotubular adenomas carpeting the entire colon. There is a family history and the symptoms start in the third or fourth decade, with abdominal pain, weight loss, diarrhoea and bloody stools.

4. A barium enema or colonoscopy is used for diagnosis. The former shows the entire colon carpeted with polyps, 2–3 mm in size with a maximal size of 2 cm. The polyps are tubular or tubulovillous. Polyps are also occasionally seen in the stomach and small bowel.

5. Histologically polyps can be tubular, villous or tubulovillous. Adenomatous, hamartomatous, hyperplastic, pseudo- and filiform polyps are the other types. Adenomas consist of 10% of all colonic polyps; 90% of them are small and < 1.5cm. Malignant conversion occurs more with villous adenomas (cauliflower appearance), and sessile and larger ones.

6. FAP is associated with hamartomatous polyps in the stomach and adenomas in the duodenum. Malignant transformation of polyps is seen, with increasing incidence with age. The risk is 12% by 5 years, 30% by 10

years and 100% by 20 years. Usually carcinoma presents at 20–40 years. Periampullary carcinoma is also associated.

7. Drugs used for treatment are sulindac and celecoxib. Flexible sigmoidoscopy is carried out every 1–2 years. Prophylactic colectomy is performed once polyps have been detected and the patient is old enough, or advanced features develop. After the development of colonic carcinoma, permanent ileostomy, endorectal pull-through pouch or Kock's pouch (distal ileum formed into one-way valve by invagination of bowel at skin site) are indicated.

8. Differential diagnoses include other polyposis syndromes:

Gardner syndrome: FAP, osteomas, desmoid tumours, thyroid cancer, cysts

Peutz–Jeghers syndrome: hamartomas, mucocutaneous lesions, cancers

Cronkhite–Canada syndrome: hamartomas, pigmentation, nail destruction, cancers

Cowden syndrome: hamartomas, papillomas, keratoses, breast/thyroid carcinoma

Juvenile polyposis

Ruvalcaba syndrome: hamartomas, penis pigmentation, macrocephaly

Turcot syndrome: brain tumours (medulloblastoma, glioma)

Lynch syndrome: hereditary non-polyposis colorectal cancer syndrome (HNPCC)

Ulcerative colitis: pseudopolyps (inflamed mucosa on a background of denuded mucosa), filiform polyp (postinflammatory, projection of submucosa covered by mucosa on all sides)

Lymphoid hyperplasia

Lymphosarcoma.

Case 1.35: Answers

1. The CT scan of the pelvis shows a large mass in the rectum. The rectal wall is thickened and there is increased density in the fat around the rectum.

MRI shows circumferential thickening of the rectum, with adjacent soft-tissue stranding. There is extension of the tumour outside the rectum on the left side, involving the mesorectal fascia.

2. Rectal carcinoma with extensive locoregional spread.

3. Rectal carcinomas are adenocarcinomas. Predisposing factors are high-fat, low-fibre diet, a family history, familial polyposis coli, Gardner syndrome, Turcot syndrome, Peutz–Jegher's syndrome, juvenile polyposis syndromes, Muir syndrome, ulcerative colitis and Crohn's disease. Colonic cancer is the most common gastrointestinal cancer. It is believed that most cancers start as an adenoma.

4. Rectal cancers may be asymptomatic or present with palpable mass, bleeding, anaemia, abdominal discomfort, change in bowel habits, obstruction and weight loss. Digital palpation, sigmoidoscopy, blood tests and LFTs are performed. Sigmoidoscopy and biopsy are used initially for diagnosis. A flexible endoscopy is performed for assessment of the rest of the colon, but when it is not possible a double contrast barium enema is performed. CT scan is used for staging of the disease. MRI and endorectal ultrasound are very useful in locoregional staging.

5. Barium enema: tumours in rectum can be polypoidal (which are seen as lobulaed masses) or annular (narrowing of lumen, with overhanging edges) or ulcerative. Large polyps with irregular margins or/and without stalk are suspicious of malignancy. Mucinous tumours are calcified. CT scan shows circumferential wall thickening or polypodidal mass. If tumour extends outside the wall, there is perirectal soft tissue stranding. Lymph nodes are seen in perirectal space. Lymphadenopathy to the pelvic side wall, metatasis to the liver, paraaortic nodes and chest are assessed. Complications of the lesion are large bowel obstruction, perforation and localised abscess formation, invasion of adjacent organs such as bladder, uterus, and vagina. 5% have synchronous cancers. Invasion of adjacent organs is assessed by loss of fat plane between the tumour and these organs. Nodes more than 10mm are considered abnormal.

6. MRI is the most useful for locoregional spread. The involvement of mesorectal fascia is the most important information for the surgeon. If the mesorectal fascia is involved, a radical surgical removal is carried out along with chemotherapy. Presence of perirectal lymph nodes and pelvic side wall nodes > 10mm alters the prognosis and treatment. Hepatic metastasis < 3cm can be treated by resection. Unresectable hepatic metastases are treated by chemoembolisation or radiofrequency ablation. Metastasis to

the adrenals and lungs can be seen. Transrectal ultrasonography is useful in the early stages where the involvement of specific layers of the wall can be assessed.

7. Differential diagnoses: lymphoma, inflammation, benign polyps, colitis, diverticulitis, carcinoid and metastasis produce rectal wall thickening.

8. Transrectal ultrasound or MRI can be used for diagnosis and local staging, CT scan is useful for assessment of metastatic spread and post operative follow up. Rectal stents are inserted for obstruction. Radiofrequency ablation and hepatic chemoembolisation are used in unresectable liver metatasis.

Case 1.36: Answers

1. The plain X-ray shows a large opacity behind the heart, with an air–fluid level. The CT scan shows loops of bowel, herniating through the oesophageal hiatus and lying in the posterior mediastinum, behind the heart.

2. Hiatus hernia.

3. Hiatus hernia is herniation of the stomach through the oesophageal hiatus. There are two types: sliding and rolling. The **sliding type** is the most common, with the oesophagogastric junction in the chest; it is caused by rupture of the phrenico-oesophageal membrane aggravated by repetitive stretching with swallowing. The **rolling type** (paraoesophageal) is a rare type (1%), with the stomach displaced into the chest, and the oesophagogastric junction in the abdomen. The majority of rolling hernias are **mixed**, where the cardia is displaced into the thorax and the greater curvature rolls up into the posterior mediastinum.

4. On the plain X-ray, a retrocardiac soft-tissue opacity or opacity with an air–fluid level might be seen. Barium swallow is used for further evaluation. In sliding hiatus hernia, the oesophagogastric junction and part of the stomach are located above the diaphragm. The distance between the B

ring and the oesophageal hiatus is > 3 cm. Tortuous oesophagus is seen joining eccentrically with the hiatus. Within the hiatus, thick folds are seen (more than six folds) with reflux oesophagitis. In true rolling hernia, the oesophagogastric junction is seen in the abdomen and a portion of the stomach in the thorax. On the CT scan, diaphragmatic hiatus > 15 mm, stomach is seen in the chest, with thick walls, and there is increased fat around the oesophagus from fat herniation.

5. Saint's triad is a combination of hiatus hernia with gastro-oesophageal reflux, diverticulosis and gallstones. Duodenal ulcer is also associated.

6. Volvulus, incarceration, obstruction, perforation, gastro-oesophageal reflux, reflux oesophagitis, Barrett's oesophagus and carcinoma are the complications. Gastric ulcer is seen in the lesser curvature in a rolling hernia.

7. Radiological differential diagnosis: Congenital short oesopahgus with intrathoracic stomach, Bochdalek hernia, large epiphrenic diverticulum of oesophagus, abscesses and cavitating neoplasms of lower lobes of lungs and mediastinum, traumatic diaphragmatic hernia and post surgical appearances of stomach/intestinal pull through procedures.

8. Nissen fundoplication or a modification of the procedure is used in the treatment of hiatus hernia. The gastric fundus is wrapped or plicated around the inferior part of the oesophagus, restoring the function of the lower oesophageal sphincter. The procedure can be done laparoscopically. The need for surgery has reduced considerably due to improved medical management of gastro-oesophageal reflux.

Case 1.37: Answers

1. AP view of barium swallow shows a focal collection of barium in the lower part of neck. Lateral view shows a large outpouching filled with barium, extending posteriorly from the lower part of hypopharynx. This is seen above the level of a contracted cricopharynx.

2. Pharyngeal pouch.

3. Pharyngeal pouch or Zencker diverticulum is a pulsion diverticulum, in which the pharyngeal mucosa herniates posteriorly between cricopharyngeus and the inferior pharyngeal constrictor muscle (Kilian's dehiscence) as a result of failure of coordination between the relaxation of cricopharyngeus during swelling and the contraction of the pharyngeal wall.

4. Clinical features are dysphagia, regurgitation, aspiration and halitosis. It is more common in much older men.

5. Barium swallow is the diagnostic procedure of choice. The pouch can be of any size. Small pouches can be obscured by the barium pool and delayed images are required to notice stasis of contrast. Large pouches are seen in lateral and AP views after the barium has passed through the rest of the oesophagus. When the pouch is very large, it might displace the oesophagus laterally.

6. Lateral pharyngeal pouches are persistent protrusions of the lateral pharyngeal wall at sites of anatomical weakness, such as the posterior thyrohyoid membrane and tonsillar fossa after a tonsillectomy. They are seen as hemispherical protrusions in the upper hypopharynx above the thyroid cartilage. On a lateral view, the pouches are seen as ovoid barium collections anteriorly in the upper hypopharynx.

7. Small asymptomatic pouches do not require treatment. Surgery is indicated when the diverticulum is large and complications develop. Surgical options are diverticulectomy with cricopharyngeal myotomy or diverticulopexy with myotomy or endoscopic division of the diverticular wall.

8. Squamous cell carcinoma is associated in 5–15%. Bezoars, tracheal fistula, vocal fold paralysis, cervical osteomyelitis and retained foreign body are complications. Hiatus hernia, laryngocele, oesophageal web, oesophageal spasm/stenosis, achalasia and gastric ulcers are also associated.

Case 1.38: Answers

1. The chest X-ray shows a soft tissue shadow in the right paravertebral region, with a clear lateral margin, extending from the root of the neck to the lower thorax. This has a mottled appearance and is a dilated oesophagus with food residues and fluid. The Barium swallow shows proximally dilated oesophagus with hold up of barium due to a smooth narrowing of the distal oesophagus.

2. Achalasia cardia.

3. Achalasia cardia is failure both of relaxation at the level of the lower oesophageal sphincter and failure of peristalsis. Most of the cases are idiopathic and caused by an abnormality of the Auerbach plexus or a defect in the dorsal nucleus of vagus. Chagas' disease is another known cause.

4. The X-ray shows dilated oesophagus and air in the oesophagus. A gastric bubble is not visualised. A paratracheal opacity is seen as a result of a fluid-filled oesophagus. Patchy alveolar opacities are seen as a result of aspiration pneumonitis. Barium shows grossly dilated oesophagus with food debris and air. Absence of peristaltic contractions in the upper oesophagus and secondary peristaltic waves are seen. There is symmetrical tapering of the distal oesophagus, with a bird-beak or pencil-tip deformity.

5. Hurst's phenomenon is temporary transit through the cardia when the hydrostatic pressure of the barium column is more than the pressure of the oesophageal sphincter. There might be sudden emptying after ingestion of a carbonated beverage. The sphincter relaxes after amyl nitrate inhalation.

6. There is a variant called rigorous achalasia, in which there are peristaltic waves; it is an early stage of achalasia.

7. Differential diagnoses: **secondary achalasia** produced by tumours (asymmetrical tapering, irregular mucosa, normal peristalsis, separation of gastric fundus from diaphragm); **benign peptic stricture** (abnormal folds, Barrett's oesophagus). Differential diagnoses for air in oesophagus in plain film: normal variant, achalasia, scleroderma, stricture, tumour after laryngectomy, intubation, thoracic surgery and mediastinitis.

8. Calcium channel blockers, anticholinergic agents, nitrates and opioids are used to relax the smooth muscle of the distal oesophagus and lower oesophageal sphincter. Botulinum toxin works by inhibiting release of acetylcholine from presynaptic terminals. Pneumatic balloon dilatation or surgical cardiomyotomy (Heller's) is used to relieve achalasia cardia, either by open surgery or laparoscopy. There is increased risk of development of oesophageal carcinoma (2–7%). Oesohagitis and aspiration pneumonia are other complications.

Case 1.39: Answers

1. This is videofluoroscopic barium swallow. The first picture shows free flow of barium from the oesophagus into the stomach during swallowing. In the second picture, barium is seen filling the oesophagus retrogradely from the stomach due to reflux.

2. Gastro-oesophageal reflux disease.

3. Gastro-oesophageal reflux is reflux of the stomach contents into the lower oesophagus, which is not equipped to handle acid overload. Normally the reflux is prevented by the lower oesophageal sphincter, phrenico-oesophageal membrane, length of subdiaphragmatic oesophagus and gastro-oesophageal angle of His. Reflux results when these defence mechanisms are overcome. The factors that determine the consequences of reflux are the frequency, volume and content of reflux, adequacy of the reflux mechanism and tissue resistance.

4. Videofluoroscopic examination with barium is used for evaluation of gastro-oesophageal reflux. Barium is administered with the patient in a supine or prone position. When the barium has passed through the oesophagogastric junction into the stomach, reflux is assessed. Normally reflux of barium is assessed in the right posterior oblique position. Provocative manoeuvres can be used for bringing out reflux, including coughing, a Valsalva manoeuvre, deep respiratory movements, swallowing saliva/water or anteflexion in an erect position. The water siphon test can be used with a combination of barium and water, which induces reflux in a prone position when drunk with a straw.

5. Another test is the radionuclide reflux test, where isotope is mixed with orange juice and the oesophageal counts are measured. Oesophageal manometry and measurement of oesophageal pH are also useful.

6. Reflux is demonstrated by the above-mentioned manoeuvres. Associated hiatus hernia is seen, which can be sliding or rolling. When reflux oesophagitis develops, it is seen in the lower third to the lower half of the oesophagus. There is segmental narrowing, granular mucosa, ulcers/erosions, superficial ulceration, prominent mucosal folds, incompetent sphincter, tertiary peristaltic contractions and transverse ridges of oesophagus (felinisation).

7. Complications of reflux: motility disorder, stricture, Barrett's oesophagus, reflux oesophagitis, carcinoma, iron deficiency anaemia, aspiration pneumonia, Mendelson syndrome and pulmonary fibrosis.

8. Mild reflux is managed by lifestyle changes (reducing weight, avoiding smoking/alcohol/cholcolates/citric acid, sleeping 3 hours after last meal, elevation of head end of bed), medications (H2 antagonists, proton pump inhibitors, prokinetic agents). Surgery is indicated when there is no response to medications or when complications develop. Fundoplication is performed, either laparoscopically or when necessary by open surgery..

Case 1.40: Answers

1. In the IVU, the renal collecting system is normal. The stomach is grossly distended and there is soft-tissue density centrally and a peripheral rim of lucency between the wall and centrally placed soft tissue density.

2. In the barium meal, the stomach is distended and there is a soft tissue mass within the lumen of the stomach, conforming to the shape of the stomach and now clearly outlined due to staining with barium.

3. Gastric bezoar.

4. Gastric bezoar is a concretion in the stomach that increases in size by accumulation of non-absorbable food or fibres (bezoar comes from the Arabic word *badzahr*, which means antidote). It is more common in those with previous surgery, altered gastrointestinal anatomy (inflammation, obstruction, malrotation, strictures), gastric motility disorders (gastroparesis, hypothyroidism, Guillain–Barré syndrome, myotonic dystrophy, medication), psychiatric complications, elderly people, hepatitis, cholestasis, cystic fibrosis, dehydration, dialysis and medications (opiates, anticholinergics, ganglion-blocking agents and antihistaminics).

5. The various subtypes are **trichobezoar** (hair), **phytobezoar** (plant and vegetable matter), **disospyrobezoars** (persimmons) and **lactobezoar** (milk). Trichobezoars are caused by swallowing of hair, which gets trapped in gastric folds, resists peristalsis and forms hair balls. In **Rapunzel syndrome**, the trichobezoar extends continuously from the stomach along the entire length of the small intestine. Lactobezoars are seen in neonates as a result of poor motility, concentrated formulas and dehydration. Other compositions are medications including the shells of medications such as bulk-forming laxatives, extended-released products, ion exchange resins, vitamins and other natural products. Clinical features are nausea, vomiting, bloating, swelling, weight loss, anorexia, intolerance to solid food and gastric outlet obstruction. Examination reveals tenderness, palpable mass or foul breath.

6. A plain X-ray shows a filling defect outlined by gas, which is amorphous, calcified granular or bubbly. A barium meal shows heterogeneous intraluminal filling defects with interstices of air within it and not attached to any wall. A CT scan is better for evaluating the bezoar, because it shows its composition of the bezoar and shows air trapped within the mass. Ultrasonography reveals an acoustic shadow surrounded by an echogenic arc of air. Complications are bleeding, obstruction, malabsorbtion and perforation.

7. Endoscopy is required for confirmation and endoscopic removal is possible, but large bezoars may require laparatomy. Diet modification, pharmacotherapy (metoclopramide, erythromycin), gastric lavage, enzymatic disruption (*N*-acetylcysteine, papain, cellulase), endoscopic therapy and surgical therapy are the treatment options.

Case 1.41: Answers

1. The barium meal shows a twisted stomach with abnormal configuration. The stomach is rotated around its long axis. The greater curvature is lying superior to the lesser curvature.

2. Gastric volvulus.

3. Gastric volvulus is twisting of one part of the stomach around another part. It is caused by unusually long gastrohepatic and gastrocolic mesenteries or by abnormality of the suspensory ligaments (hepatic, splenic, phrenic or colic).

4. Organoaxial and mesenteroaxial are the two types of gastric volvulus.

5. In **organoaxial volvulus**, the stomach is rotated around a line extending from the cardia to the pylorus along the long axis of the stomach. In **mesenteroaxial volvulus**, the stomach is rotated around transverse axis extending from the lesser to the greater curvature. A barium meal is used to diagnose the volvulus and find the type. It demonstrates the arc of twist. There might be a delay in the entry of barium into the stomach. A CT scan can be used for further evaluation.

6. The characteristic Borchardt's triad in gastric volvulus consists of epigastric pain, retching and inability to pass the nasogastric tube into the stomach.

7. Complications are ischaemia, gastric emphysema and perforation. It is associated with paraoesophageal hiatus hernia and eventration.

8. Differential diagnoses: gastric atony, acute gastric dilatation and pyloric obstruction.

Case 1.42: Answers

1. IVU shows a grossly distended loop of large bowel, which has the configuration of a caecum that has rotated and is situated in the midportion and left upper quadrant of the abdomen rather than its normal position in the right lower quadrant. Barium enema shows normal passage of barium up to the mid ascending colon. Caecum could not be filled with barium due to blockage caused by twisting of mobile caecum, which is situated more centrally in the abdomen. At the site of obstruction, a small tapered projection of barium is noted.

2. Caecal volvulus of the caecal bascule type. The term 'caecal volvulus' is a misnomer because the torsion is usually located in the ascending colon above the ileocaecal valve.

3. Caecal volvulus is twisting of the ascending colon. It is usually associated with malrotation and a long mesentery, resulting in defective peritoneal fixation of the caecum and ascending colon, which leads to abnormal mobility.

4. Although abnormal right colon mobility is found in 10–25% of patients, not all of them develop volvulus. Other features such as distal large bowel obstruction, adhesions, traction caused by appendix disease, meteorism, colonoscopy, pregnancy, post partum, postoperative state and colonic ileus have been indicated as predisposing factors.

5. The two types are: axial torsion and caecal bascule. **Axial type**: 180–360° twist along the longitudinal axis of the ascending colon. A high incidence of ischaemia is seen in this type. **Caecal bascule type**: caecum folds anteromedial to the ascending colon, with flap-valve occlusion at the site of flexion. The torsion occurs in the transverse plane.

6. In axial torsion: a distended loop of large bowel that is kidney shaped is seen, with its long axis extending from the right lower quadrant to the epigastrium of the left upper quadrant, where the caecum is visible. The haustral pattern is preserved. Distal colon is collapsed. Small bowel loops are dilated. Caecal bascule: the distended caecum is located more centrally. Small bowel loops are not dilated, as a result of passive twisting of the ileum. A barium enema shows the tapered end of the barium column pointing towards the torsion. A CT scan shows the level of twisting. Signs of ischaemia are bowel wall thickening, mesenteric fat stranding and pneumatosis intestinalis.

7. Perforation, ischaemia and abdominal compartment syndrome are complications of caecal volvulus. Caecal distension > 12 cm indicates risk of perforation. Vascular compromise can be acute or chronic. Acute torsion causes strangulation and compromise of both arteries and veins. Gradual obstruction causes venous compression as a result of raised intraluminal pressure. In abdominal compartment syndrome, increased abdominal pressure causes a fall in respiratory and cardiac function.

8. Occasionally the volvulus reduces with barium. Surgical options include caecostomy and caecopexy. Resection is indicated if the bowel is non-viable.

Case 1.43: Answers

1. ERCP shows a beaded appearance of bile ducts with multiple areas of short, irregular strictures and proximal dilations.

2. Sclerosing cholangitis. Primary sclerosing cholangitis is obliterative fibrosing inflammation of the biliary tree with multiple strictures, caused by altered bile metabolism and an increase in lithocholic acid through bacterial overgrowth.

3. Sclerosing cholangitis has a high association with inflammatory bowel disease (ulcerative colitis in 75% and Crohn's disease in 14%). This is called secondary sclerosing cholangitis. Other associations are pancreatitis, cirrhosis, chronic active hepatitis, retroperitoneal fibrosis, Peyronie's disease, orbital pseudotumour, Riedl's thyroiditis and Sjögren syndrome.

4. The most common location is the common bile duct. Intra- and extrahepatic ducts are involved in most cases. Involvement of a cystic duct, or just intra- or extrahepatic ducts is a rare presentation.

5. Cholangiography is the mainstay in the diagnosis. This can be done by percutaneous injection of contrast or after ERCP. A non-invasive method opacification of biliary tree is MRCP, where the high T2 signal of fluids is used to demonstrate bile ducts in physiological state, without need for invasive procedure. There are multifocal strictures, especially at bifurcations, with skip lesions where the bile duct calibre is normal, giving

as string of beads appearance with alternating segments of dilatation and stenosis. Small diverticula are seen. Pruned tree appearance is seen due to opacification of central ducts and no visualisation of peripheral ducts. Cobblestone appearance is seen due to nodular mucosal irregularities. Mild ductal dilatation is seen is seen proximal to affected areas. Ultrasound shows echogenic portal triads and biliary casts with wall thickening. CT scan appearances are non-specific, but it may show fatty change, inflammation and complications due to portal venous thrombosis and malignancy. MRI shows intermediate intensity in T1 and hyperintensity in T2 in periportal areas.

6. Complications are calculi, cholangitis, secondary biliary cirrhosis, portal hypertension and cholangiocarcinoma.

7. Differential diagnoses: **cholangiocarcinoma** (single short segment stricture, irregular, upstream dilatation, mass), **cholangitis** (bile duct thickening, fever), **primary biliary cirrhosis** (limited to intrahepatic ducts, less prominent strictures, crowding of bile ducts) and **AIDS cholangiopathy**.

Case 1.44: Answers

1. The X-ray of the abdomen shows multiple, irregular calcifications in the central portions of the upper abdomen. The CT scan shows an atrophic pancreas. There is a well-encapsulated, hypodense fluid collection in the tail and body of the pancreas. There is a periperal rim of calcification in the wall of the collection.

2. Chronic pancreatitis with pseudocyst formation.

3. Chronic pancreatitis is a chronic inflammatory disease of the pancreas. It is classified as chronic calcifying and chronic obstructive pancreatitis and presents with acute exacerbation of epigastric pain, jaundice, steatorrhoea and diabetes mellitus.

4. Alcoholism, congenital/acquired anomalies of pancreatic duct, sphincter of Oddi dysfunction, trauma, surgical ligation, idiopathic, renal failure and ampullary tumour are common causes. Causes of chronic calcifying pancreatitis are hereditary, juvenile tropical pancreatitis, hyperlipidaemia, hypercalcaemia and inborn errors of metabolism.

5. The X-ray shows irregular calcifications in the pancreatic area. The CT scan shows a small atrophied gland. The duct is dilated, irregular and beaded. Calcifications are seen in the gland and duct. In an acute attack, the gland is enlarged. Pseudocysts can be seen. Ultrasonography shows similar appearances with an irregular, atrophied gland, with dilated ducts and calculi. MRI shows low signal in T1 and high signal in T2. Cholangiography shows a dilated main duct, beading, string of pearls caused by multifocal dilatation and stenosis of the duct, side branch ectasia, and intraductal filling defects caused by debris, calculi or protein plugs.

6. Complications are superimposed acute pancreatitis, pseudocyst, pancreatic ascites, thrombosis of splenic/mesenteric/portal vein, pseudoaneurysm of the splenic artery and pancreatic carcinoma (2–5%).

7. Occasionally, chronic pancreatitis can involve a focal portion of the pancreas. This is difficult to differentiate from a focal pancreatic mass. In focal pancreatitis, there is a focal mass with irregular margins and upstream ductal dilatation. Differentiation might be difficult with CT, MRI or even endoscopic ultrasonography. Biopsy is required for diagnosis.

8. If there is biliary obstruction, stenting can be done. Fluid collections are drained percutaneously under radiological guidance. Guided biopsy is required for differentiating focal pancreatitis from cancer. Pseudocysts are amenable to percutaneous drainage. Surgery is required in obstinate, recurrent collections. Cystogastrostomy is a less invasive procedure of choice.

Case 1.45: Answers

1. The CT scan shows a thickened tubular structure on the right side of the pelvis, with surrounding soft-tissue stranding in the pelvis.

2. Ultrasonography done over the right iliac fossa shows a distended tubular structure, measuring 7 mm, which could not be compressed by the ultrasound probe. There is no fluid collection or gas.

3. Acute appendicitis.

4. Acute appendicitis begins when the appendiceal lumen is blocked by food/stool/parasites/barium or hyperplastic lymphoid tissue, resulting in oedematous mucosa, and leading to increased intraluminal pressure, inflammation and exudates. Growth of bacteria within the lumen enhances the inflammatory response.

5. Clinically, the symptoms start with ill-defined pain in the periumbilical region, with anorexia nausea and vomiting. Subsequently the pain moves to the right lower quadrant and becomes more intense. Tenderness is present in McBurney's point in right lower quadrant. Cough sign, Rovsing's sign, psoas sign and obturator sign are other signs of peritoneal irritation. WBC is elevated in 80–90%. WBC >15 000 cells/cm² suggests perforation. (Urinalysis can show WBCs due to bladder wall irritation. WBC >20/Hpf indicates urinary infection.) Positive triple test: CRP values of more than 8 µg/mL, WBC count of more than 11 000/mL, and neutrophils >75% are suggestive.

6. X-rays are not helpful in diagnosing appendicitis. An appendicolith is seen in 10% of cases. Other features that are suggestive, but not specific, for appendicitis are scoliosis concave to the right side, obliteration of the right psoas shadow, gas–fluid level on the right side, air in the appendix and localised ileus. Ultrasonography is the most useful modality used in diagnosis of appendicitis. The presence of a dilated (> 6 mm), non-compressible appendix has a high sensitivity and specificity in diagnosis. Other features are fluid in the appendix, an appendicolith, transverse diameter > 6 mm and focal rebound tenderness. Appendiceal abscess and phlegmon can also be diagnosed. Ultrasonography can exclude other causes of right-sided pain including ovarian cysts, renal stones and cholecystitis. A CT scan is useful in diagnosis and is a faster, reliable method with high sensitivity and specificity. The appendix is enlarged, with an appendicolith and surrounding soft-tissue stranding. No contrast enters the appendix from the caecum.

7. Perforation ensues if the diagnosis is not made early and obstruction continues. Leak of inflammatory products and bacteria into the peritoneum causes peritonitis. In adults or adolescents, the omentum walls off a perforated appendix causing a focal abscess. In young children, the omentum is not well developed, resulting in peritonitis. The risk of perforation is higher in the younger age group.

8. Appendicitis is treated with laparoscopic or open appendectomy. Non-toxic patients with a localised, walled-off abscess may be candidates for initial medical management with antibiotics, followed by an elective appendectomy.

Case 1.46: Answers

1. This is a herniogram.

2. The patient lies supine on the fluoroscopy table after emptying the bladder. After sterile preparation and local anaesthetic injection, contrast is injected in the midline supraumbilical linea alba, the midline infraumbilical region or the linea semilunaris at the lateral margin of the rectus sheath adjacent to the umbilicus. A 7- or 12-cm, 21-gauge needle is used for puncturing the peritoneum. A pop is felt. A test dose of contrast is injected to check if the needle is in the right position, which is indicated by contrast outlining bowel loops After this a guidewire is passed, the needle removed, a dilator sheath passed into the peritoneal cavity and 150 ml non-ionic contrast medium injected into the peritoneal cavity. The patient is turned prone and the head of table elevated 20–25°. X-rays are taken with the patient in prone and prone–oblique positions, supine at rest and during provocative manoeuvres, such as coughing, sniffing, and Vasalva's and Müller's manoeuvres. Elevation of the knees is done to relieve compression from obesity. Standing images are helpful. If it is negative, images are taken after the patient walks.

3. Several peritoneal folds are seen in a normal herniogram. The most lateral is the lateral umbilical ligament, which contains inferior epigastric vessels and divides the area into medial and lateral fossae. The deep inguinal ring is seen lateral to this fold and an indirect inguinal hernia originates here. A direct inguinal hernia originates medial to the lateral umbilical fold. The medial area is divided into medial and lateral areas by a medial umbilical fold, which contains the obliterated umbilical artery. Direct hernias can arise on both sides of the medial umbilical fold and more than one may be present. The midline ligament is called the median umbilical ligament and is the remnant or urachus, extending between the bladder and umbilicus. These folds might not be seen in 20%.

4. A small indirect inguinal hernial sac is outlined with contrast on the left side.

5. A herniogram is indicated when the patient has chronic inguinal pain and swelling, but clinical examinations are negative. Herniography detects occult hernia in 45% of patients, especially in obese and muscular patients in whom clinical examination is difficult. An alternative investigation is ultrasonography, which can be done dynamically. MRI is also routinely done for ruling out occult hernias. False positives can be seen. False-negative findings are rare and can result from fat plugging the orifices.

6. Complications are perforation of the bowel, injection into the stomach and left iliac vein, bowel wall haematoma, obstruction, cellulitis of the abdominal wall and septicaemia. Minor complications are puncture site haematoma, contrast reaction and abdominal pain.

Case 1.47: Answers

1. The CT scan shows a hypodense fluid collection in the right lower quadrant, which has a surrounding rim of contrast enhancement. There is soft-tissue stranding adjacent to this collection.

2. Appendiceal abscess.

3. Acute appendicitis is usually caused by obstruction to the appendiceal lumen. This results in oedema of the mucosa, which causes increased intraluminal pressure and inflammation, and exudates drain from the appendix. When the appendix is further stretched as a result of raised pressure, it perforates. This perforation is usually walled off immediately, causing a walled-off abscess. In younger children, the perforation is not walled off, due to lack of omentum, causing acute peritonitis.

4. Ultrasonography shows a right lower quadrant inflammatory mass that is a combination of appendix, mesentery, lymph nodes and abscess. The CT scan shows an irregular mass with fluid, rim enhancement and soft-tissue stranding.

5. Differential diagnoses for the radiological appearance: soft-tissue abscess, carcinoma, mucocele of appendix and appendiceal tumours. Differential diagnoses for similar symptoms: pelvic inflammatory disease, endometriosis, ovarian cyst or torsion, renal colic, degenerating uterine leiomyoma, diverticulitis, Crohn's disease, colonic carcinoma and rectus sheath haematoma.

6. A well-loculated abscess with limited symptoms is treated with intravenous antibiotics and percutaneous or transrectal drainage of the abscess. When the symptoms and WBC count subside, the patient is discharged and put on oral antibiotics. An interval appendectomy is performed after 4–6 weeks. If the abscess is multilocular or not drainable by percutaneous methods, urgent surgery is performed.

Case 1.48: Answers

1. The X-ray of the pelvis shows a large soft-tissue swelling, in the right groin area. This swelling has a mottled appearance as a result of the presence of gas.

2. The contrast enema shows a loop of large bowel herniating into the right femoral sac.

3. Right femoral hernia.

4. Femoral hernias arise from a defect in the attachment of transversalis fascia to the pubis, and are posterior to the inguinal ligament and medial to the femoral vessels. It is located in the femoral canal which is situated medial to the femoral vessels in the femoral triangle and lateral to the lacunar (Gimbernat's) ligament, bounded by the inguinal ligament anteriorly and the pectineal ligament posteriorly. Normally it contains lymphatics, loose areolar tissue and Cloquet's lymph node.

5. Femoral hernias are common in women, although, even in women, inguinal hernia is the most common type of hernia. It is more common on the right side. Hernias present with inguinal mass and medial thigh pain. Clinically a bulge is felt below the inguinal ligament, unlike the inguinal

hernia, which is located above the inguinal ligament. In femoral hernia, the neck of the sac is situated below and lateral to the medial end of the inguinal ligament, but in inguinal hernia, it is situated above and medial to the ligament. When the hernia is strangulated, there is pain, tenderness, swelling and redness, with a toxic appearance. Obstruction presents with nausea, vomiting, constipation and distension. Obesity, heavy lifting, coughing, straining, ascites, peritoneal dialysis, VP shunt, COPD and family history are predisposing factors.

6. Ultrasonography is the simplest way of diagnosing a femoral hernia. The hernia is seen medial to the femoral vein and can be elicited by coughing or a Valsalva manoeuvre. Ultrasonography differentiates a groin swelling from an abscess, lymph node or aneurysm. A CT scan shows the hernial sac situated below the inguinal ligament and medial to the femoral vessels. In incarcerated femoral hernia, the sac is situated lateral to the pubic tubercle, unlike incarcerated inguinal hernia, where the sac is situated medial to the pubic tubercle. Complications such as obstruction and strangulation can be diagnosed.

7. Complications of femoral hernia are obstruction and strangulation. It is more common than with the inguinal hernia, because they protrude through a small, defined space.

8. Repair of femoral hernia can be elective or urgent when there are complications. The surgery can be done with an infrainguinal, transinguinal or high approach.

Case 1.49: Answers

1. The barium enema shows extensive diverticular disease in the whole of the left colon and sigmoid.

2. The CT scan shows thickening of a long segment of sigmoid colon, which is studded with multiple diverticula. There is soft-tissue stranding adjacent to the sigmoid colon.

3. Sigmoid diverticulosis with diverticulitis.

4. Decreased faecal bulk, caused by a diet high in refined fibre and low in roughage, is believed to be the cause of sigmoid diverticula.

5. Overactivity of the sigmoid smooth muscle secondary to high intracolonic pressure results in herniation of the mucosa and submucosa through muscle layers. This is most common in the sigmoid colon because it is the narrowest colonic segment with the highest pressure. The herniations occur along the natural openings created by vasa recta or nutrient vessels in the colon's wall.

6. Complications are diverticulitis and bleeding. Complications of diverticulitis are abscess, perforation, obstruction and a fistula to bladder/ vagina/small bowel.

7. Diverticula are seen as outpouchings arising from the colon. They might be seen on a plain X-ray if there is remnant barium from a previous exam. Barium shows the diverticula as barium-filled outpouchings. Lateral diverticula are seen between the mesenteric and antimesenteric taeniae on opposite sides Antimesenteric taeniae are seen opposite the mesenteric side. Diverticulitis is best diagnosed with a contrast CT scan. The wall of the sigmoid colon is thickened, diverticula are thickened, and air is trapped as a result of neck thickening and increased soft-tissue density in the pericolonic soft-tissue stranding. Abscesses are seen as fluid collections with rim enhancement. Fistulous tracks and obstruction can be diagnosed.

8. Diverticulosis does not require treatment. Diverticulitis is treated with broad-spectrum antibiotics. Surgery is indicated when complications develop or there is no response to medical treatment. Percutaneous drainage of abscesses may be done under CT or ultrasound guidance.

9. The most important radiological differential diagnosis of the diverticulitis is carcinoma. Diverticulitis involves a long segment and is associated with diverticula. Tumours usually have shorter segment involvement, heaped up margins and ulcerated mucosa. However, in the presence of diverticula, carcinoma may simply produce a stricture and not produce classical appearances, and may be mistaken for a benign stricture. Colitis is another differential diagnosis, which involves a long length of the colon and has ulcerations in early stages.

Case 1.50: Answers

1. The cholangiogram shows dilatation of the right and left hepatic ducts. There is a filling defect at the confluence of the right and left hepatic ducts, beyond which no contrast is seen. The CT scan shows a hypodense enhancing mass at the junction of the right and left hepatic ducts, with proximal intrahepatic ductal dilatation.

2. Klatskin tumour, which is an intrahepatic central cholangiocarcinoma at the junction of hepatic ducts.

3. Intrahepatic cholangiocarcinoma, which is seen peripherally, is the second most common primary malignancy of the liver after HCC. Extrahepatic cholangiocarcinoma is seen outside the liver.

4. Bismuth classification of Klatskin tumour:

    Type I: main hepatic duct below bifurcation

    Type II: main hepatic duct bifurcation

    Type III: segmental bile ducts proximal to primary hepatic bifurcation affecting one liver lobe (**IIIa** – right lobe, **IIIb** – left lobe)

    Type IV: segmental ducts of both lobes.

5. Cholangiogram (percutaneous, ERCP or MRCP) shows dilatation of intrahepatic ducts and proximal hepatic ducts, and an abrupt ending with an irregular mass at the hilar region. Ultrasonography shows a hypoechoic or isoechoic central porta hepatis mass. In the infiltrative type, there is only irregularity of ducts at this location with upstream dilatation. Occasionally polypoid or nodular intraluminal mass is seen. Segmental dilatation of right and left ductal systems with non-union at the porta hepatis is a characteristic finding of Klatskin tumour. The portal vein may be encased or invaded. Lobar atrophy is seen with crowded dilated ducts, extending to the liver surface. MRI with MRCP and MR angiography (MRA) provide information on tumour size, bile duct involvement and vascular compromise, which determine the resectability of the tumour.

6. Differential diagnoses of biliary obstruction: sclerosing cholangitis (alternating areas of stenosis and dilatation), AIDS cholangitis, benign stricture, chronic pancreatitis, extrinsic tumours such as metastasis, HCC and lymphoma.

7. Most of the tumours are unresectable at the time of presentation. Surgical exploration is undertaken when there is potential for curative resection. Non-surgical intervention is used to provide palliation to malignant biliary obstruction.

8. Biliary tract drainage is indicated when there is jaundice associated with cholangitis, sepsis, pruritius, nausea, vomiting resulting in dehydration and malnutrition. Drainage can be done percutaneously or with endoscopy. Internal or external drains, internal endoprosthesis, metallic stents, radiation with intervention and metallic stents with brachytherapy are some of the techniques used. Metallic stents are commonly used. They have a large diameter lumen and self-expand to a size of 10 mm. The stent becomes incorporated into the wall of the bile duct over weeks. Stent may become obstructed later as a result of inspissated bile or tumour ingrowth through the struts and tumour overgrowth over the ends of the stent.

Case 1.51: Answers

1. In the axial view of the CT, there is a large, heterogeneous mass in the head of the pancreas, which is encasing the SMV (superior mesenteric vein) and is in contact with the SMA. There is soft tissue stranding around the pancreas. The coronal view demonstrates the invasion of the SMV and the portal vein.

2. Carcinoma of the head of the pancreas.

3. Although duct cells constitute only 4% of the pancreas, 90% of carcinomas arise from the duct cells and are ductal adenocarcinomas; they are associated with extensive scirrhous reaction with no vascularity and dense cellularity. The most common location is the head of the pancreas, followed by the body.

4. Alcohol, diabetes, hereditary pancreatitis and smoking are predisposing factors for pancreatic adenocarcinoma.

5. Pancreatic adenocarcinomas are very aggressive and usually inoperable by the time of diagnosis. They extend locally, posteriorly, anteriorly, into porta hepatis and splenic hilum. Invasion of adjacent organs such as the

duodenum, stomach, left adrenal, spleen and small bowel mesentery is common. Distal metastases to liver, lungs and bone are seen.

6. A CT scan is the imaging modality of choice for the diagnosis. It shows a focal mass with pancreatic and bile duct dilatation (double-duct sign). The pancreatic body and tail can be atrophied. If secondary pancreatitis is seen, the gland is enlarged. Ultrasonography shows a hypoechoic mass with ductal dilatation. A barium meal shows the Frostberg inverted '3' sign, which is an inverted '3' contour to the medial portion of duodenum, caused by tumour infiltrating the duodenum. Antral padding is produced by extrinsic indentation of the posteroinferior margin of the gastric antrum. Angiography shows hypovascular tumour with or without encasement of blood vessels.

7. CT and MRI are useful in diagnosing the tumour and assessing the spread and resectability. On a CT scan, spread outside the pancreas is seen as increased density in the adjacent fat. Invasion of adjacent organs is seen with infiltration of the duodenum, stomach and mesenteric root. The tumour also extends into the splenic hilum and porta hepatis. Gerota's fascia is thickened. Vascular encasement is an important feature that predicts resectability. The superior mesenteric artery and superior mesenteric vein are encased or infiltrated by the tumour. MRI is also very useful in staging the disease.

8. Focal pancreatitis (gland atrophied, ductal dilatation, biopsy required), islet cell carcinoma (more common in the tail, may be associated with endocrine symptoms, good contrast enhancement), metastasis and lymphoma are other lesions included in differential diagnoses.

Case 1.52: Answers

1. The CT scan has been done in the arterial phase. (There is bright contrast in the abdominal aorta.) The CT scan shows a large, well-defined lesion in segment 8 of the right lobe, which enhances brightly on the contrast scan. There is a central, irregular hypodensity, which is the typical appearance of a scar. In the portal phase, the lesion becomes isodense with the liver (not shown here).

2. Focal nodular hyperplasia. This is a rare, benign, congenital, hamartomatous malformation of the liver characterised by focal hepatic hyperplasia resulting from an increase in regional blood flow.

3. The exact aetiology is not known. Theories of origin include a congenital AV malformation (AVM), which triggers hyperplasia. This might be associated with haemangioma, brain tumours such as meningioma, astrocytoma, or dysplasias in other organs.

4. Oral contraceptives do not cause focal nodular hyperplasia, but they result in growth of pre-existing focal nodular hyperplasia. Adenoma is the liver lesion caused by contraceptive pills.

5. A central fibrovascular scar is the characteristic finding, which is useful in pathological and radiological diagnosis.

6. CT scan: a four-phase liver scan is performed for evaluation of liver lesions. Scans are obtained in the non-contrast, arterial (20–30 s), portal venous (60–70 s) and delayed (5 min) phases. Vascular lesions enhance in the arterial phase (focal nodular hyperplasia, adenoma, HCC, vascular metastasis, perfusion anomalies). HCC washes out the contrast in the delayed phase and becomes hypodense, whereas the other lesions do not wash out. Non-vascular metastatic lesions are hypodense in the portal phase and do not enhance in the arterial phase. MRI is also acquired in four phases. In focal nodular hyperplasia, the lesion is iso- or hyperintense on a contrast scan, enhances intensely in the arterial phase and becomes isointense in the delayed phase. The central scar is hypointense, may show calcification and shows delayed enhancement. MRI shows an iso- to hyperintense lesion in T1, hyper- to isointense in T2, and on contrast it shows intense enhancement in the arterial phase and stays isointense on delayed images. The scar shows delayed enhancement. A sulphur colloid scan shows normal uptake or hot spot caused by the presence of normal Kupffer's cells, which is a finding not seen in other liver lesions. Angiography shows a hypervascular mass, with a spokewheel pattern.

7. Focal nodular hyperplasia may rupture into the peritoneum, causing a haemoperitoneum.

8. Liver lesions are difficult to differentiate. Often, multiple imaging modalities are required for diagnosis:

    Adenoma: large tumour, no central scar, contrast enhancement features similar

    Fibrolamellar carcinoma: scar seen, but not vascular; scar does not enhance, metastasis, nodes, pain

    HCC: early arterial enhancement and washout in delayed phase, rim enhancement of pseudocapsule, variable signal in T1, haemorrhage, necrosis

    Large haemangioma: scar and necrosis can be seen, globular peripheral enhancement, with slow centripetal filling and isointense; highest T2 signal almost like a cyst.

Case 1.53: Answers

1. The X-ray of the chest (PA view) shows an opacity in the right cardiophrenic angle, which obscures the right dome of the diaphragm. On the lateral view, this is situated over the anterior aspect.

2. Morgagni's hernia.

3. Morgagni's hernia is caused by a defective development of septum transversum; herniation intraabdominal contents occurs through the space of Larrey, which is an anteromedial parasternal defect.

4. Morgagni's hernia is common on the right side (90%). The defect is very small. In infants, Morgagni's hernia is usually asymptomatic. Classically, Morgagni's hernia is seen as a unilateral, mediastinal/right cardiophrenic angle mass. It is rarely bilateral and very rarely produces respiratory distress.

5. Omental fat, transverse colon and liver are the organs that commonly herniate.

6. The X-ray shows an opacity in the right cardiophrenic angle. If there are bowel loops, they are clearly visualised. Barium will confirm the diagnosis. Large hernias can cause elevation of cardiac silhouette and bilateral bulges on either side of the lower mediastinum. CT scan is also diagnostic, particularly when the bowel is within the hernia.

7. Differential diagnoses for cardiophrenic angle mass: prominent cardiophrenic fat pad, pericardial cyst, bronchogenic cyst, lymph node, thymolipoma, varices, lymphoma, metastasis and aneurysm.

Case 1.54: Answers

1. Ultrasonography shows a well-defined, bright lesion (hyperechoic) in the right lobe of the liver. There is no biliary dilatation.

2. The CT scans have been acquired in the arterial and delayed phases. There is a right lobe liver lesion, which shows early nodular peripheral enhancement in the earlier phases and slowly fills in the centre of the lumen; it is seen as a homogeneous isodense lesion in the delayed images.

3. Cavernous haemangioma of the liver.

4. Haemangioma is the most common benign tumour of the liver. It is made up of large vascular channels lined by flattened endothelial cells, filled with slowly circulating blood, separated by thin fibrous septa. Fibrosis and thrombosis of the spaces can occur. Large haemangiomas are > 10 cm.

5. Kasabach–Merritt syndrome is haemorrhagic diathesis caused by sequestration of platelets in tumours. Haemangioma, haemangioendothelioma and angiosarcoma are tumours that produce this syndrome, which results in thrombocytopenia and purpura.

6. Ultrasonography: haemangioma is well defined and hyperechoic with posterior acoustic enhancement (bright shadows caused by increased cellular interfaces created by blood-filled spaces and septa). There is no Doppler signal. Occasionally it may be hypoechoic and inhomogeneous with scar/necrosis. CT is done with a four-phase protocol. Usually it is well defined and hypodense on plain CT. In the early arterial phase, there is circumferential nodular enhancement (enhancement of feeding vessel) and in later phases there is slow filling of the centre of the lesion from the periphery (slow flow); in later stages, there is persistence of contrast. Variations of this appearance make diagnosis difficult. MRI: the lesion is hypo- or isointense in T1 and hyperintense in T2. The characteristic feature is a high signal in T2, which gets higher even in very heavily T2-weighted sequences (light-bulb sign). A sulphur colloid scan shows a focal defect. A red blood cell (RBC) scan shows slow uptake and delayed filling.

7. Differential diagnoses include cysts, metastasis and hepatomas. With CT, cysts are also hypodense, but do not show any contrast enhancement. Hepatoma is vascular in the early phase and washes out very fast, unlike a haemangioma. Metastasis is hypodense in the portal phase and does not show centripetal filling. Cystic neoplasm and necrotic tumour are other differentials. The characteristic features of haemangioma help to differentiate from the other lesions.

8. Complications are platelet sequestration, abscess and very rarely rupture.

9. Biopsy is usually contraindicated as a result of the risk of bleeding. However, biopsy can be done with a narrow-gauge needle and if there is normal liver between the lesion and liver capsule. The needle track can be embolised with gelfoam to reduce the risk of bleeding. Small hemangiomas do not require any treatment. Large hemangiomas (>10) with symptoms require surgical resection.

Case 1.55: Answers

1. Barium follow-through shows multiple barium-filled outpouchings from the wall of the proximal small bowel.

2. Jejunal diverticulosis.

3. Jejunal diverticulosis is a pulsion diverticula resulting from increased intraluminal pressure and herniation of mucosa. It is seen in the mesenteric border of the bowel at the entrance of vasa recti. It is more common in the proximal jejunum. Ileum is involved in 15% of cases and the incidence is 2%. It is more common in men aged > 40 years. It can be associated with scleroderma, visceral myopathy, neuropathy and Ehler–Danlos syndrome. There is an association with Ehlers–Danlos syndrome.

4. The X-ray shows air–fluid levels in diverticula. Barium follow-through shows trapped barium, which might remain after the barium has cleared from the rest of the bowel. If there is a narrow neck, inflammation or stagnant secretions in the pouch, it might not be filled with barium. The size of the diverticulum ranges from a few millimetres to many centimetres. If complications such as perforation and abscess develop, a mesenteric mass, displacing the bowel loops, is seen. The diverticula can also be incidentally seen in other imaging studies such as ultrasonography or CT.

5. Clinical features are abdominal pain, flatulence, diarrhoea, steatorrhoea, malabsorption and vitamin deficiency. Complications are diverticulitis (inflammation is uncommon as a result of the fluid nature of the small bowel contents and broad opening), perforation, abscess, blind loop syndrome resulting from bacterial overgrowth, haemorrhage and obstruction caused by enteroliths. Jejunal diverticulosis is a common cause of pneumoperitoneum. Small openings in the wall of the diverticulum may allow the passage of air, but not of intestinal contents.

Case 1.56: Answers

1. The CT scan (axial and coronal views) shows multiple masses in the liver, which show contrast enhancement and central dark areas of necrosis.

2. Liver metastasis.

3. Metastasis is the most common neoplasm in an adult liver, and the liver is the second most common site for metastatic spread, after the lymph nodes. Common tumours that metastasise to the liver are tumours of the eye, pancreas, breast, gallbladder, bile ducts, colorectum and stomach.

The liver is the primary target of gastrointestinal and urological cancers, neuroblastomas, melanomas and lung cancers. In breast cancer, liver is less likely to be the primary target organ.

4. The imaging appearances of liver metastasis are varied. On ultrasonography, there are multiple hypoechoic lesions, but they can be iso-/hyperechoic. Diffuse infiltrating tumours cause hepatomegaly with coarse liver echotexture (breast, lung, melanoma, lymphoma, leukaemia). Bright metastases are seen in calcification and haemorrhage. Cystic metastasis is seen in cystadenocarcinoma (colon, ovary, stomach, pancreas) or extensive necrosis (leiomyosarcoma, squamous cell carcinoma, metastasis, testicular carcinoma). On a CT scan, most of the metastases are hypovascular. Hence they are seen as hypodense lesions in non-contrast. In the arterial phase, they are not seen clearly and, in the portal phase, they are seen as low density lesions against normally enhancing liver. Occasionally liver metastases are vascular (renal, phaeochromocytoma, melanoma, islet cell tumours and breast). These lesions enhance in the arterial phase and become isodense in the portal phase. Appearances on MRI are varied and depend on the tumour content. Haemorrhagic tumours show high signal in T1. Calcification is dark in T1 and T2. Most metastases do not show good arterial enhancement and are seen as dark areas in the portal phase.

5. Calcified liver metastasis is seen in mucinous adenocarcinoma (stomach, pancreas, colon, rectum), serous cystadenocarcinoma of ovary, breast, lung, melanoma, medullary carcinoma of thyroid, carcinoid, neuroendocrine tumour of pancreas, osteosarcoma, chondrosarcoma, testicular, renal carcinomas and lymphomas.

6. Differential diagnoses: haemangioma (solitary, slow enhancement with centripetal filling in CT/MRI, bright T2 signal in MRI); HCCs (cirrhotic liver, enhancement in arterial phase, washout in delayed images, tumour capsule); adenomas (solitary, young women on contraceptives, haemorrhage/fat common, good arterial enhancement, isodense in delayed images); liver cyst (dark on ultrasonography, hypodense on CT, low signal in T1, high signal in T2), biliary cystadenoma, biliary hamartoma, cholangiocarcinoma (solitary, slow delayed enhancement in CT and MRI); focal fatty infiltration and sparing.

7. Diagnosis is confirmed by ultrasound-/CT-guided biopsy. Treatment is with chemotherapy, cryotherapy or liver resection.

8. Many minimally invasive techniques are available for treating liver metastases: transcatheter arterial chemoembolisation, cryo-/microwave/ laser/radiofrequency/ethanol ablation.

Case 1.57: Answers

1. Plain X-ray shows gas in the wall of the caecum, ascending and transverse colon. There is also free gas outlining the bowel wall. The descending colon is normal. In the CT scan, the descending colon and small bowel loops (in the centre) are normal. On the right side, the lumen of the caecum is completely opacified by oral contrast, but there is extensive gas within the caecal wall, completely encircling the lumen.

2. Pneumatosis coli caused by ischaemia.

3. Pneumatosis intestinalis is the presence of gas in the intestinal wall. There are a wide variety of causes. The most common and the most serious is bowel ischaemia, where gas enters into bowel wall as a result of damaged mucosa. Other causes are bowel obstruction, intestinal trauma, infection, inflammation and graft-versus-host disease. Air in the bowel wall can arise from the lungs, from alveolar rupture, and extend along bronchovascular bundles to the mediastinum and retroperitoneum. COPD, cystic fibrosis and trauma are the other causes.

4. The gas usually collects in the subserosa, followed by the submucosa and muscularis, and is common in the mesenteric side. The collection can be microvesicular, in the lamina propria, or linear/curvilinear type with streaks parallel to the bowel wall. The X-ray shows small locules in bowel wall. The CT scan shows wall thickening, gas in the bowel wall, retroperitoneum and peritoneum, and portal and mesenteric veins.

5. Bowel ischaemia can be acute/chronic mesenteric ischaemia, focal segmental ischaemia or colonic ischaemia. Most cases are caused by arterial disease (occlusive/non-occlusive, thrombotic/embolic). Acute occlusion is usually embolic/thrombotic and is seen in elderly patients, especially those with cardiovascular diseases. Chronic ischaemia is caused by atherosclerosis. The superior mesenteric artery is more commonly involved. X-rays show bowel wall gas and thumbprinting as a result of

bowel mucosal oedema. A CT scan shows bowel wall thickening, absence of enhancement and gas in the bowel wall/mesentery/portal veins. With modern multidetector CT scanners, the thrombus can be seen within the contrast-enhanced vessels. CT angiography is very accurate in diagnosing the cause of bowel ischaemia, which requires emergency surgical resection.

Case 1.58: Answers

1. The lateral view of the X-ray shows a radio-opaque foreign body lodged within the upper cervical oesophagus.

2. Foreign body in the throat: part of a wishbone of a chicken.

3. Foreign body ingestion is common in children, with most children being in the 18−48 month age group. Children typically ingest objects that they pick up and place in their mouths such as coins, buttons, marbles, crayons and similar items. The oesophagus has three areas of narrowing: the upper oesophageal sphincter (cricopharyngeus), the crossover of the aorta at the level of the T4 vertebra and lower oesophageal sphincter. Of children 75% have entrapment of foreign bodies at the level of the upper oesophageal sphincter. Older children present with a foreign body sensation (scratches or abrasions to the mucosal surface of the oropharynx creates a foreign body sensation), discomfort, dysphagia or drooling. Gagging, vomiting and throat pain are seen if the foreign body moves down into the oesophagus. Chronic foreign bodies can present with poor feeding, irritability, failure to thrive, fever, stridor or pulmonary symptoms.

4. An X-ray of the neck is very useful in diagnosis of a foreign body and localising the site of entrapment. X-rays are not useful if the foreign body is not radio-opaque. Of swallowed bones 20−50% are visualised on X-rays. Coins are usually seen in a coronal alignment on an AP X-ray. If the foreign body is in the trachea, it is oriented in the sagittal plane, because tracheal rings are incomplete in the posterior aspect. Barium swallow or CT scan can be done if there is ingestion of non-opaque foreign bodies, such as plastic objects, toothpicks or aluminium soda can tabs.

5. Complications of oropharyngeal foreign bodies are abrasions, lacerations, punctures, abscesses, perforations and soft-tissue infections. Oesophageal foreign bodies can produce similar complications with pneumomediastinum, mediastinitis, pneumothorax, pericarditis or

tamponade, fistulae or vascular injuries. In stable patients, direct and indirect oropharyngeal examination and fibreoptic nasopharyngoscopy are performed and foreign bodies removed. If a foreign body is sharp, elongated or multiple, endoscopic removal is done. Airway management is indicated when patients present with airway compromise, drooling, inability to tolerate fluids, or sepsis, perforation or active bleeding. Button-battery ingestion is an emergency, because necrosis of the oesophageal wall can occur in hours, and so should be removed at the earliest opportunity. If the foreign body is located in the stomach, it can be allowed to pass with follow-up radiographs in 24–48 hours.

Case 1.59: Answers

1. The first CT scan shows a hypodense fluid collection in the left subphrenic space, surrounding the spleen. Small, bilateral pleural effusions are seen.

2. Subphrenic abscess.

3. On the second CT scan, the tip of a pigtail drain is seen within the left subphrenic abscess and the fluid collection appears smaller than on the previous CT scan.

4. Subphrenic abscesses develop after abdominal surgery; 20-40% develop after rupture of a hollow viscus or trauma. Clinical features are spiking fever, abdominal pain, tenderness and weight loss. Leukocytosis is seen. Chronic abscesses present with intermittent fever, weight loss, anaemia and non-specific symptoms.

5. On an erect abdominal X-ray, a subdiaphragmatic air–fluid level is seen. Displacement of bowel loops and ileus can be present. Abdominal ultrasound shows a loculated, septated fluid collection. Reactive pleural effusion can be seen. CT scan is the diagnostic procedure of choice for looking for abdominal abscesses. Abscesses are seen as hypodense fluid collections, which show a typical rim enhancement in the periphery. Bowel loops can be differentiated from abscesses, by giving positive oral contrast.

6. Abscesses require intravenous antibiotics and drainage.

7. A CT scan is useful for diagnosing abscesses, for assessing their relationship to neighbouring structures, for detecting complications, for surgical planning and for guidance for percutaneous drainage. Ultrasonography can also be used for guidance. Percutaneous drainage is indicated when the abscess can be safely accessed without injuring adjacent structures. The skin over the site is marked with guidance. After giving local anaesthesia, a long needle is used to puncture the skin and superficial structures. The track is dilated and a pigtail catheter placed inside the fluid collection. A follow-up CT scan can be used to confirm the position of the drain. Contrast can be injected into the drain to confirm that the abscess does not communicate with adjacent structures. Healing of the abscess is also followed up with CT or ultrasonography. Complications of the technique are haemorrhage, intraperitoneal rupture and injury to adjacent structures and fistula formation.

2

GENITOURINARY
RADIOLOGY
QUESTIONS

Case 2.1

A 45-year-old man presents with fatigue, haematuria and right-sided abdominal pain. On examination, there is a firm, non-tender mass in the right lumbar region.

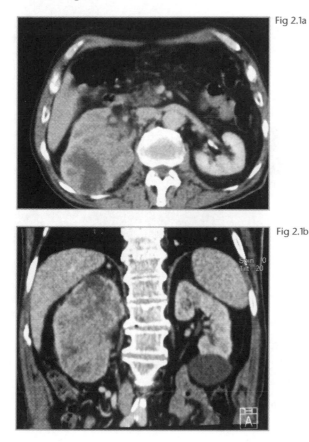

Fig 2.1a

Fig 2.1b

1. What are the findings on the CT scan?
2. What is the diagnosis?
3. What are the important factors to be assessed in the scan?
4. What further investigations are required for confirmation of the diagnosis?
5. What are the various presentations of this disease? Name one syndrome that is associated with this condition.
6. What is the aetiopathology of this disease?
7. What is the treatment of this condition?
8. Does radiology have a role in treatment?

Answers on pages 177–220

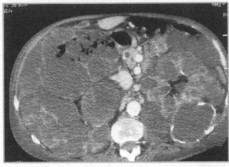
Case 2.2

A 40-year-old patient presents with fever and bilateral flank pain. On examination, the patient is febrile and tachycardic. There are bilateral masses in the lumbar region, which is tender on the right side.

Fig 2.2a

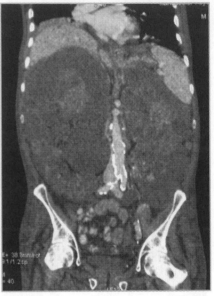

Fig 2.2b

1. What do you see on the CT scan?
2. What is the diagnosis? What complication has developed?
3. What are the associations?
4. What are the clinical presentations?
5. What are the radiological features?
6. What is the differential diagnosis?
7. What are the complications and associations?
8. What is the management?

Answers on pages 177–220

Case 2.3

A 35-year-old man was involved in a road traffic accident. He presented to A&E with severe pain in the left side of his abdomen and haematuria. On examination, his pulse was 120, BP 106/78 mmHg. There was severe tenderness and swelling on the left side of the abdomen. Multiple investigative procedures were done on this patient.

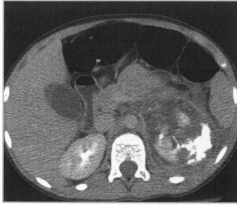

Fig 2.3a

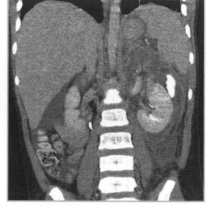

Fig 2.3b

1. What do you observe on the CT scan?
2. What is the diagnosis?
3. How is this condition graded?
4. What are the clinical features?
5. What are the radiological features?
6. What is the imaging protocol?
7. What are the complications and treatment?

Answers on pages 177–220

Case 2.4

A 53-year-old woman presented with long-standing right flank pain, haematuria and intermittent fever. On examination, she is febrile and has bilateral renal angle tenderness, without any palpable mass. A urine test demonstrated pyuria.

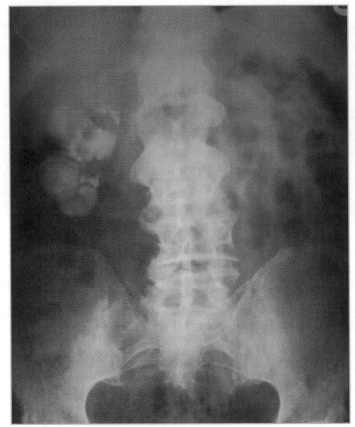

Fig 2.4

1. What do you observe on the plain X-ray?
2. What is the diagnosis?
3. What is the mode of spread of this disease?
4. What are the clinical features and pathophysiology?
5. What are the radiological features?
6. What is the differential diagnosis?
7. What are the complications?
8. What is the treatment?

Answers *on pages 177–220*

Case 2.5

A 58-year-old man presents with left flank pain, dysuria and haematuria. On examination, there is left renal angle tenderness, but no palpable mass.

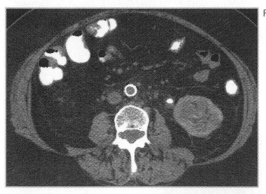

Fig 2.5a

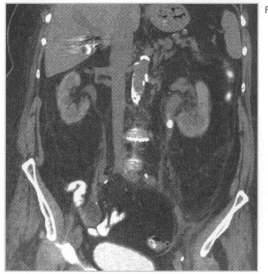

Fig 2.5b

1. What do you see on the CT scan?
2. What is the diagnosis? What complication has developed?
3. What is the aetiopathology? What are the types?
4. What are the radiological features?
5. What are the radiological features of this complication?
6. What is the radiological differential diagnosis?
7. What is the treatment?

Answers *on pages 177–220*

Case 2.6

A 42-year-old man presents with left flank pain, haematuria, fever and chills. On examination, there is tenderness in the left lumbar region, without any palpable mass.

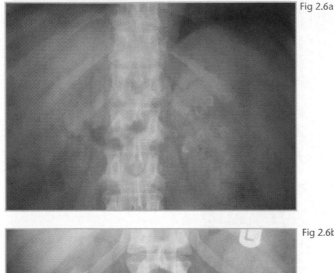

Fig 2.6a

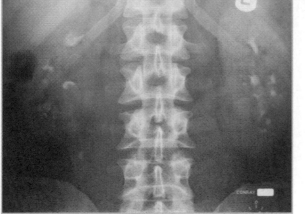

Fig 2.6b

1. What do you see on the plain film and IVU?
2. What is the diagnosis?
3. What are the pathophysiology and clinical features?
4. What are the causes?
5. What are the radiological features?
6. What are the complications?
7. What are the differential diagnoses?

Answers on pages 177–220

Case 2.7

An 11-year-old boy presents with urinary infections, dribbling and left-sided abdominal pain. He is afebrile and does not show any renal angle tenderness.

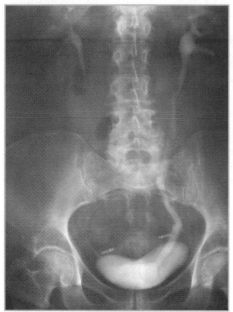

Fig 2.7a

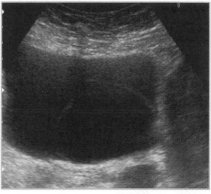

Fig 2.7b

1. What do you observe on the IVU?
2. What do you observe on ultrasonography?
3. What is the diagnosis?
4. What are the different types?
5. What are the radiological findings?
6. What is the differential diagnosis?
7. What are the complications and treatment?

Answers *on pages 177–220*

Case 2.8

A 33-year-old man involved in a road traffic accident presents with acute pain in the abdomen and pelvis and inability to void urine. The patient is hypotensive and tachycardic. X-ray showed pelvic fractures. After initial resuscitation, further imaging was performed.

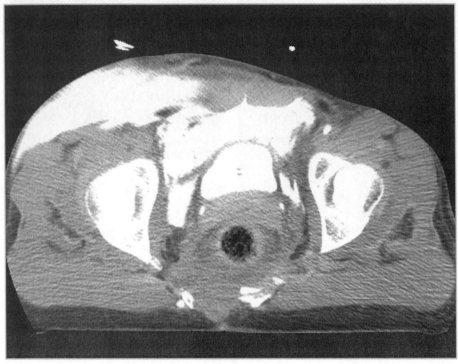

Fig 2.8

1. What is this investigation and what do you observer?
2. What is the diagnosis?
3. What are the types of this disease?
4. What is the most common location?
5. What are the radiological findings?
6. What other investigation can be performed?
7. What is the treatment?

Answers on pages 177–220

Case 2.9

A 58-year-old man presents with left flank pain, gross haematuria and weight loss. On examination, no palpable mass was felt in the abdomen.

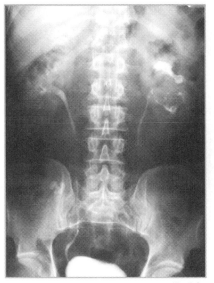

Fig 2.9a

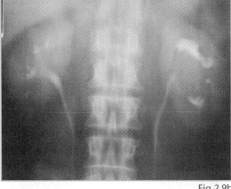

Fig 2.9b

1. What do you see on these tests?
2. What is the diagnosis?
3. What are the histological types?
4. What are the predisposing factors and clinical features?
5. What is the pattern of distribution?
6. What are the radiological findings?
7. What is the treatment?

Answers on pages 177–220

Case 2.10

A 72-year-old man presents with back pain, weight loss and urinary frequency. On examination, there is no abdominal mass. Rectal examination showed hard, irregular enlargement of the prostate gland.

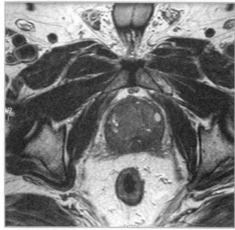

Fig 2.10a

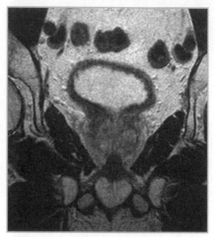

Fig 2.10b

1. What do you see on MRI of the pelvis?
2. What is the diagnosis?
3. What are the types and clinical features?
4. What is the common screening test?
5. What are the ultrasound features of this disease?
6. What is the role of MRI in this disease?
7. What is the role of biopsy?
8. What is the management of this disease?

Answers on pages 177–220

Case 2.11

A 9-year-old boy presents with pain in the lower abdomen and scrotal swelling. On examination there is a tender, hard lump in the right testis, which does not reduce or transilluminate.

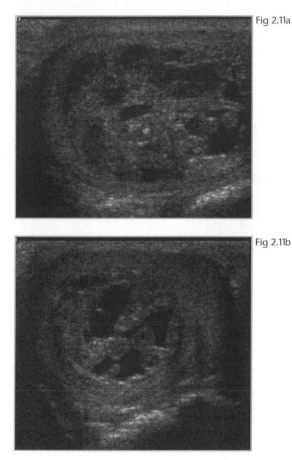

Fig 2.11a

Fig 2.11b

1. What do you observe on testicular ultrasonography?
2. What is the diagnosis?
3. What are the different types?
4. What are the clinical presentations?
5. What are the laboratory abnormalities and predisposing factors?
6. What is the mode of spread?
7. What are the radiological features?
8. What are the imaging approach and the treatment?

Answers *on pages 177–220*

Case 2.12

A 59-year-old woman presents with diffuse abdominal pain and abdominal distension. On examination, there is a large, soft, non-tender mass in the entire abdomen.

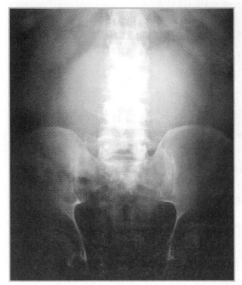

Fig 2.12a

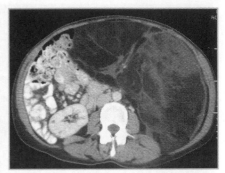

Fig 2.12b

1. What do you see on the X-ray and the CT scan of the abdomen?

2. What is the diagnosis?

3. What is the organ of origin?

4. What are the pathological subtypes?

5. What are the radiological features?

6. What is the differential diagnosis for lesions in this location? What other lesions can have similar appearance?

7. What is the treatment of this condition?

Answers on pages 177–220

Case 2.13

A 44-year-old woman presents with abdominal pain, distension and hypertension. On examination, there is no palpable mass.

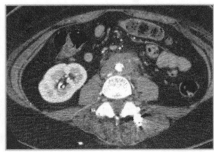

Fig 2.13b

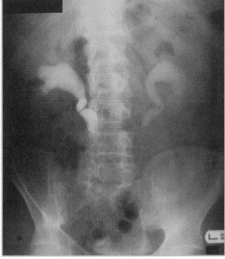

Fig 2.13a

1. What do you find on IVU and on the CT scan?
2. What is the diagnosis?
3. What is the mechanism of development of this disease?
4. What are the other causes of this disease?
5. What are the characteristic location and the associations?
6. What are the radiological features?
7. What is the differential diagnosis?
8. What is the treatment?

Answers *on pages 177–220*

Case 2.14

A 28-year-old man presents with complaints of dribbling of urine, decreased flow and dysuria. Examination of his abdomen, groin and penis is unremarkable.

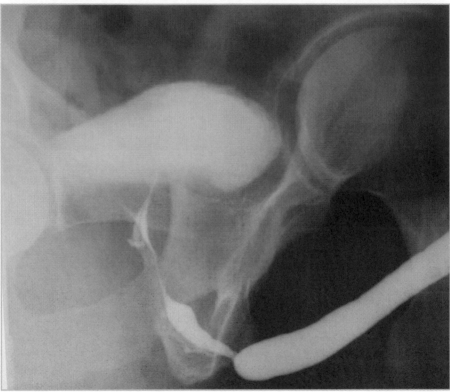

Fig 2.14

1. What is this investigation? How is it done?
2. What are the findings?
3. What is the diagnosis?
4. What are the causes?
5. What are the anatomy and most common location for this pathology?
6. What are the clinical features and pathophysiology?
7. What are the complications?
8. What is the treatment?

Answers on pages 177–220

Case 2.15

A 31-year-old woman presented with infertility, despite trying for 18 months. She has a normal menstrual cycle and flow. Clinical examination was unremarkable. Pelvic ultrasonography, follicle-stimulating hormone (FSH), luteinising hormone (LH), prolactin, testosterone and other blood tests were normal.

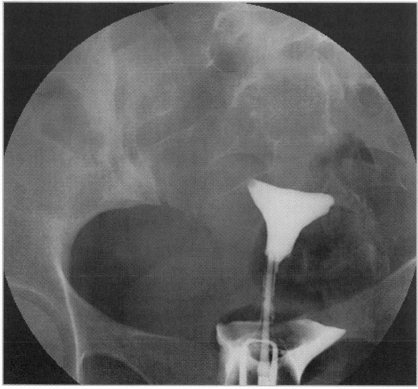

Fig 2.15a

1. What is this investigation? What are the abnormal findings?
2. What is the diagnosis?
3. What are the indications for this test?
4. What is the optimal time for this procedure?
5. How is this procedure performed?
6. What are the factors assessed in the test?
7. What are the complications and contraindications of the procedure?
8. What are the other causes of this condition?

Answers on pages 177–220

Case 2.16

A 61-year-old male patient presents with left loin pain and difficulty urinating. On examination, there is a soft mass in the left renal angle. His serum creatinine level was increased.

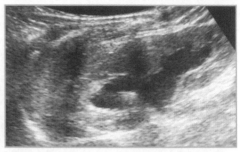

Fig 2.16b

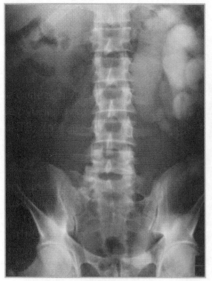

Fig 2.16a

1. What do you see on IVU (delayed film, taken after 2 hours) and ultrasound?
2. What is the diagnosis?
3. What are the causes?
4. What are the appearances on IVU?
5. What are the appearances on ultrasonography?
6. What is the differential diagnosis?
7. What is the significance of this appearance in pregnancy?
8. What is the role of radiology in treatment?

Answers on pages 177–220

Case 2.17

A 38-year-old woman presents with loin pain, fever and haematuria. On examination there is right costovertebral angle tenderness, without a discrete mass.

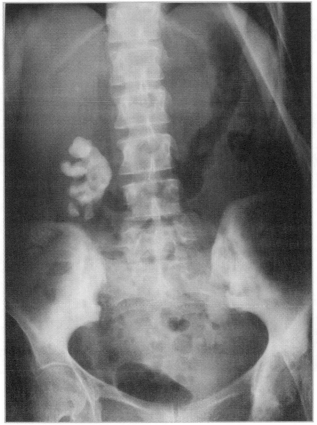

Fig 2.17

1. What do you see on the plain film?
2. What is the diagnosis?
3. What is the composition?
4. What is the causative organism?
5. What are the predisposing factors?
6. What are the radiological features?
7. What are the complications?
8. What is the treatment?

Answers *on pages 177–220*

Case 2.18

A 35-year-old woman presents with fever, chills and flank pain. On examination, a tender mass is palpable in the right renal angle. The patient is febrile with tachycardia and hypotension. There is elevation of WBCs and CRP in the blood.

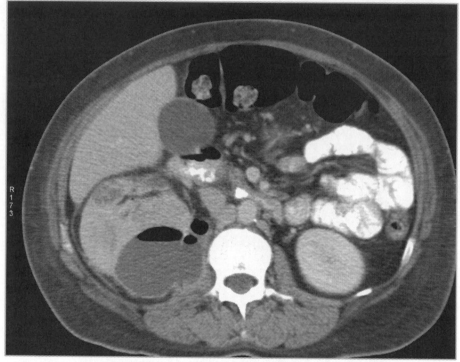

Fig 2.18

1. What do you observe on the CT scan of the abdomen?
2. What is the diagnosis?
3. What are the pathophysiology and predisposing factors?
4. What are the causative agents?
5. What are the radiological features?
6. What is the differential diagnosis?
7. What are the complications?
8. What is the treatment?

Answers on pages 177–220

Case 2.19

A 54-year-old man presents with haematuria, left-sided dull abdominal pain and a lump. On examination, the patient is anaemic with diffuse body oedema. There is a firm mass in the left lumbar region.

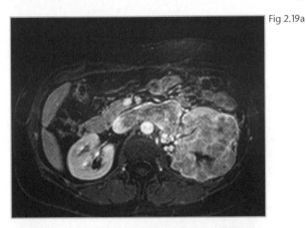

Fig 2.19a

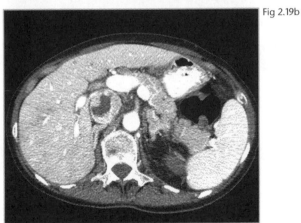

Fig 2.19b

1. What do you see on the MRI scan?
2. What is the diagnosis?
3. What additional complication can you detect on the CT scan, taken at a higher level than the MRI?
4. What are the other causes of this appearance?
5. What are the radiological features?
6. What is the staging of this disease?
7. What is the treatment?

Answers on pages 177–220

A 63-year-old man presents with three episodes of painless frank haematuria. The clinical examination is unremarkable. There is no mass in the abdomen or pelvis. On rectal examination, the prostate gland seems normal in size and consistency.

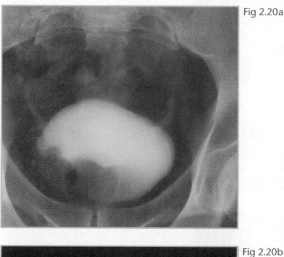

Fig 2.20a

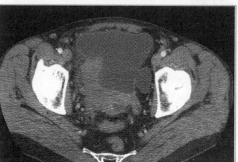

Fig 2.20b

1. What do you see in the IVU film and CT scan of the pelvis?
2. What is the diagnosis?
3. What are the types?
4. What are the clinical features?
5. What are the radiological features? What other investigations are required?
6. How do you stage the disease?
7. What are the predisposing factors?
8. What is the management of this disease?

Answers on pages 177–220

Case 2.21

A 21-year-old presents with recurrent urinary infections, dysuria and hesitancy. No abdominal or pelvis mass is palpated.

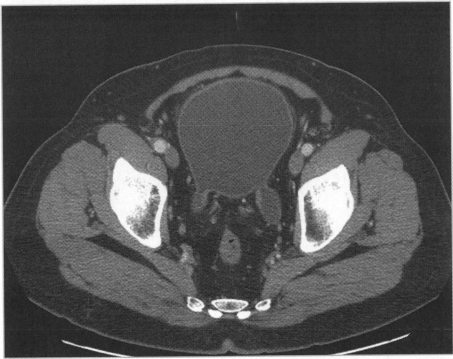

Fig 2.21

1. What do you seen on the CT scan?
2. What is the diagnosis?
3. What are the types?
4. What is the most common site?
5. What are the causes?
6. What is the appearance on radiological investigations?
7. What are the complications?
8. What is the treatment?

Answers *on pages 177–220*

Case 2.22

A 47-year-old man presents with gross haematuria. Clinical examination did not reveal any palpable mass. Ultrasonography was normal. IVU showed an obstructed left kidney. Another test was done to evaluate the ureter.

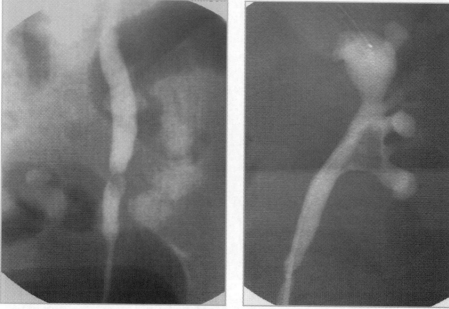

Fig 2.22a   Fig 2.22b

1. What is this procedure?
2. What are the findings?
3. How is this procedure performed?
4. What are the indications and advantages?
5. What are the disadvantages of this procedure?
6. What other tests are useful in diagnosis of this disease?
7. How is this staged and what is the treatment?

Answers on pages 177–220

Case 2.23

A 5-year-old patient presents with hesitancy and dribbling of urine. He has a long-standing spine problem and is paraplegic. On examination, he has reduced power in his lower limbs. Examination of the abdomen did not show any palpable mass.

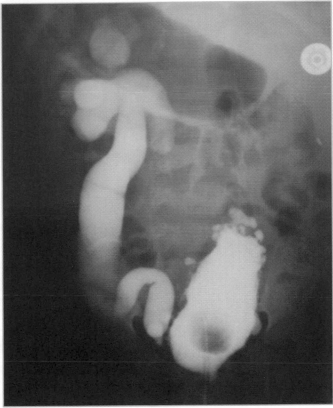

Fig 2.23

1. What do you see on this cystogram?
2. What is the diagnosis?
3. What are the causes?
4. What are the types?
5. What are the radiological features?
6. What other investigations may be required?
7. What is the differential diagnosis?
8. What is the treatment?

Answers on pages 177–220

A 69-year-old man presents with dribbling, hesitancy and poor stream during micturition. There is no fever or haematuria. On examination, no abdominal mass is palpated. Rectal examination is abnormal.

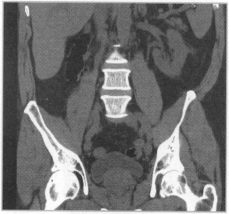

Fig 2.24a

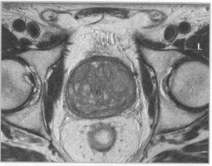

Fig 2.24b

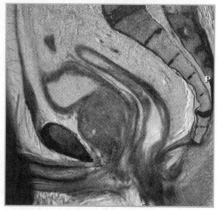

Fig 2.24c

1. What do you observe on CT and MRI of the pelvis?
2. What is the diagnosis?
3. What is the most common location?
4. What are the clinical features and pathology?
5. What are the radiological features?
6. What is the differential diagnosis?
7. What are the complications?
8. What is the treatment?

Answers on pages 177–220

Case 2.25

A 14-year-old boy presents with severe pain and swelling of the testis, fever, nausea and vomiting. On examination, the testis is swollen, red and tender.

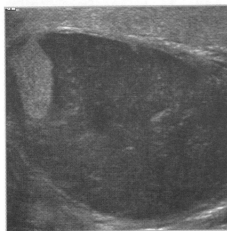

Fig 2.25a

For colour version, see *Colour Images* section from page 475.

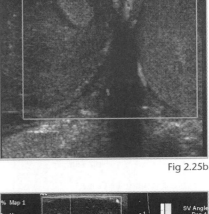

Fig 2.25b

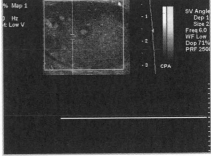

Fig 2.25c

1. What do you see on ultrasonography of the scrotum?
2. What do you see on the second and third pictures?
3. What is the diagnosis?
4. What are the predisposing factors?
5. What is the common differential diagnosis?
6. What is the role of radiology in this condition?
7. What are the complications?

Answers *on pages 177–220*

Case 2.26

A 13-year-old boy presents with fever, severe pain and swelling in his scrotum and burning micturition. On examination, he has a tender and enlarged right testicle and generalised swelling and oedema of his scrotum.

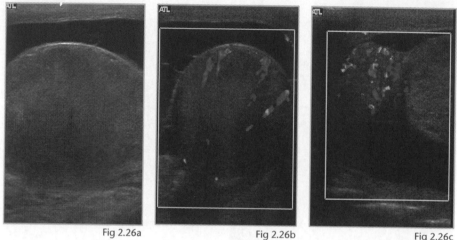

Fig 2.26a   Fig 2.26b   Fig 2.26c

For colour version, see *Colour Images* section from page 475.

1. What do you see on conventional ultrasonography and colour Doppler study of the scrotum?

2. What is the second scan and what do you see?

3. What is the diagnosis?

4. What is the aetiology and what are the clinical features?

5. What is the role of radiology?

6. What are the differential diagnoses?

7. What are the complications?

Answers on pages 177–220

Case 2.27

A 47-year-old woman comes for routine mammographic screening.

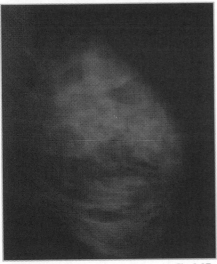

Fig 2.27a

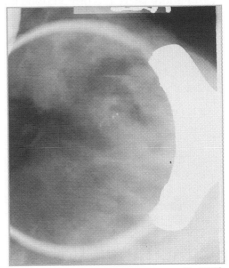

Fig 2.27b

1. What are the findings on mammography?
2. What is the likely diagnosis?
3. How is this test done?
4. What is the screening programme in the UK?
5. What are the types of early disease?
6. What are the radiological features?
7. What is the differential diagnosis?
8. What is the management?

Case 2.28

A 32-year-old woman presents with pain in the right breast and a lump. On examination, there is a firm, mobile lump in the right breast. No lymph nodes are palpable.

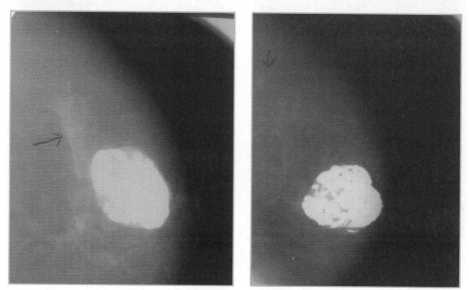

Fig 2.28a   Fig 2.28b

1. What do you observe in the mammogram? (note the area in the arrow also)
2. What is the diagnosis? Do you see any other associated lesion?
3. What is the pathology and what are the clinical features of the calcified lesion?
4. What are the mammographic features of the above condition?
5. What are the sonographic findings?
6. What are the differential diagnoses?
7. What is the treatment?

Answers on pages 177–220

Case 2.29

A 56-year-old woman presents with abdominal bloating, constipation and weight loss. On examination, there is a large, cystic mass in the lower part of her abdomen and pelvis.

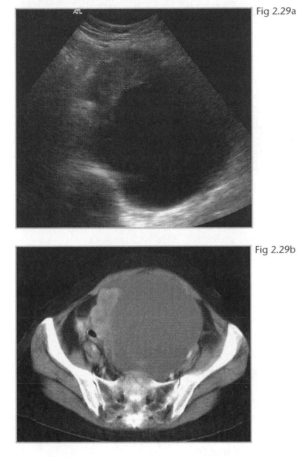

Fig 2.29a

Fig 2.29b

1. What do you see on the ultrasound and CT scans?
2. What is the diagnosis?
3. What is the classification of this disease?
4. What are the associations and radiological appearances of this disease?
5. What is the pattern of spread of this disease?
6. What is the imaging protocol?
7. What are the secondary features observed in this condition?
8. What is the staging and treatment of this disease?

Answers on pages 177–220

Case 2.30

A 35-year-old woman presents with lumpiness in both breasts with mastalgia. Fine needle aspiration cytology did not reveal malignancy.

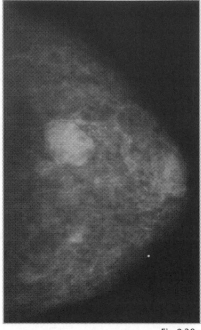

Fig 2.30a

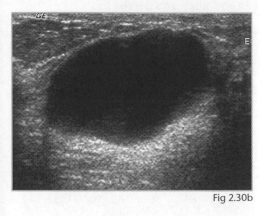

Fig 2.30b

1. What do you observe on the mammogram?
2. What is the diagnosis?
3. What are the clinical features?
4. What is the pathology?
5. What are the findings on the mammogram?
6. What is the risk of malignancy?

Answers on pages 177–220

Case 2.31

A 54-year-old woman presents with a palpable, painful lump in the right breast.

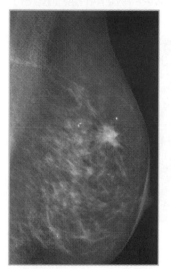

Fig 2.31a

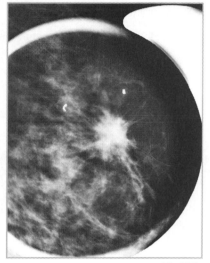

Fig 2.31b

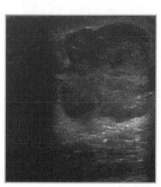

Fig 2.31c

1. What are the findings on mammography?
2. What do you observe on breast ultrasonography?
3. What is the diagnosis?
4. What are the investigations for a palpable mass?
5. What are the different types of this disease?
6. What is the treatment of this condition?

Answers on pages 177–220

Case 2.32

A 37-year-old woman presents with a chronic disease, with lower abdominal, pain, vomiting and pneumaturia. On examination, no mass is palpable in the abdomen or rectum. A barium enema and CT scan were ordered because of the clinical history of pneumaturia.

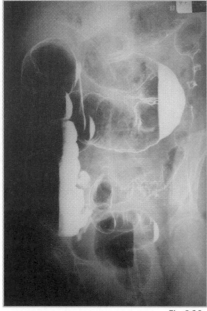

Fig 2.32a

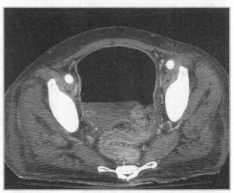

Fig 2.32b

1. What do you find on the contrast study and the CT scan?
2. What is the diagnosis?
3. What are the causes?
4. What are the clinical presentations?
5. What is the location?
6. What are the radiological procedures?
7. What other tests are required?
8. What is the treatment?

Answers on pages 177–220

Case 2.33

A 36-year-old woman presents with fever, lower abdominal pain, haematuria and leak of urine from the vagina.

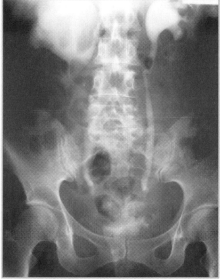

Fig 2.33a

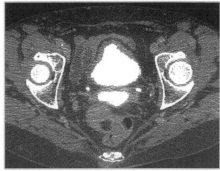

Fig 2.33b

1. What do you observe in the IVU and CT scan?
2. What is the diagnosis?
3. What are the causes and pathology of this condition?
4. What are the clinical features?
5. What are the common locations?
6. What radiological tests are required?
7. What other tests are useful?
8. What is the treatment?

Answers on pages 177–220

Case 2.1: Answers

1. CT scans of the abdomen in axial and coronal views show a normal appearing left kidney. The right kidney is enlarged and there is a large, heterogeneous mass with areas of necrosis within it.

2. Renal cell carcinoma

3. Size of the tumour, spread outside kidney, involvement of Gerota's fascia and the adrenals, regional lymphadenopathy, extension into the renal vein/IVC, and liver/lung/bony metastasis are the important factors assessed on the scan.

4. Usually a CT scan is enough to confirm a diagnosis and no further investigation such as biopsy is required. In small or indeterminate cases, an ultrasound- or CT-guided biopsy is performed. A CT scan of the abdomen and chest is done to stage the disease and identify metastases. MRI is useful in assessing vascular extension into the renal vein, IVC and right atrium.

5. The classic presentation is haematuria, abdominal mass and pain, which are seen in less than 15% of cases. Renal carcinoma can, however, present with a myriad of symptoms, including fever, anaemia, polycythaemia, hypertension, hypercalcaemia, nephrotic syndrome, weight loss, fatigue, cachexia, night sweats, hepatic dysfunction, varicocele and polyneuromyopathy. Von Hippel–Lindau syndrome is associated with renal carcinoma. In this syndrome, the tumours are bilateral, multicentric and occur at a younger age.

6. Renal cell carcinoma arises from the proximal tubular epithelium. Oncocytoma, a rarer variety, is thought to arise from the distal tubule. RCC is more common in males and in the sixth decade. Smoking, obesity, cadmium, asbestos, petroleum products and analgesic nephropathy are predisposing factors. Histologically they are divided into: clear cell, chromophilic, chromophobic, collecting duct variety and oncocytic types. Abnormal chromosome 3 has been identified in the majority of RCCs.

7. Definitive treatment is radical nephrectomy, which can be done by a transperitoneal/retroperitoneal/thoracoabdominal/laparoscopic route. Resection of lymph node and thrombus is performed if present.

Palliative treatments:

– nephrectomy: for symptomatic relief

– chemotherapy: renal tumours are refractory. Gemcitabine can be tried

– hormonal therapy: megesterol was used, but was not of much benefit

– immunotherapy: interferons, IL-2, lymphokine activated killer cells, tumour infiltrated leukocytes, BCG, stem cell transplantation

– radiotherapy: for local symptoms, bone/brain metastasis.

8. Radiofrequency ablation under ultrasound or CT guidance is performed in small tumours confined to the kidney or tumours in a solitary kidney. Embolisation is useful to reduce vascularity of a large tumour before surgery, if the tumour is in a solitary kidney or as a palliative measure.

Case 2.2: Answers

1. The CT scan shows bilaterally enlarged kidneys. Both the kidneys have been replaced by multiple cysts of varying sizes. Cysts in the posterior aspect of the left kidney show calcified walls. In addition, there are multiple locules of gas seen within the cysts located anteriorly in the right kidney.

2. Autosomal dominant polycystic kidney disease (ADPKD). The presence of gas indicates that some of cysts have become infected. Adult polycystic kidney disease is an autosomal dominant condition (1/1000). Cysts arise from the nephrons and the collecting tubules. Islands of normal parenchymal renal tissue are interspersed between the cysts. Haematuria is one of the presentations and can result from either calculi (in 10%) or associated renal cell carcinoma, and warrants ultrasonography or a CT scan.

3. The *ADPKD* gene is located in the short arm of chromosome 16. This has 100% penetrance and variable expressivity. It is associated with cysts in the liver, pancreas, spleen, lung, thyroid, ovaries, testis, uterus, seminal vesicles, epididymis, and bladder. Other associations are berry aneurysms in the circle of Willis, aortic aneurysm, aortic regurgitation, bicuspid aortic valve, coarctation, mitral regurgitation, colonic diverticulosis and mitral valve prolapse.

4. ADPKD presents in the fourth or fifth decade, and in all patients by age 60. Presenting features are hypertension, renal failure, haematuria, proteinuria, abdominal pain and renal mass.

5. A plain X-ray can show calcifications or calculi and enlarged renal contours. On IVU, the kidneys are enlarged and renal pelvis is compressed and elongated. The calyces are stretched over the cyst and may cause the typical spider leg deformity. Ultrasound shows bilaterally enlarged kidneys, with multiple cysts of varying sizes. CT scan shows the cysts, which may be calcified. Normally they are hypodense. Hyperdense cysts indicate haemorrhage or infection. A Swiss-cheese nephrogram refers to the appearance of multiple small cysts with smooth margins. The kidneys become smaller with onset of renal failure. Associated renal cell carcinoma can be detected. On MRI scan, the cysts are hypointense in T1 and hyperintense in T2.

6. Differential diagnoses: **multiple simple cysts** (no family history, not diffuse), **von Hippel–Lindau disease** (associated pancreatic cysts, haemangioblastomas, phaeochromocytoma), cysts of renal failure (kidneys small and non-functioning), **infantile polycystic kidney disease** (small cysts, hyperechoic on ultrasonography), **tuberous sclerosis**, **medullary cystic disease** and **multicystic dysplasia**.

7. Complications of cysts: infection, haemorrhage, rupture. Other complications: calculi, infection, renal cell carcinoma. Death could result from hypertensive disease, uraemia, cerebral haemorrhage caused by aneurysm rupture or hypertension and cardiac complications. ADPKD is associated with cardiac valvular abnormalities (mitral valve prolapse), berry aneurysms and colonic diverticula.

8. Cysts without complication are followed with ultrasonography to detect renal tumours and other complications. Screening with MRA is done to detect aneurysms. If MRA is negative, it is repeated every 5 years. If MRA is positive, a conventional angiogram is done. If aneurysm > 6 mm, it needs endovascular treatment or surgical clipping. If aneurysm < 6 mm, follow-up with angiogram is done after 2 years. Renal failure requires dialysis and transplantation.

1. Axial and coronal contrast enhanced CT scans of the abdomen show a normal appearing right kidney. The left kidney outline is poorly defined in the axial scan and there is diminished enhancement of the parenchyma in the anterior and lateral aspects. More importantly there is dense contrast in the collecting system, extending outside the kidney in the left perinephric space due to extravasation.

2. Grade 4 renal trauma with renal haematoma, perinephric haematoma and contrast extravasation from the collecting system.

3. Renal trauma grading system:

   Grade 1: subcaspsular haematoma

   Grade 2: superficial renal lacerations with perinephric haematoma

   Grade 3: deep renal laceration without extension to collecting system.

   Grade 4: deep laceration with extension to the collecting system/ thrombosis of segmental artery with infarction

   Grade 5: traumatic occlusion of main renal artery/renal artery avulsion/ shattered kidney.

4. Blunt trauma accounts for 90% of renal injuries. It is associated with other organ injury in 75%. Soft tissue bruising, flank pain and tenderness may be present. Haematuria is the main sign (seen in 95%), which may be prompt or delayed. About 25% of those with gross haematuria have significant renal injury. Around 25% of those with renal vascular pedicle injury have no haematuria. Meteorism, resulting in abdominal distension within 24–48 hours due to retroperitoneal haematoma, can be present.

5. Radiological features of various types of renal injury:

   Contusions: high density in non-contrast, low density in contrast enhancement

   Subcapsular haematoma: crescenteric fluid collection.

   Perinephric haematoma: surrounds kidney

   Infarct: wedge-shaped, hypodense, non-enhancing area

   Laceration: linear hypodensity

Fracture: laceration connects two cortical surfaces

Laceration with involvement of collecting system: extravasation of contrast in delayed images

Active haemorrhage: contrast enhancement within haematoma; active leak of contrast during arterial phase, same density as aorta

Shattered kidney: multiple renal lacerations

Occlusion of renal artery: no contrast in renal artery, hypodense kidneys

Avulsion of renal artery: haematoma in the vicinity of the renal artery and absence of renal parenchymal enhancement

Thrombosis of renal vein: hypodense filling defect in renal vein, hypodensity in kidney

Avulsion of pelviureteric junction (PUJ): massive contrast extravasation from the PUJ.

6. Ultrasonography is the fastest method of diagnosis, but CT is the most effective technique because it shows arterial bleed and collecting system injuries. Injury to other organs and bowel can also be assessed. Minor injuries can be followed up with renal ultrasonography.

7. Renal failure and Page's kidney (post-traumatic renovascular hypertension) are the complications. Minor injuries and haemodynamically stable patients are observed without any intervention. Active bleeding can be managed by embolisation of the renal artery or surgery. Most of the urine leaks close spontaneously. Surgical exploration is needed (<10% of patients) for progressive blood loss or expanding abdominal mass. Transperitoneal approach is used to excluded injury to adjacent organs.

Case 2.4: Answers

1. The plain X-ray shows dense, amorphous calcification of the entire right kidney.

2. Tuberculosis of the right kidney. Calcified granulomas in the kidney are producing a pseudocalculous appearance.

3. Renal TB is caused by *Mycobacterium tuberculosis*. The urogenital tract is the second most common site of TB involvement after the lungs. Infection spreads haematogenously from a distant focus which is often not identified.

4. During initial seeding, *Mycobacterium tuberculosis* lodges in the periglomerular capillaries, with a resulting immune reaction that produces caseating granulomas in the cortex. The organisms spill from the nephrons and are trapped in the narrow segment of the loop of Henle; this results in ulcerous lesions of the papilla, which erode into the calyces. The collecting system is hence affected by contiguous spread from the renal parenchyma to the urothelium. Haematogenous spread directly to the collecting system is unusual. Clinically the salient features are sterile pyuria, dysuria, urgency, frequency, haematuria and a past history of renal TB; 75% are unilateral.

5. An X-ray might show features of pulmonary TB (pulmonary findings are seen in < 50% of patients with renal TB). An X-ray is useful only in later stages, when the kidney goes into the autonephrectomy phase, in which it is small, scarred and non-functioning with extensive dystrophic calcifications. Parenchymal calcifications are seen. IVU may show early stages of abnormality. The earliest change is an irregular feathery appearance of the papilla as a result of erosion. Small cavities are subsequently seen from the calyx into the papilla. Strictures of the infundibulum and pelvis are seen as dilated calyces. A phantom calyx indicates incomplete visualisation of calyx as a result of stenosis. Kinking of the renal pelvis and thick collecting system are other features. The kidneys are scarred in later stages and small with distortion of the collecting system, although they are large in the early stages. Tuberculomas are seen that displace the collecting system. Ultrasonography and CT show cavities, granulomas, distorted collecting system, scars, strictures and calcifications.

6. Differential diagnoses are renal abscess, renal tumours, pyelonephritis and xanthogranulomatous pyelonephritis. The extensive calcification in a small kidney is, however, fairly specific for renal TB.

7. Complications are autonephrectomy with loss of renal function, extension of infection to pararenal space and psoas and extension to adjacent organs. Renal TB often extends to ureters, bladder and seminal vesicles.

8. Anti-tuberculous therapy is initiated once the diagnosis of renal TB is established. Dilatation of ureteral strictures caused by tubercular granulomas and fibrosis may be necessary during treatment. Surgery is required for severe cases, not responding to medical treatment.

Case 2.5: Answers

1. The axial CT scan shows a dense opacity in the proximal left ureter, at the pelviureteric junction, which is surrounded by soft tissue stranding in the periureteric space. This is also seen in the coronal CT scan. There is proximal dilatation of the left renal collecting system.

2. Left ureteric calculus. The patient has developed left hydroureteronephrosis.

3. The predisposing factors of renal calculi are: dehydration, decreased urinary citrate, repeated UTIs, inadequate urinary drainage, prolonged immobilisation, vitamin A deficiency, hyperparathyroidism and hypercalcuria. Based on composition, renal stones can consist of calcium oxalate, struvite, calcium phosphate, uric acid, cystine and xanthine.

4. **Radiological features**:

   X-rays: more than 60% of stones are radio-opaque, but small stones may be missed (30% of stones are missed).

   Opacity of stones: opaque (calcium, struvite), mildly opaque (cystine), lucent (uric acid) non-opaque (xanthine, matrix, indinavir stones).

   Shape of stones: staghorn – struvite; spiculated/mulberry – calcium oxalate; milk of calcium – calcium carbonate seed calculi – diverticulum, cyst or hydronephrosis.

   IVU: is useful in outlining the renal tract. Delayed films may show site of calculus, in case of obstruction.

   Common sites of obstruction: pelviureteric junction (PUJ), vesicoureteric junction (VUJ), iliac vessel crossing.

   Non-contrast CT scan of abdomen and pelvis: shows stones, with other indirect signs such as periureteral, perinephric (oedema in the bridging septa due to increased lymphatic pressure) and peripelvic stranding. To differentiate stone in UVJ and a stone passed into the bladder, a scan is done in the prone position so that a free stone falls down into the bladder. Ureteric rim sign is thickening of the ureter around impacted ureteric calculus due to oedema. The most common differential diagnosis is phlebolith. CT scan is very useful in assessment of other structures, which might cause abdominal pain.

5. Radiology of obstruction: IVU shows dilated ureter and the site of obstruction. There might be a delayed nephrogram or non-visualisation of the collecting system. Delayed films are required to identify the site of obstruction. Ultrasound shows a dilated collecting system with high resistive index on the Doppler scan. A ureteral jet is not seen on the affected side. The CT scan shows a dilated ureter and collecting system. Perinephric and periureteral stranding indicate obstruction. The higher the degree of obstruction, the higher the degree of stranding. Focal collection of urine can be seen as a result of extravasation due to forniceal rupture. The kidneys are enlarged.

6. Differential diagnoses of ureteric calculus are: phleboliths, calcified lymph nodes, foreign bodies and GIT, gallstones and appendiceal concretion.

7. Small calculi (<5 mm) can be safely observed, as they are likely to pass unless they are impacted. Stones in the PUJ are removed by nephrolithotomy, under antibiotic cover. Calculi in the distal ureter may be removed endoscopically with a Dormia basket. Calculi in the mid-ureter can be removed ureteroscopically or pushed up in the kidney and removed by lithotripsy. Lithotripsy of ureteric stones can be performed *in situ*, provided there is no obstruction.

Case 2.6: Answers

1. The plain film shows small specks of calcification in the renal medulla on the left side. The IVU shows abnormal deformed calyces, with contrast extravasation from calyces within the renal papillae.

2. Acute renal papillary necrosis.

3. Renal papillary necrosis is ischaemic necrosis of the renal medulla secondary to interstitial nephritis or vascular obstruction. There are three stages:

Necrosis *in situ*: the necrotic papillae detach but remain within the bed, unextruded

Medullary type (partial papillary slough): single cavity in papilla with the long axis paralleling the long axis of papilla and communicating with calyx — bilateral or unilateral.

Papillary type: total papillary slough.

Papillary necrosis presents with flank pain, dysuria, fever, chills, hypertension, proteinuria, pyuria, haematuria and leukocytosis.

4. The causes of renal papillary necrosis are analgesic nephropathy, diabetes mellitus, pyelonephritis, renal obstruction, sickle cell disease, TB, trauma, renal vein thrombosis, cirrhosis, coagulopathy, dehydration, haemophilia, acute transplant rejection, portpartum state and high-dose urography. Unilateral papillary necrosis indicates obstruction, renal vein thrombosis or acute bacterial nephritis.

5. On plain radiograph, calcification of sloughed renal papillae may be noted within renal outlines. IVU shows a normal or small kidney. Occasionally, the kidney is large as a result of obstruction or infection. The renal contour is smooth or wavy. The earliest sign is a subtle area of contrast extending from the fornix parallel to the long axis of the papilla. Cavitation of the papilla, central or eccentric, widened fornix, club-shaped calyx, rind shadow of papilla, filling defect in calyx, pelvis or ureter (sloughed papilla), decreased density of contrast in nephrogram and deceased parenchymal thickness are other features. Ultrasonography can show multiple, cystic spaces within renal medulla.

6. Sloughed renal papillae within renal collecting system may result in obstructive uropathy. There is also a higher incidence of transitional cell carcinoma and squamous cell carcinoma.

7. Differential diagnoses: **hydronephrosis** (does not show necrotic papilla), **congenital megacalicosis** (normal renal function), **postobstructive renal atrophy, renal TB.**

1. The IVU shows normal kidneys. The bladder is distended with contrast. There is a large bulbous contrast filled structure within the left side of the bladder, arising from the distal end of the left ureter.

2. Ultrasonography shows a distended, rounded hypoechoic structure arising from the posterior wall of the urinary bladder.

3. Simple ureterocele of the left ureter.

4. Ureterocele is cystic ectasia of a subepithelial segment of an intravescial ureter. Ureteroceles can be **simple** or **ectopic.** Simple ureterocele is seen in normal patients with a single ureter and is caused by congenital prolapse of a dilated distal ureter into the bladder lumen at the usual location of the trigone. It is often an incidental finding. Ectopic ureterocele is located in a ureteric orifice that is distal to the normal trigone, either within or outside the bladder. Most of them (80%) are associated with the upper moiety of a duplex kidney; 20% occur in a single non-duplicated system

5. IVU shows a normal or renal duplex collecting system. There is early filling of the bulbous terminal ureter – the classic cobra-head appearance, with a radiolucent halo resulting from an oedematous ureteral wall. Voiding cystourethrography (VCU) shows a round or oval defect near the trigone, which becomes less prominent with bladder distension. Ultrasonography shows a fluid-filled distal ureter inside or outside bladder.

6. **Pseudoureteroceles** are caused by obstruction of a normal ureter, which mimics a ureterocele. Causes are tumour (bladder tumour, phaeochromocytoma) and oedema (impacted stone, cystitis, instrumentation, schistosomiasis). This also produces a cobra-head appearance with a thick, irregular halo, but there is no protrusion of the ureter into the bladder.

7. Obstruction (due to poor drainage or prolapse into bladder neck/ contralateral ureter), infection and stones are complications. In symptomatic patients with complications, diathermy incision of the uretocele is performed endoscopically.

Case 2.8: Answers

1. This is a CT cystogram (contrast instillation into bladder through a catheter), showing bright contrast in the bladder. Contrast is also seen in the prevesical space, paravesical space and anterior abdominal wall. No contrast is noted in the peritoneal cavity.

2. Extraperitoneal rupture of the bladder.

3. Bladder rupture occurs after blunt injury to the pelvis and is usually associated with pelvic fracture in 70% of the cases. There are two major types: **intraperitoneal rupture** and **extraperitoneal rupture.** Occasionally a combined type is seen. Classification:

   Type I: partial tears of mucosa

   Type II: intraperitoneal rupture (10–20%)

   Type III: interstitial (partial-thickness laceration of intact serosa)

   Type IV: extraperitoneal (most common)

   Type V: combined.

4. Extraperitoneal rupture is seen close to the bladder base anterolaterally. It is caused by a pelvic fracture or avulsion tear at the fixation points of the puboprostatic ligaments. Intraperitoneal rupture is commonly seen at the dome of the bladder, which is intraperitoneal and the weakest location, without reinforcing tissue. It is caused by an invasive procedure such as cystoscopy, surgery or a stab wound, or by blunt trauma with a rise in intravesical pressure.

5. Type I injuries present with haematuria, but not detectable imaging. Cystogram is performed after injecting 350–400 ml contrast through a catheter in the bladder and imaging in multiple planes. In extraperitoneal rupture, there is flame-shaped contrast extravasation into the perivesical fat, best seen in post-void films. Inferiorly this collection can extend into the thigh or scrotum because of disruption of the inferior fascia of the urogenital diaphragm (perineal membrane). When there is breach of the Scarpa and Camper fascia, urine is seen in the rectus sheath or under the

skin. In intraperitoneal rupture, there is contrast extravasation into the peritoneal cavity and outlining of the bowel loops. Washout studies are done after contrast has been drained. If there is retention of contrast, the bladder is irrigated with sterile water. If there is still residual contrast enhancement, it indicates bladder wall injury.

6. A CT cystogram is a better investigation. Contrast is introduced through a catheter in the bladder. Alternatively it can be injected intravenously and delayed images of the pelvis are taken after 20 minutes with clamping of the catheter. This enables accurate identification of the site of rupture and the type of rupture, and assesses other organs and bony injuries. Upper urinary track and kidneys are also assessed. A CT cystogram is also very useful in type III injuries, which are intramural or partial-thickness laceration. CT cystography shows intramural contrast within the bladder wall. A negative cystogram does not exclude rupture. Occasionally the contrast irritates the detrusor muscle, which goes into spasm and temporarily seals off the site of rupture, giving a false-negative result.

7. Treatment: extraperitoneal rupture is managed with catheter drainage of the bladder for 7–10 days and obtaining a cystogram. Healing of the tear is confirmed with contrast cystogram prior to removal of the catheter. Intraperitoneal tears usually involve the posterior part of the bladder dome. They are managed by surgical repair and catheter drainage of the bladder for 2–3 weeks.

Case 2.9: Answers

1. IVU (intravenous urography, first picture) shows a soft tissue mass in the left renal pelvis, which is distorting and stretching the collecting system. This is best illustrated in the homogram (second picture).

2. Transitional cell carcinoma (TCC) of the right renal pelvis.

3. Of urothelial tumours 90% are TCCs, 1–7% squamous cell carcinomas (SCCs), and 1% adenocarcinomas and inverted papillomas.

4. Smoking, coffee, analgesic abuse, plastic, tar, petrochemical industries, chronic infections, irritation, calculi, cyclophosphamide and Lynch syndrome II are predisposing factors. Haematuria, flank pain, dysuria, weight loss, anorexia, flank mass and bone pain are common presenting symptoms.

5. Renal pelvis is involved in 60%, a ureter in 35%, both a renal pelvis and a ureter in 7% and bilateral in 2–5%. TCCs spread in a cephalad-to-caudad fashion. Lymphatic spread is to para-aortic, paracaval, common iliac and internal iliac nodes. Haematogenous seeding occurs to the liver, lung and bone.

6. IVU is useful for evaluating the upper tract. A filling defect is seen in the ureter, with irregular margins, with upstream dilatation. Similar changes are seen in the renal pelvis. There is dilatation of the ureter below the tumour, which is called the goblet sign. CT scan is useful in diagnosis. TCCs are seen as irregular filling defects within the renal pelvis and ureters. They are hypodense with contrast enhancement and show surrounding soft tissue stranding. CT is useful for assessing spread outside the ureter. MRI and MR urography are increasingly used in diagnosis and assessment of spread. Voided samples for cytopathology, cystoscopy, ureteropyeloscopy and percutaneous nephroscopy are useful in diagnosis.

7. Superficial tumours can be treated with mitomycin C, thiotepa or BCG. Advanced tumours require chemotherapy or radiation. Nephroureterctomy with excision of the bladder cuff is the conventional surgical treatment of patients with renal pelvis TCC, regionally extensive disease, high-grade or high-stage lesion. Tumour resection can also be done with ureteroscopy or percutaneously. (There is risk of tumour seeding with percutaneous surgery.)

Case 2.10: Answers

1. MRI in axial and coronal planes shows a mass in the peripheral zone of the prostate gland (normally the periphery of the prostate, which has glandular elements that are bright on T2-weighted images). There is stranding in the periprostatic soft tissue.

2. Prostate carcinoma. Normally, in T2-weighted images, the prostate is dark in the centre as a result of fibrous stroma and bright in the periphery as a result of glandular elements. Carcinoma is more common in the peripheral zone and, when it develops, the bright signal in the peripheral zone is lost.

3. Prostate cancer is the second most common malignancy in males after lung cancer. It is seen above the age of 45 years. The Gleason score grades the cancer pathologically. The carcinoma can be latent, incidental, and occult or present clinically; 70% occur in the peripheral zone; 20% are seen in the transition zone and 10% in the central zone. Clinically, they are asymptomatic, but in advanced cases they can present with obstructive symptoms, haematuria, bone pain, anaemia and renal failure.

4. Prostate-specific antigen, which is produced by prostatic epithelium, is elevated in prostate cancer and correlates with the tumour volume. Benign conditions that produce elevated PSA are: benign prostatic hyperplasia (BPH), prostatitis, prostatic massage and prostate intraepithelial neoplasia. PSA is not elevated if the tumour volume is <1 mL. Of prostate cancers, 20% have normal PSA. Occasionally normal older men have a high PSA. However, a PSA >10 nmol/mL is suggestive of prostate cancer.

5. Ultrasound is an excellent method for assessment of local disease. The tumour is visualised better on transrectal ultrasonography, which shows irregular enlargement with deformed contour and heterogeneous texture. The lesion can be hypo-, iso- or hyperechoic. Ultrasound-guided six quadrant biopsy is performed from different portions of the gland for tumour detection.

6. MRI is not used for primary diagnosis, but it is useful for assessing local and regional spread. Early stage tumour is seen as a low signal intensity mass in the peripheral zone, which normally shows a high signal due to the presence of glands. When the tumour extends outside the capsule, the neurovascular bundle becomes asymmetrical, rectoprostatic angle is obliterated and a low signal lesion is seen in the seminal vesicle. Haemorrhage from biopsy can mimic a tumour, so MRI is not done immediately after biopsy.

7. Ultrasound-guided biopsy is indicated for patients with an elevated PSA and enlarged prostate. If the biopsy is positive, staging is done with MRI to assess extracapsular extension. A bone scan is done for skeletal metastasis.

8. Low-grade tumours can be observed. If the disease is confined to the gland and life expectancy > 15 years, radical prostatectomy can be done. If disease is inside the capsule and life expectancy < 15 years or if outside capsule, but no metastases, radiotherapy is used. Androgen deprivation (orchiectomy, leuproline, diethylstilbestrol), cryosurgery and chemotherapy are used in advanced disease and metastasis.

Case 2.11: Answers

1. There is a large heterogeneous mass, with solid and cystic components, in the right testis. There is no hydrocele.

2. Teratoma of the right testis.

3. Testicular cancers are the most common tumours in males between 15–35 years, accounting to 1.5% of all male cancers.

   Classification:

   Germ cell tumours

   – seminoma

   – non-seminomatous tumours (embryonal cell carcinoma, teratoma [differentiated, malignant intermediate, malignant anaplastic, malignant trophoblastic], epidermoid cyst, yolk sac tumour, choriocarcinoma)

   Sex cord and stromal tumours: Leydig cell tumour, Sertoli cell tumour, gonadoblastoma

   Secondary tumours: metastasis, lymphoma, leukaemia

4. Testicular tumours present with a painless enlarging testis, with mass, pain or heaviness in the lower abdomen. They can present with gynaecomastia, virilisation or metastasis. Seminomas are seen in older adults. The tumours seen in children are teratomas, embryonal cell carcinomas, yolk sac tumours, Sertoli's cell tumours (oestrogen secreting) and Leydig cell tumours (androgen secreting).

5. α-Fetoprotein is elevated in yolk sac tumours. β-Human chorionic gonadotrophin (βhCG) is elevated in choriocarcinoma and seminoma. Lactate dehydrogenase (LDH) correlates with bulk of tumour. There

is increased risk in undescended testis, gonadal dysgenesis and family history. Peak age is 25–35 years.

6. Metastasis spreads along the testicular lymph drainage to the left para-aortic nodes, interaortocaval node and then to the mediastinal and left supraclavicular nodes. Haematogenous metastasis is seen early in choriocarcinoma and also in teratomas.

7. Testicular tumours are best diagnosed by ultrasonography, which shows homogeneous or heterogeneous soft-tissue tumours with increased vascularity. Seminomas are usually homogeneous. Teratomas are heterogeneous, with solid and cystic components. Calcification can be present. Doppler ultrasonography shows intense vascular flow in the tumour.

8. The tumour staging is done using CT, which is useful for finding enlarged retroperitoneal nodes. A CT scan of the chest is done for exclusion of pulmonary metastasis. Occasionally MRI is done in indeterminate cases. Treatment is with orchiectomy and chemotherapy, depending on the stage.

Case 2.12: Answers

1. The X-ray of the abdomen shows a large mass in the central abdomen, which is displacing the bowel loops around it. CT scan of the abdomen shows a large mass in the left side of the retroperitoneum, which is predominantly made up of fat (note the very low density of the tumour), but also contains fibrous strands and solid soft tissue components. The bowel loops are all displaced to the right side by the mass.

2. Retroperitoneal liposarcoma.

3. This tumour arises from undifferentiated mesenchyme in the retroperitoneum. The common locations are anterior to the spine, psoas muscle, paraspinal region and posterior pararenal space.

4. Liposarcoma is a slow-growing malignant tumour. The retroperitoneum is a common site for this tumour. Histologically, it can be well differentiated,

pleomorphic, anaplastic or myxoid. **Well-differentiated** tumour is difficult to differentiate from a lipoma. **Myxoid** tumour has lot of myxomatous connective tissue. **Pleomorphic** and **anaplastic** types are the most aggressive. They are common in men in the 40- to 60-year group and present with abdominal pain, weight loss, anaemia, palpable mass and abdominal distension.

5. The appearances of liposarcoma depend on the histological type. Well-differentiated tumours have a diffuse fat density. Soft-tissue density with CT is 20–50 HU. Fat has a density < 0 HU. Well-differentiated tumours have a low density similar to normal fat. The only way of differentiating from a benign lipoma is the presence of soft-tissue components. Intermediate- and high-grade tumours have varying amounts of soft-tissue and fatty components. Myxoid tumours have a combination of fat and myxomatous tissue, giving a fluid density, and can be confused with cystic tumours. High-grade tumours have a pure soft-tissue mass and it is difficult to diagnose liposarcomas. Calcification can be seen in 10%. MRI shows a high signal in T1- and T2-weighted images and fat suppression in STIR sequences. Angiography shows a hypovascular mass.

6. Differential diagnosis for retroperitoneal tumours: lymphoma, leiomyosarcoma, fibrosarcoma, malignant fibrous histiocytoma, neurofibrosarcoma and neurofibroma. Differential diagnosis for fat containing lesions in abdomen: lipoma, hernia, omental infarct and fat necrosis.

7. Surgical resection with chemotherapy is the treatment of choice.

Case 2.13: Answers

1. IVU shows bilateral hydronephrosis and dilatation of proximal ureters, which are medially displaced and taper gradually near the lumbosacral junction. The CT scan shows a hypodense soft tissue mass in the midline of retroperitoneum, with encasement of midline vessels and left ureter.

2. Idiopathic retroperitoneal fibrosis.

3. Primary retroperitoneal fibrosis is an autoimmune disease that is an immune response to ceroid – a byproduct of aortic plaque that leaks into the retroperitoneum.

4. Malignancy with desmoplastic response (carcinoid, lymphoma, metastases), drugs (methysergide, ergotamine, hydralazine, methyldopa, amphetamines, lysergic acid diethylamide or LSD), fluid collection, aneurysm, radiation and polyarteritis nodosa are other causes of retroperitoneal fibrosis.

5. The characteristic location is the midline of the retroperitoneum around the aortic bifurcation. Proximally it can extend up to the renal hilum. It usually does not extend below the pelvic brim, but occasionally extends behind the bladder and rectosigmoid. It is associated with other fibrosing conditions such as mediastinal fibrosis, orbital pseudotumour, Riedel's thyroiditis, sclerosing cholangitis and Peyronie's disease. It is seen in men aged 30–60 years.

6. IVU shows the classic triad with bilateral hydroureteronephrosis above the level of L4–5, marked medial deviation of the ureters in the middle third and gradual tapering of the ureter. Ultrasonography shows a hypoechoic periaortic mass. CT shows a periaortic hypodense mass, which might show contrast enhancement in the acute stage. MRI shows low-to-medium signal intensity in T1 and T2. The signal depends on the amount of fibrous tissue. Uptake is seen on a gallium scan when there is active inflammation.

7. Differential diagnoses include retroperitoneal lymphadenopathy caused by lymphoma, TB or metastasis, and retroperitoneal sarcomas.

8. Treatment of the causative factor, steroids and treatment of obstruction with nephrostomy or ureteral stents are used in the management of retroperitoneal fibrosis.

Case 2.14: Answers

1. This is a retrograde urethrogram. An 8 or 10 French urethral catheter is placed in fossa navicularis and the balloon is inflated with 1–3 ml sterile water until the balloon occludes the urethral lumen. A scout film is obtained; 10 ml iodinated contrast is injected into the catheter under fluoroscopy and images of the anterior urethra are taken. High pressure during the injection can lead to contrast extravasation. An alternative to this procedure, but less useful, is the anterograde cystourethrogram, where the bladder is distended with contrast and the catheter removed. The patient is asked to void and images are taken before, during and after voiding.

2. There is smooth narrowing of the membranous urethra.

3. Urethral stricture.

4. Urethral strictures can be traumatic, inflammatory, infectious (sexually transmitted infection [STI] such as gonorrhoea), ischaemic, malignant or congenital, and lead to scar formation and narrowing of the urethral lumen. Posterior urethral stricture results from a distraction injury secondary to trauma or surgery.

5. The urethra is divided into anterior and posterior segments. The anterior urethra includes the meatus, fossa navicularis, penile urethra and bulbar urethra. The posterior urethra includes the membranous and prostatic urethra. The anterior urethra lies within the corpus spongiosum, with the penile urethra lying more centrally, and the bulbous urethra more dorsally. The prostatic urethra extends from the bladder neck to verumontanum, and the membranous urethra from verumontanum to the urogenital diaphragm. The most common location is the bulbar urethra.

6. Urethral strictures occur after an injury to the urothelium or when the corpus spongiosum causes formation of scar tissue. A congenital stricture results from inadequate fusion of the anterior and posterior urethra and is short. Common presentations are obstructive voiding symptoms such as dribbling, hesitancy, decreased force of stream, incomplete emptying of bladder and intermittency.

Genitourinary Answers

Genitourinary Radiology **195**

7. Complications of urethral strictures are obstruction, with proximal reflux and infections.

8. Surgical treatment is indicated for severe voiding symptoms, bladder calculi, post-void residual urine, urinary tract infection and failure of conservative management. Diagnosis can be confirmed with flexible cystourethroscopy. Treatment consists of internal urethrotomy. Urethral stents, primary repair or repair with grafts or pedicled skin flaps is used. Complications of surgery are recurrence, bleeding, infection, dehiscence, fistula and extravasation of irrigation fluid into perispongial tissues, with increasing fibrosis.

Case 2.15: Answers

1. This is a hysterosalpingogram. The uterus is normal. However, very little contrast is noted in the fallopian tubes and there is no contrast spilling from the tubes into the peritoneum.

2. Bilateral tubal block.

3. Hysterosalpingogram is opacification of the uterus and fallopian tubes. It is mainly done for work-up for infertility and for congenital anomalies

4. The procedure is performed only on days 6–12 after the last menstrual period (LMP).

5. The patient is placed in the lithotomy position. Under aseptic technique, a 6 Fr catheter is inserted into the cervical canal using a speculum. Once the tube is inside the cervix, the balloon is inflated; 4–10 ml contrast is injected into the uterus under fluoroscopy.

6. The shape of the uterus and fallopian tubes is assessed. Any congenital anomalies are identified. The most important factor to be assessed is peritoneal spill. If no peritoneal spill occurs, delayed films are taken and, if there is still no spill, it indicates tubal blockage.

7. Complications are pain, infection (in patients with hydrosalpinx, peritubal collections), contrast allergy (venous or lymphatic extravasation) and radiation. Antibiotics are administered for 10 days if dilated fallopian tubes or peritubal adhesions were identified. This is to prevent development of a tubo-ovarian abscess. Contraindications are active uterine bleeding/periods, active infection, pregnancy and uterine surgery within the last few days.

8. Other causes of infertility are:

   Ovulatory: (thyroid disorders, prolactinoma, excessive androgens, diabetes, stress, lifestyle changes)

   Cervical: (stenosis, abnormal mucus, STD, antibodies to sperm)

   Pelvic: (adhesions, endometriosis, infections)

   Uterine: (thin lining, polyps, fibroids, septum, blocked tube) and unexplained (10%).

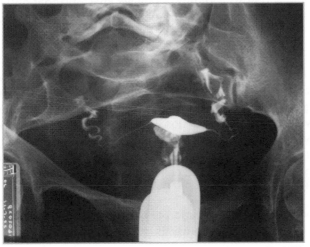

Fig 2.15b

Case 2.16: Answers

1. This is a delayed film on IVU. There is no contrast in the right kidney. The left kidney is enlarged and there is massive dilatation of the left pelvicalyceal system and proximal ureter. Ultrasound shows mild dilatation of the left renal pelvis and calyces.

2. Left hydronureteronephrosis caused by obstruction.

3. Hydronephrosis is aseptic dilatation of the collecting system. Obstruction can be caused by intrinsic, intramural or extrinsic pathologies. The common cause of acute obstruction is passage of calculus/blood clot, instrumentation, suture, sulfonamides or pregnancy. Chronic obstruction results from PUJ obstruction, tumours (ureteric and extrinsic), retroperitoneal fibrosis and tumours, pelvic mass, bladder outlet masses (BPH, prostate carcinoma), urethral polyps/neoplasms/strictures, posterior urethral valve and ureterocele.

4. In acute obstruction, the kidney is a normal size, with an increasingly dense nephrogram, delayed opacification of the collecting system, dilated collecting system and ureter with blunting of the calyceal angle. Delayed films show the level of obstruction. In chronic obstruction, the kidney is large, with wasted parenchyma, decreased radiological density, a thin band of dense contrast surrounding the calyces, delayed opacification of collecting system and a dilated collecting system.

5. Ultrasonography shows separation of the renal sinuses and dilated collecting system. Hydronephrosis is graded into three types:

    Grade **1**: mild separation of central sinuses, ovoid

    Grade **2**: rounded separation of collecting system

    Grade **3**: severe.

    The amount of dilatation depends on the duration of obstruction, renal output and presence of decompression. Doppler ultrasonography shows a high resistive index > 0.77, which helps in differentiation from false-positive cases. In the bladder a ureteral jet is not seen. The complications of hydronephrosis are pyonephrosis, contrast extravasation and papillary necrosis.

6. Differential diagnoses for dilated collecting system without obstruction: full bladder, overhydration, medications, diabetes insipidus, after IVU, reflux, pregnancy, postobstructive, postinfective, postsurgical, megaureter, megacalycoses, extrarenal pelvis, parapelvic cysts and sinus vessels. Occasionally, false-negative appearances are seen in hyperacute obstruction, dehydration, spontaneous decompression or staghorn calculus filling the pelvis.

7. Hydronephrosis is seen in 80% of pregnant women as a result of the effect of progesterone on smooth muscle relaxation and compression of the ureter at the pelvic brim by an enlarged uterus. This dilatation is physiological, common on the right side, seen up to the pelvic brim and resolves within a few weeks of delivery.

8. Percutaneous nephrostomy is done to relieve obstruction. Under ultrasound and fluoroscopic guidance a needle is advanced into the lower pole calyx and a drainage tube introduced.

Case 2.17: Answers

1. The X-ray shows a large, branching, radio-opacity conforming to a calyceal configuration, in the right side.

2. Staghorn calculus in the right kidney.

3. Although any type of urinary stone can form staghorn calculi, 75% are composed of struvite (magnesium ammonium phosphate with carbonate–apatite and matrix). These are also called triple phosphate/infection/phosphatic/urease stones. They can also be composed of a mixture of calcium oxalate and calcium phosphate.

4. Struvite stones are invariably associated with infections, especially with urease-producing bacteria, such as *Ureaplasma urealyticum* and *Proteus* spp., staphylococci, or *Klebsiella*, *Providencia* or *Pseudomonas* spp. These agents lead to hydrolysis of urea into ammonium and hydroxyl ions, which combined with alkaline urine facilitates stone formation. They have varying amounts of matrix that protect the bacteria from antibiotics.

5. Predisposing factors are urinary diversion, catheters, neurogenic bladder, vesicoureteral reflux (VUR), anatomical abnormalities and urinary infections.

6. Stones that involve the renal pelvis and extend into at least two calyces are called staghorn calculi. IVU shows the calculus as a filling defect in the pelvis or obscured by contrast. If there is scarred infundibulum, treatment is done with percutaneous nephrostomy. If the infundibulum is large, lithotripsy is possible. Ultrasonography demonstrates calculus and hydronephrosis. A CT scan without contrast is used for evaluation of flank pain.

7. Complications are obstruction and infection. Staghorn calculus is associated with xanthogranulomatous pyelonephritis.

8. Complete surgical removal of stones is required in all patients except those who have significant comorbid conditions that preclude surgery. Treatment with antibiotics, a low-phosphorous, low-calcium diet, aluminium hydroxide gel, urease inhibitors and urinary acidification is attempted. These calculi are effectively broken by ESWL as a result of multiple laminations. Repeated therapy required in 50% because of the large stone burden. Percutaneous nephrolithotomy is used when there is infundibular scarring.

Case 2.18: Answers

1. The CT scan shows a well-defined, hypodense lesion in the posteromedial aspect of the interpolar region of the enlarged right kidney. Gas is seen within this cystic lesion.

2. Renal abscess.

3. Infection can reach the kidney haematogenously from other foci in the body, or by contiguous spread from adjacent structures, or ascending infection from the urinary tract (the most common). Infection is common in diabetics and immunosuppressed individuals and it is more common in patients with urinary stasis and structural anomalies like PUJ obstruction or renal calculus. Urine culture and blood culture may be positive. Clinical features are renal angle tenderness, flank pain, pyuria, haematuria, fever and chills. Negative urinalysis and culture are seen in 20%.

4. Ascending infection is associated with *E. coli* and *Proteus* spp. Haematogenous infection is caused by *Staph. aureus*.

5. Ultrasonography or CT is used for diagnosis. A CT scan shows a well-defined hypodense lesion with a thick, enhancing wall and central non-enhancement as a result of liquefaction. Gas may be present. There is soft-tissue stranding into the adjacent perinephric space. MRI shows low signal in T1, high signal in T2 and peripheral rim enhancement after administration of contrast.

6. Differential diagnoses for cystic renal mass: cystic renal cell carcinoma, complicated renal cyst, renal TB, haematoma, hydatid cyst, polycystic kidney, medullary cystic disease and congenital multicystic kidney.

7. Spread to adjacent structures, perinephric abscess, psoas abscess, pyonephrosis and septicaemia are the complications.

8. A renal abscess requires intravenous antibiotics and hydration. If there is no clinical improvement, percutaneous drainage is done under CT or ultrasound guidance. Perirenal abscess and infected urinoma require drainage. Occasionally, large and complicated abscesses require surgical débridement. Nephrectomy is done for symptomatic xanthogranulomatous pyelonephritis.

Case 2.19: Answers

1. MRI shows a large mass in the left kidney, which shows heterogeneous contrast enhancement. The left renal vein is expanded and there is a hypointense mass extending into it.

2. Renal cell cancer with tumour extension into the left renal vein.

3. The CT scan, done proximal to the MR scan, shows expansion of the IVC and a thrombus within it. This patient has left renal cancer and tumour extension to the left renal vein and IVC.

4. Other causes of renal vein thrombosis are thrombophlebitis, dehydration, nephrotic syndrome from membranous glomerulonephritis, sickle cell disease, systemic lupus erythematosus (SLE), trauma, amyloidosis, neoplasm, abscess, aneurysm, hypercoagulable state, pyelonephritis and low-flow states.

5. In renal carcinoma with renal vein thrombosis, a CT scan shows a hypodense filling defect in the corticomedullary phase. There is an abrupt change in the calibre of the vein. Collateral veins are seen around the kidney. If the thrombus enhances, it is likely to be a malignant tumour thrombus rather than a bland thrombus in association with renal cell caner. Doppler and MRI are also useful in evaluating the renal vein thrombosis. The extent of thrombus into the IVC and right atrium should be assessed, since the treatment varies. In patients without renal cancer, the changes of the renal vein thrombosis depend on the rapidity of occlusion, extent of occlusion, collaterals and site of occlusion. Doppler ultrasonography shows less pulsatile venous flow and collaterals. The main renal vein is not visible, and the resistive index is elevated. CT shows a prolonged nephrographic phase, thick renal fascia, collaterals and haemorrhage. MRI can be used for assessment of renal vein thrombosis.

6. The Robson modification of the Flocks and Kadesky system is commonly used in clinical practice:

    Stage I: tumour confined within the kidney capsule

    Stage II: tumour invading perinephric fat but still contained within Gerota's fascia

    Stage III: tumour invading the renal vein or IVC (IIIA), the regional lymph node (IIIB) or both (IIIC)

    Stage IV: tumour invading adjacent viscera (excluding ipsilateral adrenal) or distant metastases.

7. Treatment of renal vein thrombosis involves treatment of the primary cause, symptomatic treatment with a diuretic, angiotensin-converting enzyme (ACE) inhibitors, anticoagulation and atorvastatin to decrease the rate of progression of kidney disease. In patients with renal carcinoma, renal vein involvement without metastasis, a radical nephrectomy is performed with early ligation of the renal artery but no manipulation of the renal vein. If the IVC is involved, its vascular control is obtained above and below the thrombus, thrombus is resected intact and the IVC closed.

Genitourinary Answers

1. IVU shows an irregular filling defect within the bladder, predominantly on the right side. The CT scan shows a large soft tissue mass arising from the base of the bladder posteriorly and extending in the bladder lumen on the right side.

2. TCC of the bladder.

3. TCC (90%), SCC (5%) and adenocarcinoma (2%) are the common histological subtypes of bladder cancer.

4. Painless haematuria is the most common presentation; 90% of bladder cancers present with haematuria. All patients with gross painless haematuria should be considered to have bladder cancer unless proven otherwise, and investigated.

5. Cystoscopy is required for direct visualisation and biopsy of the lesion. MRI of the bladder is done to assess locoregional spread. IVU and ultrasonography are useful to look for synchronous tumours in the upper urinary tract. The tumour is seen as a within-bladder filling defect on IVU. On ultrasonography/CT, a polypoidal mass or diffuse, irregular, wall thickening is noted.

6. TNM staging is used.

   Ta: confined to epithelium

   T1: invasion into lamina propria

   T2: invasion into muscularis propria

   T3: invasion of perivesical fat

   T4: involvement of adjacent organs

   N1: One lymph node <2 cm

   N2: One lymph node 2–5 cm/multiple lymph nodes <5 cm

   N3: Lymph node >5 cm

   M1: metastasis.

7. Smoking, aromatic amines, acrolein, analgesics and artificial sweeteners are recognised predisposing factors for TCC. Long indwelling catheters, bladder stones and schistisomiasis of bladder predispose to SCCs.

8. In superficial bladder cancers, endoscopic resection of the tumour is performed. In tumours with muscle wall invasion and invasion of adjacent organs, radical cystoprostatectomy in men and anterior pelvic exenteration in women are performed, with urinary diversions. Bladder-sparing surgery is done in some centres with endoscopic resection, external beam radiation and chemotherapy. In superficial bladder cancers, intravesical BCG may be used. Intravesical chemotherapy (valrubicin) is useful in resistant cases. External beam radiation increases survival in muscle-invasive disease. A methotrexate, vinblastine, Adriamycin (doxorubicin) and cisplatin (M-VAC) combination is used in treatment of metastatic bladder cancer.

Case 2.21: Answers

1. The CT scan shows posterior outpouchings arising from the posterolateral aspect of the bladder on both sides.

2. Bladder diverticulum.

3. Bladder diverticulum can be a primary congenital type or an acquired secondary diverticulum.

4. Bladder diverticulum occurs at sites of anatomical weakness. The weakest area is the ureteral meatus and most diverticula originate at this location. The other location is the posterolateral wall. Diverticulum in this location is called **Hutch's diverticulum.**

5. **Primary** diverticulum is idiopathic or congenital and can occur with or without vesicoureteric reflux. Hutch's diverticulum is associated with reflux.

   Secondary (acquired) diverticulum is caused by bladder outlet obstruction or is postoperative or associated with syndromes (prune-belly, Menkes, Williams, Ehlers–Danlos and Diamond–Blackfan syndromes).

6. IVU or voiding cystourethrography (VCUG) is used for diagnosis. They both show contrast-filled outpouchings from the posterolateral wall of the bladder.

7. Complications are calculus in diverticulum, SCC (1–7%), obstruction and VUR.

8. Asymptomatic diverticula do not require active treatment. Congenital diverticulum is removed surgically. For secondary diverticula, the bladder outlet obstruction is corrected.

Case 2.22: Answers

1. This is retrograde urography. (See catheter in the ureter passed retrogradely.)

2. There is stricture, with an irregular filling defect (dark area) in the distal ureter. The proximal collecting system is not dilated, but there is another filling defect in the renal pelvis. This patient has multicentric TCCs in the distal ureter and renal pelvis.

3. In retrograde urography, radio-opaque contrast is introduced directly into the ureter and collecting system, through cystoscopy and ureteral catheterisation. Sedation or general anaesthesia is required. The procedure can be performed with fluoroscopy or standard X-rays.

4. Retrograde urography is useful for detailed examination of the pelvicalyceal collecting system, ureters and bladder. This technique allows better visualisation of the collecting system than IVU by increasing the distension of the urinary collecting system. This technique is used when CT or MRI is unsuccessful, there is proximal obstruction and IVU shows no visualisation of the ureter, in cases in which the degree, type, cause and length of ureteral obstruction must be defined, or when patients are allergic to intravenous contrast. Overall retrograde urography is more than 75% accurate in establishing the diagnosis of urothelial cancer.

5. Overdistention and backflow may distort calyces and obscure detail. Risk of infection is higher than that with other types of urography and the procedure is more invasive, so that sedation or general anaesthesia is required. Acute ureteraloedema and secondary stricture formation are rare.

6. A multiphase CT scan is useful for assessing ureters. It is obtained in non-contrast, early arterial and delayed phases. This is useful for diagnosis and to assess spread of tumour outside the ureter and involvement of adjacent structures. TCCs present as irregular masses, are hypovascular and do not enhance as much as the rest of the kidney. MR urography is another non-invasive way of assessing urothelial tumours. Ureteroscopy with biopsy or cytology brushings is 95% accurate for assessing urothelial tumours.

7. Staging of ureteral tumours:

   Tis: Carcinoma *in situ*

   Ta: Superficial/papillary

   T1: Lamina propria invasion

   T2: Muscularis propria invasion

   T3: Peripelvic/periureteral/renal invasion

   T4: Contiguous organ involvement.

   Treatment of superficial tumour: topical instillation of the chemotherapeutic agents mitomycin C, thiotepa or BCG. Segmental ureterectomy coupled with ureteral reimplantation is indicated for patients with low-grade/stage tumours in the distal ureter. Recurrence rate is high. Nephroureterectomy with excision of the bladder cuff is indicated in higher-grade lesions. Chemotherapy and radiation are used in metastasis and muscle invasive tumours with local spread.

Case 2.23: Answers

1. The cystogram shows a grossly abnormal bladder which is shaped like a fir tree, with trabeculations and sacculations. There is also vesicoureteric reflux on the right side, with gross dilatation of the ureter and collecting system of the right kidney.

2. Neurogenic bladder.

3. Causes:

Supraspinal: vertebrovascular accident, brain tumour, Parkinson's disease, Shy–Drager syndrome

Spinal: injury, multiple sclerosis (MS), syrinx, myelomeningocele

Peripheral nerve lesions: diabetes, syphilis, herpes zoster, polio, herniated disc, pelvic surgery, pernicious anaemia.

4. Neurogenic bladder is a malfunctioning bladder resulting from any type of neurological disorder:

Detrusor hyperreflexia: suprapontine upper motor neuron (UMN) lesion, overactive bladder

Detrusor dyssynergia: suprasacral spinal lesion; detrusor and sphincter contract at same time, causing urinary retention

Detrusor hyperreflexia with impaired contractility: synergic, but not enough detrusor contraction; retention with irritative voiding symptoms

Detrusor instability: overactive symptoms without neurological impairment; normal sphincter

Overactive bladder: urgency, frequency, neurological or non-neurological

Detrusor areflexia: lower motor neuron (LMN) lesion, inability of detrusor to empty.

5. The X-ray may show spinal defects in children with a congenital neurogenic bladder. IVU or cystogram shows distended bladder, which can be in the shape of a pine or fir tree, with trabeculations. IVU also assesses upper urinary tract abnormalities. Ultrasound is useful for assessing residual urine.

6. Other tests: urinalysis, urine culture, urine cytology, renal function, voiding diary, pad test, post-void residual volume, uroflow rate, filling cystometrogram, voiding cystometrogram, cystogram, electromyography, cystoscopy, videourodynamics.

7. Differential diagnoses for abnormally shaped bladder are: pelvic lipomatosis, pelvic masses, pelvic lymphadenopathy, pelvic haematoma.

8. Treatment: antimicrobial therapy, spinal surgery, urethral occlusive devices, catheterisation and urinary diversions.

Case 2.24: Answers

1. The coronal view of the CT scan shows an enlarged prostate gland that is indenting into the bladder base. MRI of the pelvis shows smooth symmetrical enlargement of the prostate. The central part of the gland is hypertrophied and it is seen compressing the peripheral zone.

2. Benign prostatic hyperplasia (BPH).

3. BPH is seen in the central portions of the glands. The transitional and periurethral zones are proximal to verumontanum, which forms the lateral lobes and the median lobe. The peripheral zone is involved in adenocarcinoma of the prostate.

4. Patients present with obstructive symptoms, such as incomplete emptying, frequency, intermittency, urgency, weak stream, straining and nocturia.

5. BPH is diagnosed clinically. Ultrasound-guided biopsy is done when the prostate is enlarged and irregular, the PSA is high and there is high clinical suspicion of prostate carcinoma. Ultrasonography and CT show an enlarged homogeneous prostate gland. Calcification may be seen. The enlarged gland is round, oval or pear shaped. IVU is indicated if patients present with haematuria, a history of urolithiasis, high creatinine, high post-void residual volume and urinary infections. IVU shows indentation of the bladder neck as a result of median lobe hypertrophy. When bladder outlet obstruction is present, there is proximal dilatation of the collecting system. Other investigations include flow rate, residual urine, pressure–flow studies and endoscopy of the urinary tract.

6. Prostate carcinoma: affects peripheral zone. The gland is enlarged, hard and irregular. In MRI, there might be extension outside the prostate to involve adjacent structures. PSA >10 nmol/mL is suspicious of cancer and >30 nmol/mL is diagnostic.

7. Acute retention of urine, chronic retention, bilateral hydronephrosis and renal impairment, haemorrhage, urinary infection and bladder diverticular formation are the complications.

8. Treatment is with medication: α blockers/androgen deprivation/ phytotherapeutic agents, 5-α reductase inhibitors. Surgical procedures are TURP (transurethral resection of prostate), open prostatectomy, bladder neck incision, laser, transurethral microwave therapy, transurethral needle ablation of prostate and high intensity focused ultrasound.

Case 2.25: Answers

1. Ultrasonography of the scrotum shows an enlarged right testis that is diffusely of low echogenicity.

2. The second and third images are obtained with colour Doppler ultrasound. The second picture is an axial view, which shows hypoechoic right testis and a normal left testis, which has normal echogenicity and capsular blood flow. The third scan, a Doppler ultrasound of the right testis, shows no spectral wave form in a blood vessel within the testis, suggestive of avascularity.

3. Acute testicular torsion.

4. Acute testicular torsion is a urological emergency and the most common scrotal disorder in children. It is common in the neonatal period and puberty. Predisposing factors are a bell-and-clapper deformity (high insertion of tunica vaginalis on the cord), loose mesorchium between the testis and epididymis, and loose attachment of testicular tunics to the scrotum. There is a tenfold increased incidence with undescended testis. Trauma, sexual activity, exercise, active cremasteric reflex and cold weather are other factors. Torsion presents with sudden severe pain, swelling, erythema, tenderness, low-grade fever, nausea and vomiting. The testis is swollen, oedematous and erythematous. The testis lies horizontally and there is loss of the normal cremasteric reflex.

5. The most common differential diagnosis is epididymo-orchitis. Phren sign (relief of pain on elevation of the testis) is negative (in epididymitis the pain is relieved). CBC may be normal or show elevated WBCs. Differentiation of these two entities is crucial, since torsion requires emergent surgery and epididymo-orchitis is managed with antibiotics. Another differential is a torsion of a testicular appendage. The most common type is torsion of the appendix of testis (pedunculated hydatid of Morgagni). The testis has normal flow, but the appendage is oedematous. Amputation of the appendage is curative.

6. Usually testicular torsion is a clinical diagnosis. Ultrasound can be done if clinical examination is indeterminate. Ultrasound is normal in the early stages (<6 hours), but after that shows diffuse hypoechogenicity. The testis and epididymis are enlarged. Twisted spermatic cord is rarely seen. Scrotal skin is thickened and there is reactive hydrocele. Doppler ultrasound does not show any flow within the testis or epididymis. Loss of spermatic cord Doppler flow is demonstrated. A false negative result is seen in incomplete torsion <360°, or torsion de torsion sequence. Scintigraphy shows decreased perfusion and there is a round cold area in the region of the testis. In the acute stage, nubbin sign is present (bump of activity extending medially from the iliac artery due to increased blood flow in the spermatic cord with abrupt termination). In late stages, doughnut/rim sign is seen due to increased peritesticular flow and a cold area in the centre.

7. The testis usually turns medially up to 180°. Diminished blood flow is seen in <180° torsion after 1 hour. Absent blood flow is seen in any degree of torsion after 4 hours. Testicular atrophy is the major complication. Other complications are infection, infertility and cosmetic deformity. Analgesics are administered. Manual detorsion can be attempted and it involves twisting the testicle outwards and laterally. This can be done within the first hour or so. Definitive treatment is detorsion and orchiopexy. A totally infracted testicle should be removed.

Case 2.26: Answers

1. Ultrasonography shows a swollen and oedematous right testis and epididymis, with a reactive hydrocele of the tunica vaginalis.

2. The second and third scans are colour Doppler scans, which show intense vascularity in the epididymis and the testis.

3. Acute epididymo-orchitis

4. *E. coli, Staph. aureus, Neisseria gonorrhoea, Chlamydia trachomotis* and *Proteus mirabilis* are common organisms that cause epididymitis. It is usually an ascending urinary infection, but can be blood-borne. Initially, the epididymis is involved, which is followed by global or focal involvement of the testis. Clinical features are fever, pain, swelling, tenderness and erythema of the scrotum. Symptoms of UTI and prostatitis may coexist.

5. On ultrasound, the epididymis is enlarged and shows low echogenicity. If the head is enlarged it suggests a haematogenous spread. If the tail is enlarged, it suggests an ascending infection with reflux from the urine. The spermatic cord is enlarged. Thick tunica albuginea can be seen. The testis has low echogenicity when it is involved. Reactive fluid collection can be seen. Colour Doppler ultrasound shows an increased number and concentration of vessels in the affected region. The peak systolic velocity is increased. Scintigraphy shows increased perfusion of the spermatic cord vessels and increased activity of the scrotal contents, which can be curvilinear and lateral if only the epididymis is involved, and central if the testis is also involved. There is no uptake if there is torsion.

6. The most common clinical condition that can be confused with epididymitis is a testicular torsion. Phren sign (relief of pain on elevation of testis) is positive (unlike torsion, where there is no relief). Elevated WBCs are seen. Differentiation of these two entities is crucial, since torsion requires emergent surgery and epididymo-orchitis is managed medically with antibiotics. Ultrasound helps in differentiation from torsion, which has no vascular flow within it, but there is increased vascularity in epididymo-orchitis. Other differential diagnoses are testicular abscess (increased perfusion, no uptake centrally), tumours (increased perfusion, decreased uptake, raised tumour markers, ultrasound shows focal mass) and hydrocele (no uptake).

7. Complications are orchitis, abscess, testicular infarction, chronic epididymo-orchitis, atrophy, hydrocele, pyocele and Fournier's gangrene.

Case 2.27: Answers

1. Mammography shows a cluster of fine calcification in the right breast. The second film is a magnification view, which demonstrates the area of microcalcification with more clarity.

2. Ductal carcinoma *in situ*.

3. A mammogram is performed with compression. Routinely, craniocaudal and mediolateral oblique views of both breasts are obtained. Further views are obtained if the lesion is indeterminate.

4. Screening mammogram is done for women older than 50 years at 3-yearly intervals. Screening is started earlier at 30 years, if the patient has a first degree relative with breast cancer in the premenopausal years.

5. Carcinoma *in situ* can be ductal carcinoma *in situ*, lobular carcinoma *in situ* or intracystic papillary carcinoma *in situ*.

6. The main mammographic feature of a ductal carcinoma *in situ* is microcalcification, which is irregular and clustered and heterogeneous. Occasionally it is associated with an area of thickening or ill-defined mass. Ductal carcinoma *in situ* is a heterogenous group of malignancies originating from the extralobular terminal duct without invasion of the basement membrane. Almost all comedo types of DIS have microcalcification.

7. Breast calcification is seen in a wide variety of disease. Ductal calcification is 0.1–0.3 mm, irregular, mixed linear and punctate, and is also seen in epithelial hyperplasia, atypical ductal hyperplasia and secretory disease. Lobular microcalcification is smooth, round, similar in size and density, and seen in cystic hyperplasia, adenosis, sclerosing adenosis, hyperplasia and lobular carcinoma *in situ*.

8. Ductal carcinoma *in situ* is managed by excision or local excision with radiotherapy. Mastectomy is performed when it is widespread or involves the nipple. Postoperative follow-up for 5 years is advised in these cases.

Case 2.28: Answers

1. The mammogram shows a well-defined, lobulated, smooth mass with dense calcification. An area of architectural deformity and speculation noted in the area marked with the arrow.

2. Calcified fibroadenoma. There is an associated soft tissue lesion (arrows), which turned out to be carcinoma.

3. Fibroadenoma is composed of proliferative fibrous stroma and epithelial structures. It is the most common benign solid tumour in women and the third most common breast lesion in children after fibrocystic disease and carcinoma. There are three types: intracanalicular, pericanalicular and combined. It is seen at a mean age of 30 years. It enlarges at the end of menstrual cycle and during pregnancy, and regresses after the menopause. It is usually 1–5 cm. Giant adenomas may be >5 cm. It is bilateral in 4% of patients. Clinically, it presents as a smooth, palpable, mobile, non-tender mass.

4. A mammogram shows a well-defined, smooth round, or oval mass, with halo sign. Popcorn calcification is the characteristic appearance. Occasionally calcifications can be peripheral, of pleomorphic linear or branching pattern.

5. Ultrasound of fibroadenoma shows a well-defined, round or oval, homogenous, well-defined mass. Posterior acoustic enhancement is seen. The length to depth ratio is usually >1.4. Mass is freely mobile. Calcification produces distal acoustic shadow.

6. The most common differential diagnosis is a carcinoma. Carcinomas have spiculated margins and punctate calcifications on mammography. In ultrasound, they are heterogeneously hypoechoic, with acoustic shadowing and length to depth ratio <1.4 (oval). Other differential diagnoses for well-circumscribed lesions in mammogram are: cyst, sclerosing adenoma, papilloma, galactocele, sebaceous cyst, medullary carcinoma, mucinous carcinoma and papillary carcinoma.

7. Fibroadenomas do not require excision unless they become very large, for cosmetic reasons, or if they are associated with suspicious cytology. In this particular case, the treatment primarily should be for the carcinoma of the breast.

Case 2.29: Answers

1. Ultrasonography shows a large lesion in the right ovary, which is predominantly cystic, but has a peripheral solid mass. The CT scan shows a large tumour, predominantly cystic, with solid components, arising in the right side of the pelvis.

2. Malignant ovarian tumour.

3. Classification of ovarian tumours:

   Epithelial **tumours**: serous, mucinous, endometrioid, clear cell, undifferentiated, Brenner's tumour

   Germ **cell tumours:** teratoma, dysgerminoma, endodermal sinus tumour, mixed germ cell tumour, choriocarcinoma, embryonal carcinoma

   Metastases (breast, colon)

   Sex **cord stromal tumours**.

4. Ovarian cancers are the 5th leading cause of cancer in women. Peak incidence is at 50–60 years. Malignancy increases with age. It is associated with breast cancer, Lynch syndrome, nulliparity, early menarche, late menopause and family history. Ultrasound is the first test used in evaluation of the ovarian tumours. Features of malignancy are: thick irregular walls with thick septations or papillary projections; solid components; postmenopausal ovaries >9 cm^3; colour flow in the wall, septa, papillary nodules and solid components; low-resistance Doppler flow pattern, ascites, lymph nodes, metastasis, pseudomyxoma and peritoneal metastasis. CT scan is used for staging. The primary tumour can be characterised which shows features similar to ultrasound. Extension to adjacent organs, and lymph nodes in the pelvis and abdomen, and metastases to the lung and liver are evaluated. MRI can be used for characterisation of primary tumour and local staging.

5. The tumour can spread directly to adjacent structures such as the bowel, bladder and uterus. Peritoneal spread occurs as a result of transcoelomic spread. Lymphatic spread occurs to pelvic side wall and para-aortic nodes. Haematogenous spread to the liver, lung, adrenals and bones is seen.

6. Ultrasonography is used to identify a mass and differentiate solid and cystic lesions. CT is used to confirm diagnosis, assess locoregional extent, for liver and lung metastasis and retroperitoneal nodes, and for secondary features. CT is also used for follow-up after surgery or chemotherapy.

7. Secondary features are: **ascites** (indicates malignancy), in lesser sac, loculated; **peritoneal implants** – soft tissue nodules on surface of liver, spleen, with scalloping of liver and spleen surface; **omental implants** – seen as thickened, nodular, calcified omentum; **mesenteric deposits**, **pseudomyxoma peritonei** (high-density ascites, calcifications, scalloping of abdomen organs), **lymphadenopathy, bowel invasion, hydronephrosis, liver, lung** and **bony metastasis.**

8. Treatment depends on the staging of the cancer. Tumour is staged by the FIGO (International Federation of Gynaecology and Obstetrics) protocol.

   Stage I: limited to the ovary

   Stage II: extension to the pelvis

   Stage III: Extension to the abdomen

   Stage IV: haematogeneous metastasis.

   Staging is done with staging laparatomy with abdominal hysterectomy, bilateral salphingo-ophrectomy, omentectomy, random peritoneal biopsy and lymph node biopsy; 50–70% present at stage III or IV at diagnosis. Chemotherapy is given for advanced stages.

Case 2.30: Answers

1. The mammogram shows a large, well-defined, lobulated, smooth mass. Breast parenchyma appears marginally dense and inhomogeneous. Ultrasound of the mass shows a well-defined, fluid-filled cystic lesion.

2. Fibrocystic disease with breast cyst. The terminology of benign breast diseases is confusing. To simplify, the term aberration of normal development and involution (ANDI) has been coined, to included fibrocystic disease, fibroadenosis, chronic mastitis and mastopathies.

3. Fibrocystic changes are the most common diffuse breast disorder, seen at age 35–55 years. It is an exaggeration of normal cyclical proliferation, with involution of the breast and incomplete absorption of fluid by apocrine cells. It is usually asymptomatic in macrocystic disease but there is pain and tenderness in microcystic disease. There are multiple nodules. Symptoms occur with ovulation and regress with pregnancy and the menopause.

4. The pathological features include:

A. Stromal fibrosis: overgrowth of fibrous connective tissue.

B. Cystic changes : micro- or macrocystic dilatation of ducts.

C. Epithelial hyperplasia.

D. Ductal papillomatosis.

5. Mammographic features include: round or ovoid cysts with smooth margins, lobulated multilocular cysts, or multinodular pattern or teacup-like curvilinear calcification, or psammatous calcification, or punctate calcifications within one or more lobes. Ultrasound shows ductal dilation, cysts or nodules. Differential diagnoses include: simple cysts, fibroadenoma and galactocele.

6. There is an increased risk of malignancy, if there is atypical hyperplasia, scelerosing adenosis or papilloma with fibrovascular core.

Case 2.31: Answers

1. Mammography shows a small, dense spiculated mass in the upper quadrant of the right breast, which is better demonstrated on the magnified view. Few specks of calcification are noted adjacent to this mass.

2. Ultrasound of the breast shows a well-defined, heterogeneous, soft tissue mass.

3. Carcinoma of the breast.

4. **History and clinical examination** of the breasts and axillae:

   Mammography: craniocaudal, mediolateral oblique, localised views with compression and magnification. Analysis of mass or masses, tumour calcification, skin thickening, architectural deformity and axillary nodes are undertaken. Spiculation, microcalcification, architectural distortion, asymmetric thickening/ducts, skin thickening/retraction, nipple retraction and axillary nodes are suggestive of cancer.

   Ultrasound: is useful in young patients with dense breasts, difficult mammography, to determine cystic or solid nature, to evaluate for axillary lymph node metastasis.

   Cytology/biopsy: FNA is the least invasive and is very accurate. Trucut or core biopsy under local anaesthesia gives better histological diagnosis. Needle biopsy of palpable axillary nodes is indicated to rule out metastasis. Small, impalpable lesions may be amenable to needle biopsy under ultrasound or stereotactic mammographic guidance.

   MRI: useful tool in suspected multifocal small breast carcinomas, postoperative and postradiation recurrence of carcinoma in the breast. Tumours show rapid increase in signal intensity after dynamic contrast injection, followed by plateau with early washout.

   CT, bone scan, PET scan, PET-CT: to assess distal metastatic spread.

   Triple assessment is designed for patients with suspected carcinoma of breast, where clinical assessment is combined with radiological imaging and tissue sampling with fine needle or core biopsies.

5. Types of breast carcinoma are:

   Ductal carcinoma: spiculated mass, calcification

   Infiltrating lobular carcinoma: spiculated mass, microcalcification

   Tubular carcinoma: well-differentiated, dense nodule, spiculated

   Medullary carcinoma: well-defined, lobulated, non-calcified.

   Mucinous/colloid: well-circumscribed lobulated, pleomorphic

   Papillary carcinoma: well-defined, round, oval, microcalcification

   Paget's disease: initially in nipple, then surrounding spread

Inflammatory carcinoma: diffuse increase density, stromal coarsening, thickened ligaments, skin thickening.

6. Surgery, chemotherapy, radiation and hormonal therapy are indicated depending on the stage, grade and hormone receptor status of the tumour. Sentinel node biopsy of the axillary nodes under radiological imaging will reduce morbidity following breast surgery.

Case 2.32: Answers

1. Barium enema films taken in lateral decubitus position show normal contrast visualisation of the colon. A gas–fluid level is seen behind the rectum and sigmoid colon, in the urinary bladder lumen. The CT scan shows a distended bladder with an air fluid level within it. There is a loop of rectum/sigmoid on the left side, which is seen directly communicating with the lumen of the bladder.

2. Rectovesical fistula.

3. Rectovesical fistula is an abnormal communication between the bladder and rectum. The pathological process is always in the intestine. Diverticular disease, Crohn's disease, trauma, surgery, radiation and malignancy are the common causes. Colorectal cancer is a common cause. Bladder cancer is rarely, if ever, associated with fistula, probably because of earlier detection. Ovarian, prostate and cervix cancers are known to be associated

4. Suprapubic pain, frequency, dysuria and tenesmus (Gouverneur syndrome) are the common symptoms. Occasionally, it may be asymptomatic. Intermittent pneumaturia and faecaluria can be seen, are non-specific and seen in 60% only. The differential diagnoses for pneumaturia are infection with gas-forming organisms, diabetes and instrumentation. Pneumaturia is more likely in Crohn's disease or diverticulitis than cancer. Faecaluria is pathognomonic and seen in 40%.

5. A fistula is located in the posterior wall of the bladder.

6. A barium enema demonstrates a fistula and delineates diverticular disease from cancer. A CT scan with rectal contrast is the most sensitive test for detecting colovesical fistula. It demonstrates small amounts of air or contrast in the bladder, localised thickening of the bladder wall or a gas-containing mass adjacent to the bladder. Instead of oral contrast, rectal contrast is given. Three-dimensional CT is very useful in delineating the anatomical relationships. Cystography shows contrast outside the bladder, but is less likely to demonstrate a fistula. **Herald sign** is a crescenteric defect in the upper margin of the bladder seen on an oblique view and indicates a perivesical abscess. Ultrasonography can show an echogenic beak sign, which connects the peristaltic bowel lumen and bladder. MRI is very useful in showing a fistulous connection.

7. Cystoscopy, colonoscopy and laparoscopy are useful in indeterminate cases.

8. Definitive treatment is resection of the involved segment of bowel and primary re-anastomosis, with or without closure of the bladder defect, which heals with temporary urethral catheter drainage. Conservative management is indicated in poor surgical candidates.

Case 2.33: Answers

1. IVU shows normal left pelvicalyceal system and large right pelvicalyceal system. There is very little contrast within the bladder, but contrast is seen within the vagina. The CT scan shows dense contrast not only in the bladder lumen, but also in a distended vagina (posterior to the bladder).

2. Vesicovaginal fistula (VVF) and right hydroureteronephrosis.

3. VVF is an abnormal fistulous tract between the bladder and vagina. Common causes are prolonged obstructed labour (leading to pressure necrosis, oedema, tissue sloughing), post-surgical (hysterectomies, urological and gastrointestinal surgery), pelvic infections (TB, syphilis, lymphogranuloma venereum), vaginal trauma, erosion with foreign bodies and congenital. Risk factors are prior pelvic or vaginal surgery, pelvic inflammatory disease, ischaemia, diabetes, arteriosclerosis, carcinoma, endometriosis, uterine myomas, infections and pelvic abscess.

4. Uncontrolled leakage of urine into the vagina, pain, ileus, fever, local infections, skin excoriation, abnormal urinary stream and haematuria are the clinical features.

5. Usually the communication is between the anterior wall of vagina and the posterior wall of bladder. Less frequently there is communication between the bladder and cervix or between the ureter and vagina/uterus/cervix or between the urethra and vagina.

6. A cystogram can demonstrate communication between the bladder and vagina. IVU is used to exclude ureteral injury, which is associated in 10–15% of cases. If suspicion is high for ureteral injury or fistula and IVU is negative, retrograde urography should be performed at the time of cystoscopy and examination under anaesthesia. A fistulogram may be possible. Colour Doppler ultrasonography with ultrasonic contrast instilled in the bladder can show jet phenomenon – through the bladder wall towards the vagina.

7. Indigo carmine can be injected intravenously during pelvic surgery and leak into the pelvis can be assessed. In the double-dye test, a patient ingests pyridium and indigo carmine/methylene blue is instilled into the bladder via a urethral catheter. Pyridium turns urine orange and methylene blue turns it blue. A tampon is placed in the vagina. If it turns orange, it is a ureterovaginal fistula, blue a VVF and blue/orange a combination of VVF and ureterovaginal fistula. Combined vaginoscopy/cystocopy can be performed to localise the communication site.

8. If fistulae are diagnosed early after surgery, an indwelling catheter is placed for 30 days. Small ones resolve or decrease in size. Larger fistulae require surgical correction.

3
MUSCULOSKELETAL RADIOLOGY
QUESTIONS

Case 3.1

An 11-year-old girl, presents with pain and deformity of the back. On examination she has difficulty on lateral bending and there is tenderness in the midthoracic and lumbar spine.

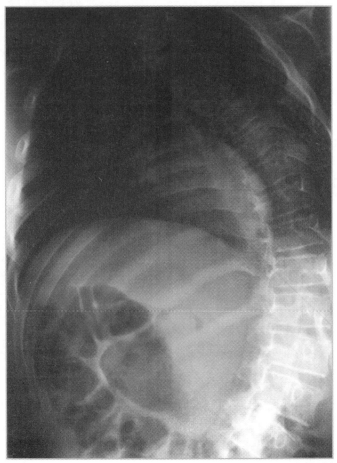

Fig 3.1

1. What does the AP X-ray of the spine show?
2. What is the diagnosis?
3. What are the types of this disease?
4. What is the role of radiology?
5. Does this patient need treatment?

Answers on pages 271–331

Case 3.2

A 71-year-old man falls down the stairs and has severe pain and tenderness in his left hip. On examination, the femur is externally rotated and there is restriction of movement.

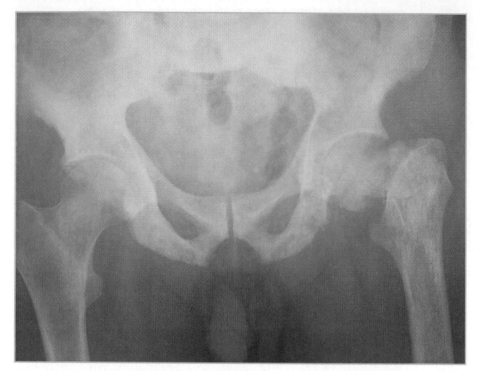

Fig 3.2

1. What are the findings on this X-ray?
2. What is the diagnosis?
3. What is the mechanism of injury?
4. What are the radiological features?
5. What is the imaging protocol?
6. What are the prognostic indicators?
7. What are the complications?
8. What is the treatment?

Answers on pages 271–331

Case 3.3

A 47-year-old man was involved in a major road traffic accident and presents to A&E in an unconscious state. On examination, he is tachycardic and hypotensive. There are multiple bony injuries in the body. After stabilisation he was investigated.

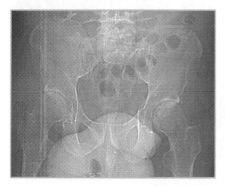

Fig 3.3a

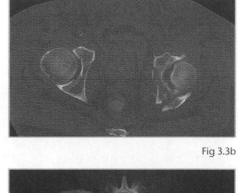

Fig 3.3b

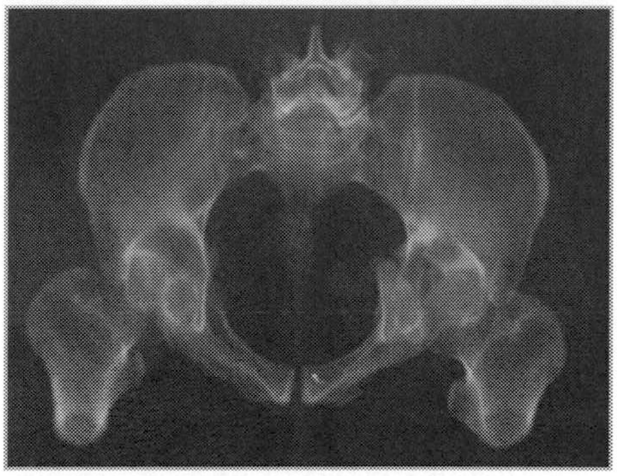

Fig 3.3c

1. What are the findings on the X-ray and the CT scan?
2. What are the important components of the acetabulum?
3. How do you classify these fractures?
4. What are the common types?
5. What is the mechanism of injury?
6. What are the other associated injuries?
7. What are the complications?
8. What are the investigations required?
9. What are the important factors to be noted on a CT scan?

Answers on pages 271–331

Case 3.4

A 74-year-old woman presents with backache. On examination, there is tenderness in the lower dorsal and upper lumbar vertebrae with severe restriction of movement.

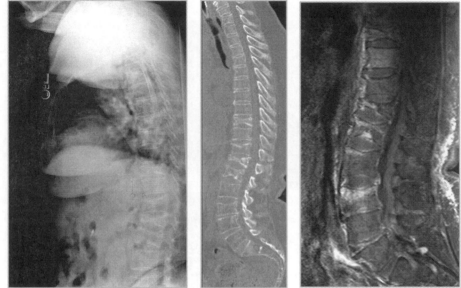

Fig 3.4a   Fig 3.4b   Fig 3.4c

1. What are the findings on the X-ray, the CT scan and MRI?
2. What is the diagnosis?
3. What are the causes?
4. What are the radiological features?
5. What is the role of MRI?
6. What are the other investigations that might be required in this patient?
7. What are the complications?
8. What is the role of radiology in treatment?

Answers on pages 271–331

Case 3.5

A 37-year-old construction worker fell from scaffolding and is unable to move. On examination, he has pain and tenderness in the lower spine, with severe restriction of movement. There are multiple fractures in his lower limbs.

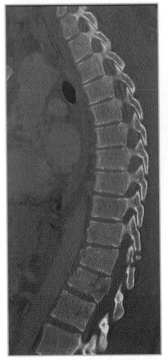

Fig 3.5a

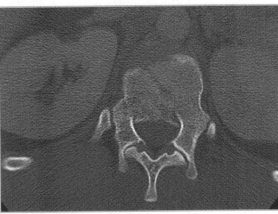

Fig 3.5b

1. What are the findings on the CT scan?
2. What is the diagnosis?
3. What is the mechanism?
4. What is the classification of fractures in this location?
5. What are the radiological features?
6. What are the other types of fracture in this region?
7. What are the complications and the treatment?

Answers *on pages 271–331*

Case 3.6

A 27-year-old man was involved in a road traffic accident and presents with pain and tenderness in the cervical spine. On examination, the lower cervical spine is tender and there is limitation of movement.

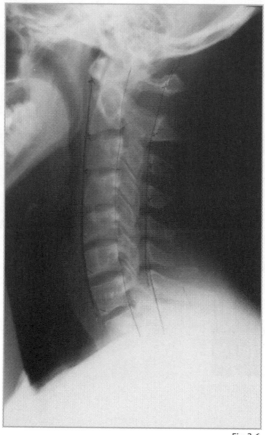

Fig 3.6

1. What do you observe on the X-ray of the cervical spine?
2. What are the lines that have been marked on the X-ray?
3. What is the diagnosis?
4. What is the mechanism of injury?
5. What are the radiological features?
6. What are the other injuries seen with the same mechanism?
7. What is the treatment?

Answers on pages 271–331

Case 3.7

A 35-year-old woman was involved in a high-velocity motor traffic accident and brought in unconscious.

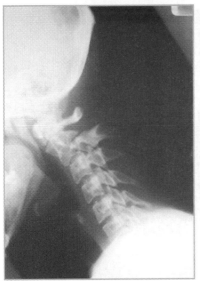

Fig 3.7a

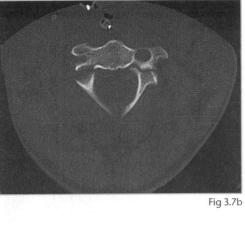

Fig 3.7b

1. What do you see on the X-ray and the CT scan of the cervical spine?
2. What is the diagnosis?
3. What is the mechanism?
4. What are the radiological features?
5. What are the other injuries that may be encountered in this location?

Answers on pages 271–331

A 26-year-old woman twists her ankle and falls down. On examination, there is swelling and tenderness in the right ankle.

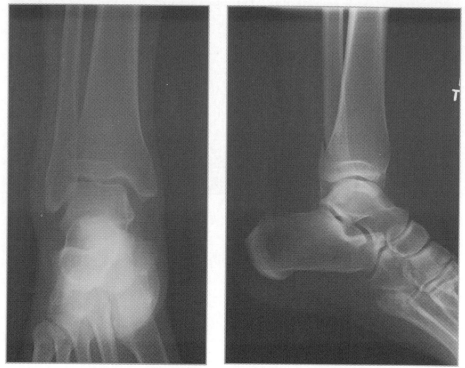

Fig 3.8a   Fig 3.8b

1. What are the findings on the X-ray?
2. What is the diagnosis?
3. What are the types of fracture based on the mechanism?
4. What are the other types of fracture in this region?
5. What are the complications and treatment?

Answers on pages 271–331

Case 3.9

A 37-year-old woman presents with pain, tenderness and restricted movement of the right shoulder joint. On examination, she has limited abduction and external rotation. There is no palpable mass.

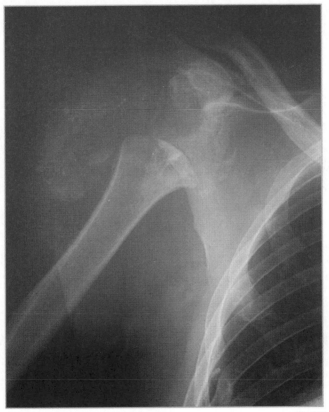

Fig 3.9

1. What are the findings on the X-ray?
2. What is the diagnosis?
3. What is the pathology of this disease?
4. What are the causes?
5. What are the two types of this condition?
6. What are the radiological features?
7. What is the differential diagnosis?
8. What are the different sites affected by this disease?

Answers *on pages 271–331*

A 41-year-old woman presents with severe pain in her abdomen, back and hips. On examination she has flexion deformity and tenderness in both her hips. Ultrasound examination was not helpful because of bowel gas.

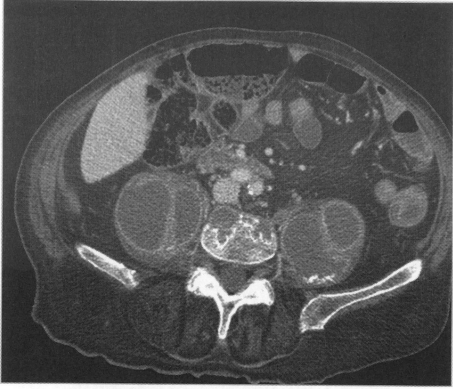

Fig 3.10

1. What do you find on the CT scan?
2. What is the diagnosis?
3. What are the causes?
4. What is the causative organism?
5. What are the clinical features?
6. What are the imaging findings?
7. What are the differential diagnoses?
8. What are the treatment and the role of radiology in management?

Answers on pages 271–331

A 15-year-old girl presents with severe pain in her left shoulder. On examination the shoulder is very warm, red and tender. Lab analysis shows an elevated WBC count. A series of radiological tests was ordered.

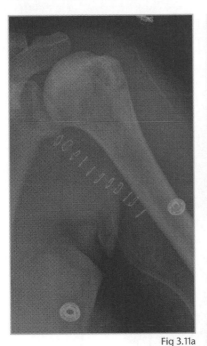

Fig 3.11a

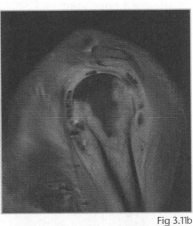

Fig 3.11b

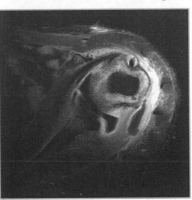

Fig 3.11c

1. What do you see on the X-ray of the left shoulder?
2. What is the second test and what do you see?
3. What is the diagnosis?
4. What are the causes and the pathophysiology of the disease?
5. What is the clinical course?
6. What are the radiological features?
7. What are the differential diagnosis and the complications?
8. What is the treatment?

Answers *on pages 271–331*

An 11-year-old boy presents with fever, severe pain and swelling of his right leg. On examination he is febrile. His right leg is swollen, red and tender. The swelling is bony hard on palpation and there is severe restriction of movement of the right knee joint.

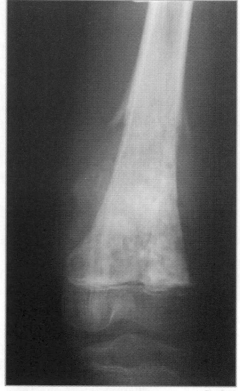

Fig 3.12

1. What are the findings on the plain film?
2. What is the diagnosis?
3. What are the clinical features?
4. What are the radiological features?
5. What are the complications?
6. What is the differential diagnosis?
7. What are the variations in the presentation?
8. What is the treatment?

Answers on pages 271–331

Case 3.13

A 25-year-old man presents with severe knee pain and restriction of movement after being injured in a football match. On examination, the anterior drawer test is positive.

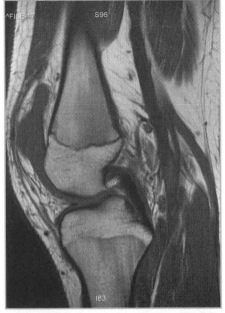

Fig 3.13a

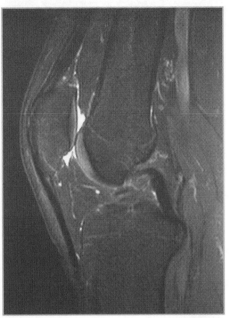

Fig 3.13b

1. What is this investigation? What is missing on this scan?
2. What is the diagnosis?
3. What is the mechanism of injury?
4. What is the anatomy of the injured structure?
5. What other injuries are associated? What are the clinical features?
6. What are the radiological findings?
7. What tests are done to elicit this abnormality?
8. How is this managed?

Answers on pages 271–331

Case 3.14

A 56-year-old patient with a chronic medical condition presents with pain in the foot. The X-rays below were done with a 1-year interval.

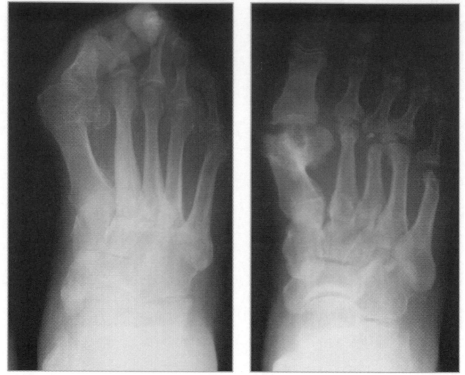

Fig 3.14a   Fig 3.14b

1. What are the findings on the X-rays?
2. What is the diagnosis?
3. What is the pathophysiology?
4. What are the pathological changes in a diabetic foot?
5. What are the radiological features?
6. What is the role of imaging?

Answers on pages 271–331

Case 3.15

A 45-year-old man presents with right knee pain and locking, after injuring himself in a football match. On examination, the joint is tender and clicking sounds were heard. There is restriction of joint movement and McMurray's test is positive.

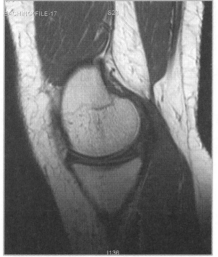

Fig 3.15a   Fig 3.15b

1. What do you see on MRI?
2. What is the diagnosis?
3. What is the anatomy of the structure?
4. What is the mechanism of this lesion?
5. What are the types?
6. What is the appearance on MRI?
7. What is the differential diagnosis?
8. What is the treatment?

Answers on pages 271–331

Case 3.16

A 36-year-old man, who recently joined a gym, presents with severe pain near his left ankle, particularly on standing. On examination, there is tenderness and swelling over the back of the ankle, with restriction of flexion.

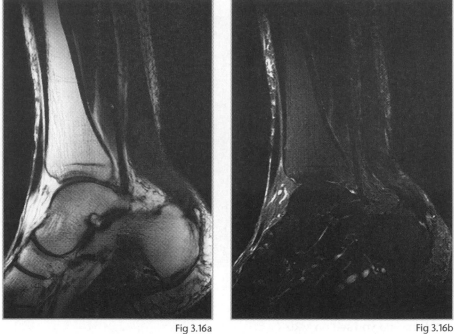

Fig 3.16a   Fig 3.16b

1. What do you see on MRI?
2. What is the diagnosis?
3. What is the anatomy of the structure?
4. What is the mechanism and the risk factors of this lesion?
5. What are the types?
6. What is the appearance on ultrasonography and MRI?
7. What is the differential diagnosis?
8. What is the treatment?

Answers on pages 271–331

A 39-year-old woman presents with left knee pain and discomfort. On examination, there is a soft lump with tenderness in the posterior aspect of the knee. There was no pulsation.

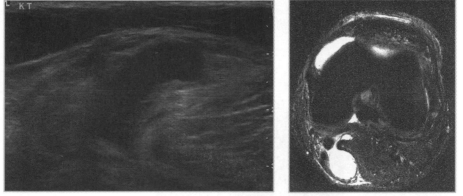

Fig 3.17a   Fig 3.17b

1. What do you see on the ultrasound and MR scans?

2. What is the diagnosis?

3. What is the origin of this condition?

4. What is the common location?

5. What are the causes?

6. What are the types?

7. What are the radiological features?

8. What are the complications?

9. What is the differential diagnosis?

10. What is the treatment?

Answers *on pages 271–331*

A 41-year-old man falls down stairs and presents with severe pain and inability to move his right foot. On examination, there is severe pain and tenderness in his midfoot and movement is restricted.

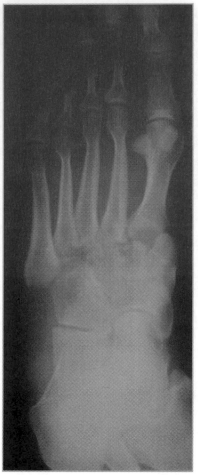

Fig 3.18

1. What are the findings on the X-ray?
2. What is the diagnosis?
3. What is the mechanism?
4. What is the normal alignment of joints at this level?
5. What are the radiological features?
6. What is the treatment?

Answers on pages 271–331

Case 3.19

A 37 year old fell down on to outstretched hands and presents with severe pain and tenderness in the right shoulder. On examination, there is restricted abduction and external rotation.

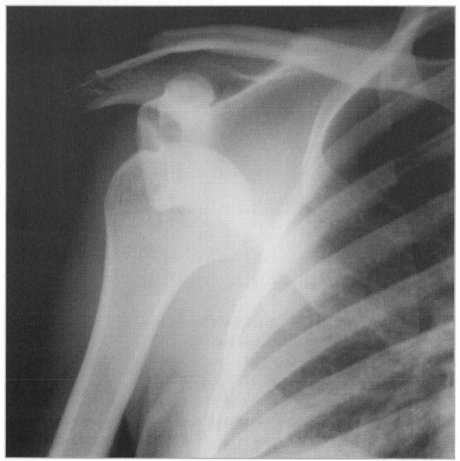

Fig 3.19

1. What are the findings on the X-ray?
2. What is the diagnosis?
3. What is the mechanism?
4. What are the radiological features?
5. What are the other injuries which may be sustained with similar trauma to the shoulder?
6. What are the complications and the treatment?

Answers *on pages 271–331*

A 27-year-old man was involved in a motor vehicle accident and is unable to move his right leg. Clinical examination demonstrated restricted movement of the right knee joint, with massive effusion.

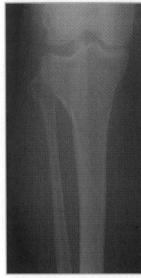

Fig 3.20a

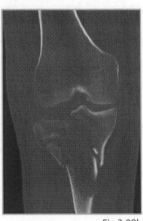

Fig 3.20b

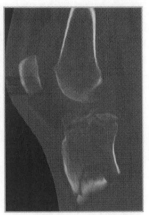

Fig 3.20c

1. What are the findings on the X-ray and the CT scan?
2. What is the commonly used classification?
3. What is the most common type?
4. What is the mechanism of injury?
5. What are the associated complications?
6. What are the investigations required for diagnosis and management?
7. What are the important factors to be noted on the CT scan?
8. What is the treatment?

Answers on pages 271–331

Case 3.21

A 28-year-old man banged his left hand against the wall and developed swelling and pain. On examination there is severe tenderness and restriction of movement of his left hand.

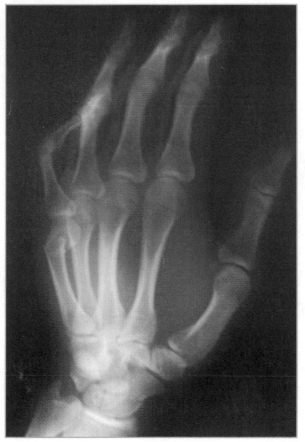

Fig 3.21

1. What are the findings on this X-ray?
2. What is the diagnosis?
3. What is the mechanism of injury?
4. What are the radiological features?
5. What are the treatment and the complications?

Answers on pages 271–331

Case 3.22

A 17 year old falls from a motorcycle and presents with severe pain and swelling of the right forearm. On examination, there is severe tenderness and restricted movement of the proximal forearm.

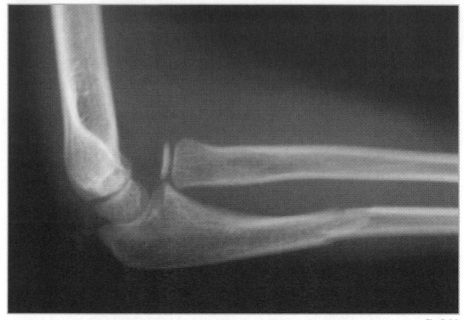

Fig 3.22

1. What are the findings on this X-ray?
2. What is the diagnosis?
3. What is the mechanism of injury?
4. What are the radiological findings?
5. How does it differ from Galeazzi's fracture?
6. What are the treatment and complications?

Answers on pages 271–331

Case 3.23

A 27-year-old man was involved in a motor vehicle accident and presented with severe pain in his abdomen, pelvis and legs. On examination his left leg is externally rotated and abducted and there is tenderness in his left hip.

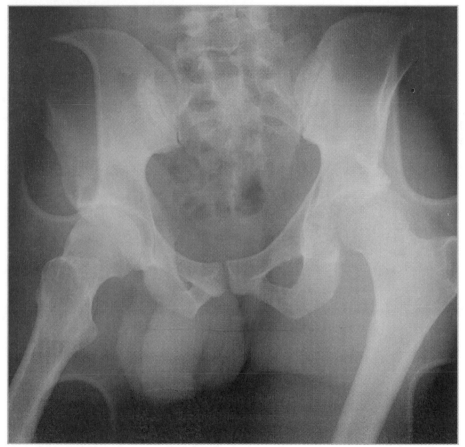

Fig 3.23

1. What do you observe on the plain X-ray of the pelvis?
2. What is the diagnosis?
3. What are the types of this disease and their mechanisms?
4. What is the classification?
5. What are the complications and the treatment?

Answers *on pages 271–331*

Case 3.24

A 26-year-old woman jumped from the second floor of her house and landed on her left foot. She is brought to the hospital with swelling and bruises in her back and left foot. On examination, she has tenderness and restriction of movement of her feet.

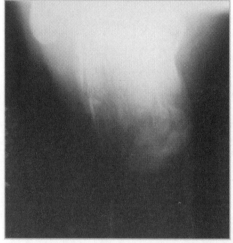

Fig 3.24a

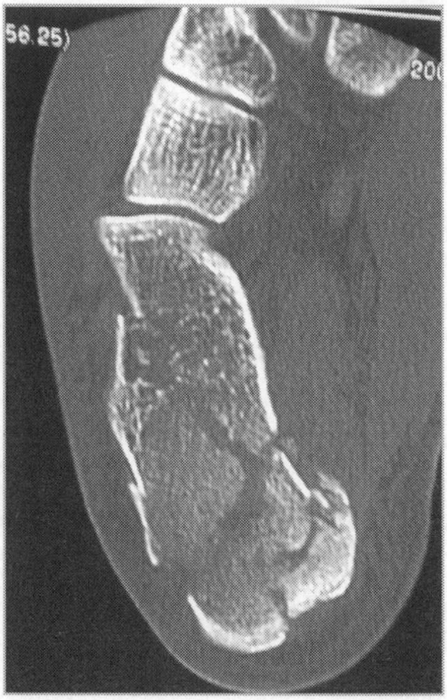

1. What are the findings on the X-ray?
2. What do you observe on the CT scan?
3. What is the diagnosis?
4. What is the mechanism?
5. What are the radiological features?
6. What is the role of CT in this patient?
7. What is the treatment?

Fig 3.24b

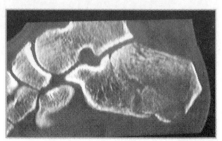

Fig 3.24c

Answers on pages 271–331

A 67-year-old woman fell down onto her outstretched hands and presents with swelling, tenderness, deformity and restricted movement of the left wrist joint.

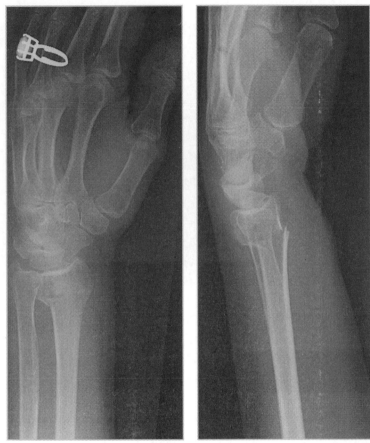

Fig 3.25a   Fig 3.25b

1. What are the findings on this X-ray?
2. What is the diagnosis?
3. What is the mechanism of injury?
4. What are the radiological features?
5. What is the differential diagnosis?
6. What are the complications?
7. What is the treatment?

Answers on pages 271–331

Case 3.26

A 10-year-old boy presented with pain in the right leg, which limits his movement. On examination, tenderness was elicited over the proximal tibia, with limitation of joint movement. No warmth or tenderness was noticed. The laboratory tests were normal.

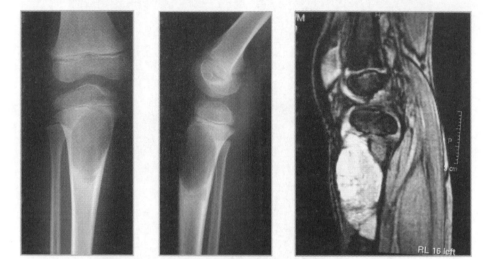

Fig 3.26a   Fig 3.26b   Fig 3.26c

1. What do you observe on the plain X-ray and on MRI of the leg?
2. What is the diagnosis?
3. What are the clinical features?
4. What are the predisposing factors?
5. What are the common locations?
6. What are the radiological features?
7. What are the complications and treatment?
8. What are the differential diagnoses?

Answers on pages 271–331

Case 3.27

A 10-year-old boy presented with severe pain, tenderness and limitation of movement of the left leg. On examination the proximal portion of the left leg was warm, tender, with a bony swelling and restriction of joint movement.

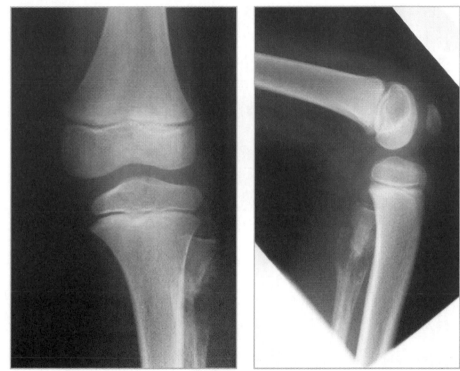

Fig 3.27a   Fig 3.27b

1. What do you observe on the plain film of the left leg?

2. What is the diagnosis?

3. What are the clinical features?

4. What are the common locations?

5. What are the radiological features?

6. What is the differential diagnosis?

7. What are the prognostic factors?

8. What is the treatment?

Answers on pages 271–331

A 61-year-old woman presents with backache and headache. On examination, there is tenderness in the lumbar and dorsal spine with limitation of movement. Blood tests reveal anaemia and leukopenia. Abnormal proteins were noted in the blood and urine.

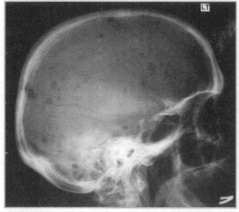

Fig 3.28a

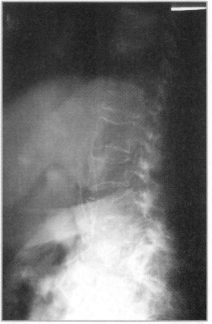

Fig 3.28b

1. What do you see on the X-ray of the spine and skull?
2. What is the diagnosis?
3. What is the origin of this lesion?
4. What are the types of presentation and the locations?
5. What are the clinical features?
6. What are the radiological features?
7. What is the differential diagnosis?
8. What is the associated syndrome?

Answers on pages 271–331

A 75-year-old woman presents with diffuse bone pain, especially in the hip and spine. On examination, there is tenderness in the spine with restriction of movement.

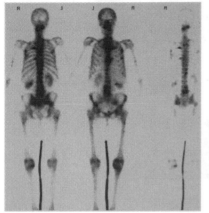

Fig 3.29a

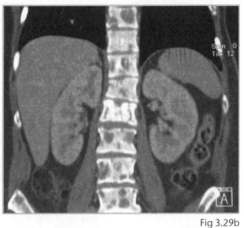

Fig 3.29b

1. What are the findings on the bone and CT scans?
2. What is the diagnosis?
3. What are the causes of this disease?
4. What are the different appearances of this disease?
5. What are the differential diagnoses?

Answers on pages 271–331

Case 3.30

A 37-year-old man had a fall and he presents with severe pain in his knee. Examination revealed a tender knee and restricted movement.

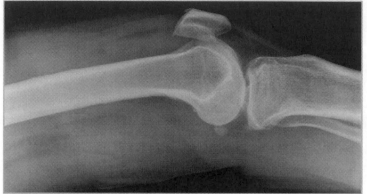

Fig 3.30a

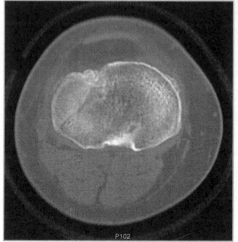

Fig 3.30b

1. What is the view on figure 3.30a?
2. What do you observe?
3. What is the underlying condition?
4. What do you observe on the CT scan?
5. What is the pathophysiology?
6. What are the appearances on CT and MRI?
7. What are the other areas where it is seen?
8. What is the importance of this sign?

Answers on pages 271–331

Case 3.31

A 61 year old presents with diffuse bone pain and an enlarging head. On examination, there is tenderness in the pelvis and spine. Serum calcium and phosphorus are normal, but ALP is elevated. The PSA is normal.

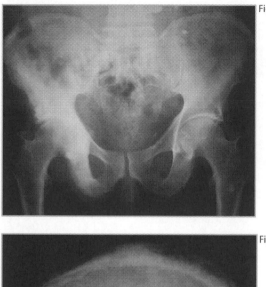

Fig 3.31a

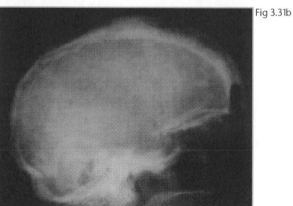

Fig 3.31b

1. What do you see on the X-rays of the pelvis and skull?
2. What is the diagnosis?
3. What is the aetiology of this lesion?
4. What are the different radiographic phases?
5. What are the clinical features?
6. What are the locations and the radiological features?
7. What is the differential diagnosis?
8. What are the complications and the treatment?

Answers *on pages 271–331*

A 39-year-old male patient with Crohn's disease develops right hip pain, which is worse on walking. On examination there is limitation of movement of the right hip joint.

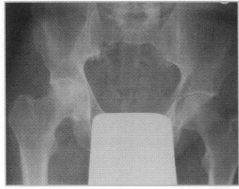

Fig 3.32a

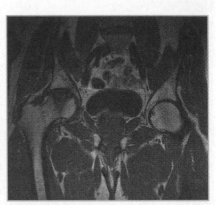

Fig 3.32b

1. What do you observe on the X-ray of the pelvis?
2. What do you see on MRI of the pelvis?
3. What is the diagnosis?
4. What are the causes?
5. What are the radiological features and differential diagnosis?
6. How is this disease staged and what are the prognostic factors?
7. What are the complications?
8. What is the treatment?

Answers on pages 271–331

Case 3.33

A 6-year-old boy fell down stairs. He presents with pain and swelling. On examination, his elbow is swollen, tender and deformed with restricted flexion and extension.

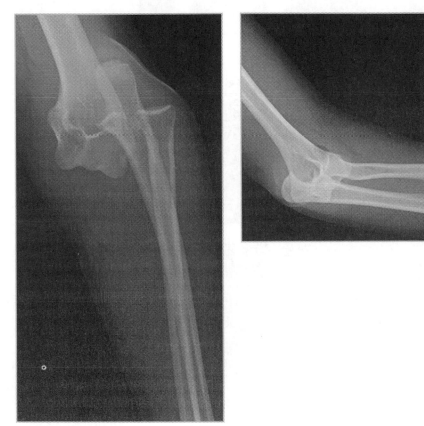

Fig 3.33b

Fig 3.33a

1. What are the findings on the X-ray?
2. What is the diagnosis?
3. What is the mechanism?
4. What are the radiological features?
5. What are the complications and treatment?

Answers on pages 271–331

Case 3.34

A 16-year-old girl presents with back pain, fever, nightsweats and weight loss. On examination, severe tenderness was elicited in the dorsolumbar junction.

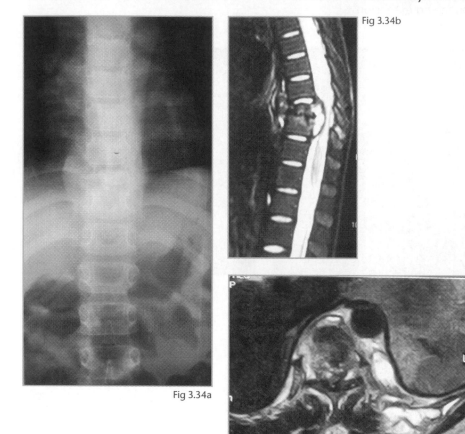

Fig 3.34b

Fig 3.34a

Fig 3.34c

1. What do you see on the X-ray of the spine and on MRI?
2. What is the diagnosis?
3. What are the pathophysiology and the mode of spread?
4. What are the common locations?
5. What are the clinical features?
6. What are the radiological features?
7. What is the differential diagnosis?

Answers *on pages 271–331*

A 38-year-old woman fell off her motorbike and presented with facial injury. On examination, there is swelling and bruising of her face. The left eye is swollen and there is mild proptosis.

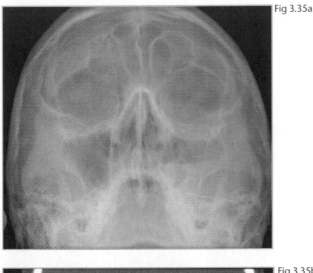

Fig 3.35a

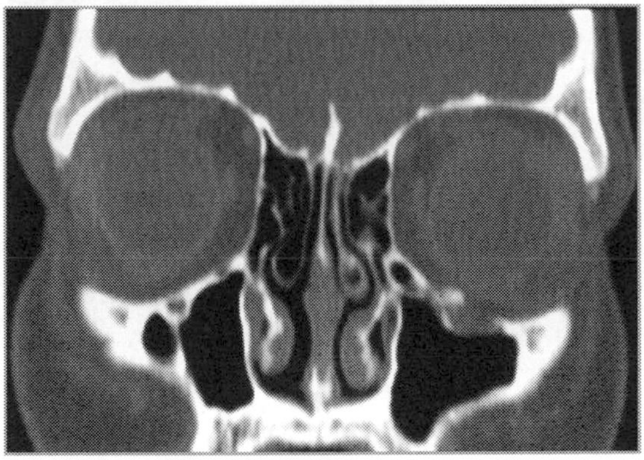

Fig 3.35b

1. What are the findings on the X-ray and the CT scan?
2. What is the diagnosis?
3. What is the mechanism?
4. What are the radiological features?
5. What is the important factor that decides treatment?
6. What are the complications?
7. What is the treatment?

Answers on pages 271–331

A 27-year-old man fell down and presented with severe pain and swelling of the left wrist. On examination, the left wrist is swollen, red and tender with limited flexion and adduction.

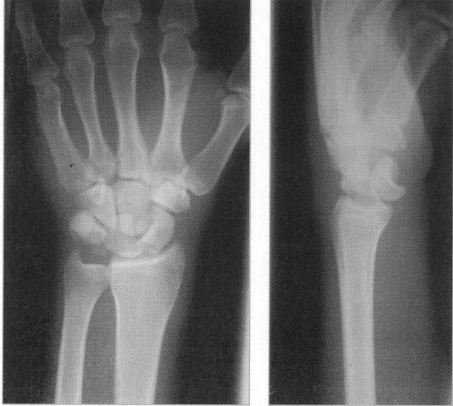

Fig 3.36a   Fig 3.36b

1. What are the findings on the X-ray?
2. What is the diagnosis?
3. What is the mechanism?
4. What are the radiological features?
5. What are the types of instability resulting from fracture in this region?
6. What are the complications and the treatment?

Answers on pages 271–331

A 6-year-old boy falls from a tree onto his outstretched hands. He presents with severe pain in his right arm and forearm; his arm is flexed and there is swelling, tenderness and limitation of movement.

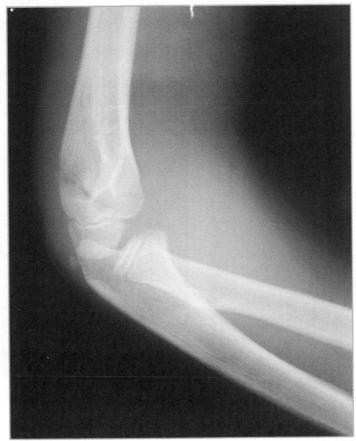

Fig 3.37

1. What are the findings on this X-ray?
2. What is the diagnosis?
3. What is the mechanism of injury?
4. What are the important things to look for on the X-ray?
5. What is the treatment and what are the complications?

Answers on pages 271–331

Case 3.38

A 9-year-old girl injured her left hand when playing. On examination the left thumb is painful and tender, with limited movement.

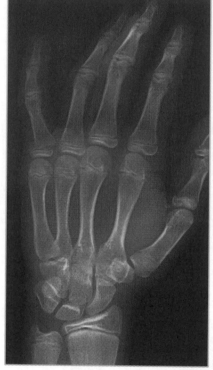

Fig 3.38a

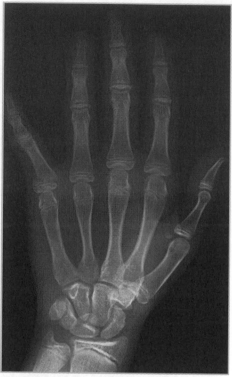

Fig 3.38b

1. What are the findings on this X-ray?
2. What is the diagnosis?
3. What is the mechanism of injury?
4. What are the types of this injury?
5. What is the treatment?

Answers on pages 271–331

A 29-year-old man was assaulted in a pub and presented with severe pain, swelling and restricted movement of his left thumb.

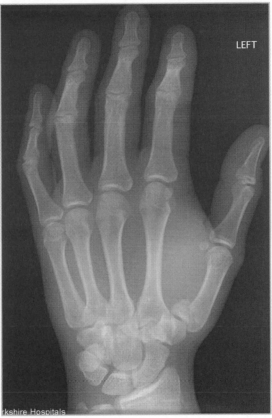

LEFT

rkshire Hospitals

Fig 3.39

1. What are the findings on this X-ray?
2. What is the diagnosis?
3. What is the mechanism of injury?
4. What are the radiological features?
5. What is Rolando's fracture?
6. What is the treatment?

Answers on pages 271–331

A 45-year-old man complains of severe pain on elevation of his right shoulder. On examination, there is no palpable mass, but there is restriction of abduction and forward flexion.

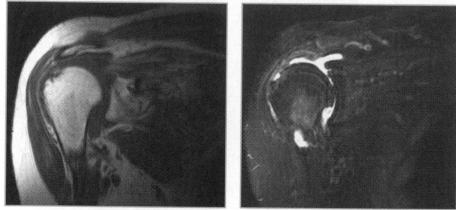

Fig 3.40a   Fig 3.40b

1. What do you see on MRI?

2. What is the diagnosis?

3. What is the anatomy?

4. What is the mechanism of development?

5. What is the characteristic location?

6. What are the clinical features?

7. What are the imaging features on MRI and the differential diagnosis?

8. What other investigation can be performed?

9. What is the treatment?

Answers on pages 271–331

Case 3.41

A 22-year-old woman fell while running for a bus and presents with pain and swelling of her left wrist and hand.

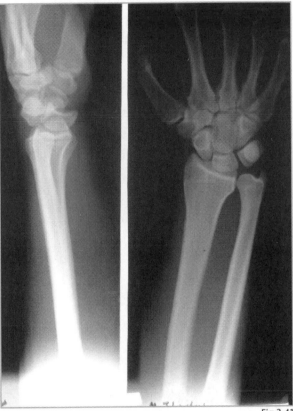

Fig 3.41

1. What are the findings on the X-ray?
2. What is the diagnosis?
3. What is the mechanism?
4. What are the radiological features?
5. What are the other types of fracture in this region?
6. What are the complications and the treatment?

Answers on pages 271–331

A 31 year old falls down and has pain, swelling and tenderness in his left wrist. On examination, there is tenderness in his left anatomical snuffbox and there is restriction of movement about the wrist joint.

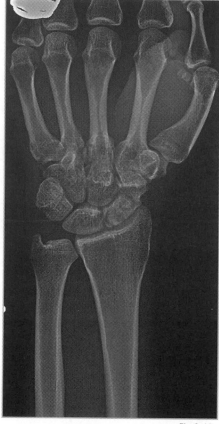

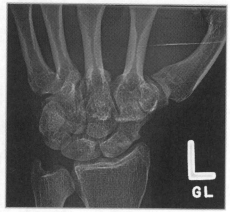

Fig 3.42b

Fig 3.42a

1. What are the findings on this X-ray?
2. What is the diagnosis?
3. What is the mechanism of injury?
4. What are the radiological features?
5. What is the imaging protocol?
6. What are the prognostic indicators?
7. What are the complications?
8. What is the treatment?

Answers on pages 271–331

Case 3.43

A 57-year-old man presents with severe pain and swelling in his right arm. On palpation, a hard, fixed mass is palpated in the lateral aspect of the right arm. Movement is painful.

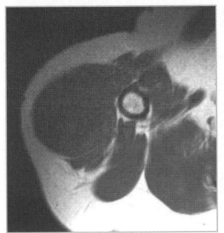

Fig 3.43a

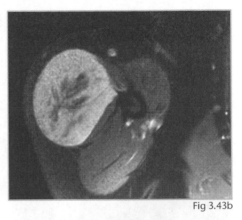

Fig 3.43b

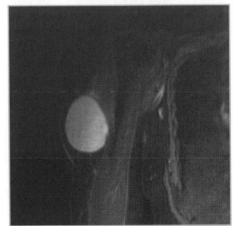

Fig 3.43c

1. What are the findings on MRI?
2. What is the diagnosis?
3. What are the pathological types of this lesion?
4. What are the clinical features?
5. What are the radiological findings?
6. What is the role of imaging in this disease?
7. What is the treatment?
8. What is the role of imaging after treatment?

Answers on pages 271–331

A 71-year-old patient with known prostate cancer presented with pain in his neck and back, radiating to his arm, and inability to move all his limbs. On examination, there is weakness in the arms and legs, with increased reflexes.

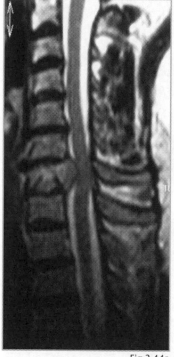

Fig 3.44a

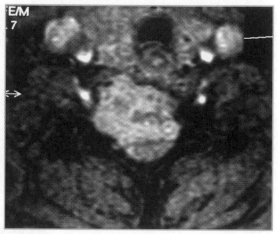

Fig 3.44b

1. What are the findings on MRI?
2. What is the diagnosis?
3. What are the causes of similar neurological symptoms?
4. What are the clinical features?
5. What are the MRI features?
6. What is the treatment in this case?

Answers on pages 271–331

Case 3.45

A 14-year-old boy presents with pain on the right side of the neck and pain and paraesthesiae in his arm and forearm. An elevated arm stress test is positive.

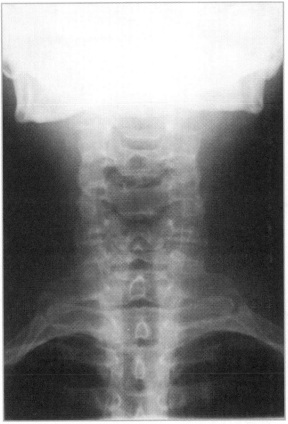

Fig 3.45

1. What do you observe on the chest X-ray?
2. What is the diagnosis?
3. What are the types?
4. What are the radiological features?
5. What are the aetiology, clinical features and complications?
6. What is the treatment?

Answers *on pages 271–331*

A 51-year-old woman presents with back pain radiating along the left posterior thigh, leg and lateral aspect of the foot. On examination, there is no spinal tenderness. There is weakness of left ankle plantar flexion and hamstrings. Ankle jerk is diminished. Loss of sensation is noted along the lateral foot and heel on the left side.

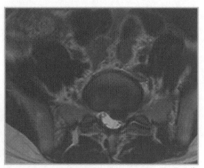

Fig 3.46b

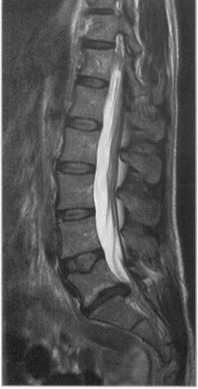

Fig 3.46a

1. What do you see on the MRI?

2. What is the diagnosis?

3. What are the aetiology and the pathophysiology of this disease?

4. What are the common sites of this disorder?

5. What are the different morphological types of this lesion?

6. What are the radiological findings?

7. Which nerve root is affected in a lesion at the L3–4 disc level?

8. What are the complications?

Answers on pages 271–331

A 35-year-old man presented with pain in the left leg, which limits his movement. On examination, tenderness was elicited over the proximal tibia, with limitation of joint movement.

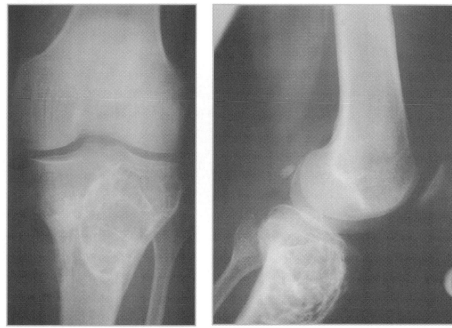

Fig 3.47a   Fig 3.47b

1. What do you observe on the plain film of the leg?
2. What is the diagnosis?
3. What are the clinical features?
4. What are the pathological features?
5. What are the common locations?
6. What are the radiological features?
7. What are the complications and the treatment?
8. What is the differential diagnosis?

Answers on pages 271–331

Case 3.1: Answers

1. The X-ray shows an extensive lateral bending deformity in the dorsolumbar region, which is concave to the right side.

2 Idiopathic scoliosis. Scoliosis is the presence of one or more lateral rotatory curves of the spine in the coronal plane > 10°. Scoliosis can be postural or structural. Structural scoliosis can be: **congenital** (failure of formation, failure of segmentation, combination), **idiopathic**, **mesodermal** (neurofibromatosis [NF], osteogenesis imperfecta, mucopolysaccharidosis [MPS], Marfan syndrome), n**euromuscular** (spinal dysraphism, myelomeningocele, syringomyelia, Chiari malformation, polio, arthrogryposis, motor neuron disease, congenital hypotonia), **radiation, dysplasia, infections, tumours**.

3. Idiopathic scoliosis is the most common type (80%). There are three types:

Infantile: up to 3 years, boys, thoracic, convex to left

Juvenile: 4–9 years, dorsolumbar, convex to left

Adolescent: > 10 years – maturity; most common, female, thoracic, convex to right.

4. An X-ray is used to confirm diagnosis, exclude underlying causes, assess the severity of curves, monitor progression, assess skeletal maturity and determine suitability for surgery. Bone scans are useful for painful scoliosis to exclude underlying tumours or infections. CT with sagittal and coronal reconstructions is useful for assessing segmentation anomalies and to find the true extent of rotation and rib deformities. MRI is used for assessing spinal and neurological abnormalities, which might preclude surgery. On an X-ray, apical vertebra refers to the vertebra that is displaced most. End-vertebrae are the superior and inferior vertebrae in the curve. A neutral vertebra is not rotated. A primary curve is the structural curve and a secondary one is the non-structural curve that develops as compensation for the primary curve. There are many indices used to grade scoliosis. The most common is the Cobb and Webb technique (lines are drawn tangential to the superior and inferior end-vertebrae. The Cobb angle is formed at the intersection of these lines. Cobb classification of scoliosis:

I: < 20°; II: 21–30°; III: 31–50°; IV: 51–75°; V: 76–100°; VI: 101–125°; VII: > 125°.

Vertebral rotation is assessed by the Nash–Moe technique. Skeletal maturity is assessed by the Risser technique, which evaluates the level of ossification of the iliac wing apophysis. If the apophysis is completely fused, the patient is skeletally mature and the curve unlikely to progress further. Routine views obtained are posteroanterior (PA) and lateral views of the entire spine, including the pelvis, to visualise the iliac apophysis and lateral bending views for assessing compensatory curves.

5. Scoliosis produces cosmetic deformity, disability, pain, cardiovascular compromise, respiratory failure and restrictive lung disease. Scoliosis progresses with age and the rate of progression depends on the cause and the patient's growth. Progression stops when maturity is attained, especially if the curve is < 30°. When the curve is < 25° in an immature skeleton or 30° in a mature person, management is regular follow-up and radiography. Curves < 25° require treatment when they are rapidly progressive. Curves of 25–50° are managed as for orthotic disease. Spinal fusion is required for curves > 50°.

Case 3.2: Answers

1. There is a transverse fracture line in the neck of the left femur, with overlapping of the bony fragments and deformity.

2. Fracture of the neck of the femur.

3. Fracture of the neck of the femur is caused by a fall producing a direct blow, with lateral rotation of the extremity, where the head is firmly fixed by the anterior capsule and iliofemoral ligaments, while the neck rotates posteriorly. The posterior cortex impinges on the acetabulum and neck fractures. The fracture is more common in elderly people, even after trivial falls or twisting injury. In young people, they are the result of high-impact trauma or a stress fracture, due to repetitive stress on the neck of the femur by unusual activity.

4. The X-ray shows a fracture line through the neck of the femur. Garden's classification of femoral neck fractures:

   Grade I: incomplete or valgus-impacted fracture

   Grade II: complete fracture without bone displacement

Grade III: complete fracture with partial displacement of fracture fragments

Grade IV: complete fracture with total displacement of fracture fragments.

Tension fractures are located in the superior aspect of the femoral neck, whereas compression fractures are located in the inferior aspect. The standard examination of the hip is an AP view and cross-table lateral view.

5. Occasionally a fracture line is not seen in both these views, but if there is high clinical suspicion, evaluation with MRI or CT is indicated to rule out fracture. A bone scan is also very sensitive. Fracture of the lesser trochanter usually indicates metastatic lesion.

6. **Modified Pauwel's method of classification**: the fracture is classified as transverse, horizontal or vertical. Most of horizontal fractures have non-union. Normally a convex outline of femoral head joins the concave outline of the femoral neck, producing an 'S' or a reversed 'S' curve. The outline of the femoral neck is never tangential to the outline of a femoral head in a reduced femoral neck fracture. Fractures with posterior communication have a bad prognosis. This is best assessed on a lateral view.

7. Avascular necrosis (11%): increased incidence when fracture is displaced; non-union (10–30%).

8. Treatment of femoral neck fractures is with cannulated screws or pins, open reduction, hemiarthroplasty or total hip replacement.

Case 3.3: Answers

1. The X-ray of the pelvis shows a comminuted fracture in the left acetabulum. The axial and three-dimensional CT scan of this patient shows fracture of both the anterior and posterior columns of the left acetabulum.

2. The acetabulum has two columns and walls (anterior and posterior), a dome and a quadrilateral plate.

3. There are 10 patterns of acetabular fractures (Judet and Letournel et al). Elementary patterns include anterior wall, posterior wall, anterior column, posterior column and transverse fractures. Associated patterns include both columns, posterior column with posterior wall, transverse column with posterior wall, and T-shaped and anterior column with posterior hemitransverse fractures.

4. Fractures of both columns are the most common type of acetabular injury.

5. Most acetabular fractures occur in the setting of significant trauma secondary to either a motor vehicle accident or a high-velocity fall. Blunt force is exerted on the femur, passes through the femoral head and is transferred to the acetabulum. The direction and magnitude of the force and the position of the femoral head determine the pattern of acetabular injury.

6. Abdominal, pelvic, spinal and cranial injuries are associated.

7. Complications are nerve injury (gluteal, femoral and sciatic nerves), infection, thromboembolism, osteonecrosis, chondrolysis and osteoarthritis.

8. An AP view of the pelvis and oblique views are necessary for acetabular fractures. A CT scan with three-dimensional reconstruction is the most sensitive method for assessment of fractures. This helps in assessing the important components of the fracture, which is useful for surgical planning.

9. Extent of fracture in relation to the columns, walls, dome and quadrilateral plate is assessed on a CT scan. The orientation of the fracture is also assessed.

Case 3.4: Answers

1. The lateral X-ray and sagittal view of the CT scan show decreased density of the vertebrae. There are also moderate wedge compression fractures of T9 , L1 and L2 vertebrae. This is confirmed by MRI, which does not show any soft-tissue mass in the vertebral body, but does show multiple spinal fractures.

2. Osteoporosis with wedge compression spinal fractures.

3. Types of osteoporosis:

Type I: postmenopausal, **Type II**: senile
Idiopathic, **Secondary**

- **Endocrine**: steroids, Cushing's disease, hyperthyroidism, hypogonadism, acromegaly
- **Nutrition**: malabsorption, scurvy, alcoholism
- **Drugs**: heparin, steroids
- **Genetic, metabolic disorders**: osteogenesis imperfecta, Marfan's syndrome, Ehler–Danlos syndrome, homocystinuria, hypophosphatasia, Wilson's disease, alkaptonuria, Menkes syndrome

4. In the spine, the bones are diffusely osteopenic, with resorption of the horizontal trabecula and coarsely thickened vertical trabecula. **Empty box vertebra/picture framing**: increased density of endplates as a result of resorption of spongy bone. Vertebral body compression fractures are very common. They can be wedge, biconcave or true compression fractures. There is no osteophyte formation.

5. MRI is useful for diagnosing osteoporotic fracture in the setting of backache. The most important use is to differentiate a benign osteoporotic fracture from an acute traumatic fracture, or more importantly a malignant fracture. Features of metastatic compression fractures are a convex posterior border of the vertebral body, abnormal signal intensity of the pedicle or posterior element, an epidural mass, an encasing epidural mass, a focal paraspinal mass and other metastases. In osteoporotic compression fracture there is a low signal intensity band in T1 and T2, with normal signal in the body and retropulsion of posterior bone fragment and multiple other fractures.

6. In patients with osteoporosis, bone density is measured to predict the risk of developing fractures which helps in receiving appropriate treatment. This can be done with single photon absorption or dual photon absorption using radionuclide or dual energy X-ray bone densitometry. This can also be done with a CT scan or ultrasonography (calcaneum).

7. Fractures, pain and deformity are the main complications in osteoporosis. Secondary complications are related to immobility due to fractures in the elderly, namely pulmonary thromboembolism and nosocomial infections.

8. In severe osteoporotic compression fracture with pain, percutaneous vertebroplasty is done under fluoroscopic or CT guidance. Vertebroplasty is a procedure aimed at preventing vertebral body collapse by injecting polymethylmethacrylate (PMMA) cement into the vertebral body. Indications are painful compression fractures refractory to conservative therapy. Ideal candidates are those who present within 4 months of fracture, with midline non-radiating back pain increasing with weight bearing, which is exacerbated by palpation of the spine.

Case 3.5: Answers

1. The CT scans of the lumbar spine in axial and sagittal views show a comminuted fracture of the L1 vertebra that is compressed. In the axial view, there is a retropulsion of the bony fragment, which is seen extending into the spinal canal.

2. Burst fracture of a lumbar vertebra.

3. Burst fracture is caused by a fall from a height, which results in axial loading to the intervertebral disc and causes increased nuclear pressure and hoop stresses in the annulus. This in turn causes high shear stress on the vertebral endplate at the inner border of the annulus, away from the disc's centre. It involves compressive failure of the vertebral body with failure of both anterior and middle columns. A large central posterior superior fragment occurs as a result of these forces.

4. Fractures can be classified as isolated process fractures (spinous or transverse process), type A (compression and burst), fracture dislocations (traumatic spondylolisthesis) and Chance fracture. A burst fracture can be stable (no neurological damage, intact posterior arch, < 50% anterior body collapse) or unstable (neurological deficit, > 50% vertebral height loss).

5. The X-ray shows a comminuted vertebral body fracture. There is a loss of height of the vertebral body anteriorly and laterally. L1–3 pedicles are usually comminuted or detached. L4 and L5 pedicles are intact. The cephalad third of the vertebral body is fixed with central retropulsion of bone into the canal. The middle column can be disrupted at L4–5 but, if posterior elements are intact or have only longitudinal fracture, injury is stable.

6. Chance fracture is a distraction injury from anterior hyperflexion across a restraining seatbelt. This results in horizontal splitting of the vertebra, with horizontal disruption of the intervertebral disc and rupture of the ligaments. These patients have associated bowel and colon injuries. Other injuries in the lumbar spine are simple wedge compression fractures, fracture dislocations, transverse process fractures, spinous process fractures and pars interarticularis fractures.

7. Neurological deficit is seen as a result of spinal cord compression. The neurological injuries arising from lumbar burst fractures are less common and have a better prognosis than neurological injuries arising from a thoracolumbar burst fracture. Burst fractures with no neurological damage are managed conservatively with bedrest and bracing of the lumbar spine. A total contact orthosis is worn for 4–6 months. Surgical decompression is indicated for burst fractures with neurological damage.

Case 3.6: Answers

1. There is an oblique fracture of the C7 spinous process.

2. Alignment of the vertebrae on the lateral film is the first aspect to note in a patient with suspected cervical spine injury. The **anterior spinal line** is drawn along the anterior margin of the vertebral bodies and the **posterior spinal line** along the posterior margin. **The spinolaminar**

line is drawn along the junction of laminae and spinous processes. All these lines and the tips of the spinous processes (C2–7) should be aligned. Any malalignment should be considered evidence of ligamentous injury or occult fracture, and cervical spine immobilisation should be maintained until a definitive diagnosis is made.

3. Clay shovellers' fracture

4. Clay shovellers' fracture is a hyperflexion injury, resulting in sudden exertions of muscular attachments. It is a stable injury. It can be seen at C6 or T1.

5. The lateral view of the cervical spine shows an oblique fracture in the spinous process. The other bones and soft tissues are normal. A CT scan is indicated for cervical spine injury if there is suspicion of an unstable injury or neurological deficit. If the avulsion fracture is not limited to the spinous process, but extends into the lamina, there is greater potential for spinal cord injury. A CT scan can rule out associated facet fracture or unilateral jump facet.

6. **Flexion teardrop fracture**: avulsion of anteroinferior quadrant of the vertebral body.

   Simple **wedge fracture, anterior subluxation** and **bilateral facet lock** are other flexion injuries in cervical spine.

7. Clay shovellers' fracture is treated conservatively. A hard collar is worn for at least 10 days. Following this, a cervical collar is worn until good callus has formed.

Case 3.7: Answers

1. The X-ray of the cervical spine shows fracture through C2 with anterior subluxation of C2 on C3 displacement. The CT scan shows fractures through both pedicles of C2 vertebra.

2. Traumatic spondylolisthesis of C2, also called hangman's fracture. Hangman's fracture is a bilateral pedicle fracture of C2, along with distraction of C2 from C3 secondary to complete disruption of the disc

and ligaments between C2 and C3. Traumatic spondylolisthesis differs in the degrees of disc and ligamentous disruption and secondary C2–3 distraction.

3. Hangman's fracture is caused by a combination of hyperextension and distraction. The mechanism of the traumatic spondylolisthesis fracture pattern is primarily hyperextension with varying degrees of axial compression and lateral flexion. Without the primary distraction force, there are varying degrees of disc and ligamentous disruption and secondary C2 displacement.

4. Classification of hangman's fracture:

   Type I fractures: bilateral pedicle fractures with < 3 mm of anterior C2 body displacement and no angulation. The mechanism of this injury is hyperextension with concomitant axial loading and a force sufficient to cause the fracture, but not enough to disrupt the anterior longitudinal ligament (ALL), posterior longitudinal ligament (PLL) or the C2–3 disc. The integrity of the C2–3 disc, ALL and PLL determines the stability of the injury and, with these elements intact, the injury is considered stable. Commonly associated concomitant injuries are C1 posterior arch fractures, C1 lateral mass fractures and odontoid fractures.

   Type II fractures: these demonstrate significant displacement and angulation. The mechanism is hyperextension with concomitant axial loading, followed by flexion with concomitant axial compression, resulting in bilateral pedicle fractures with slight disruption of the ALL and significant disruption of the PLL and C2–3 disc. This injury is considered unstable. A wedge compression fracture of C3 is the most common associated injury.

   Type **IIA fractures**: no anterior displacement, but there is severe angulation. The mechanism for this injury is flexion with concomitant distraction. The resultant injury pattern is bilateral pedicle fractures with C2–3 disc disruption and some degree of insult to the PLL. This is an unstable fracture. X-rays show increased C2–3 interspace.

   Type **III fractures**: these show severe displacement and severe angulation. The mechanism of this injury is flexion with concomitant axial compression. X-rays show bilateral pedicle fractures with C2–3 disc disruption, but also concomitant unilateral or bilateral C2–3 facet dislocations. Varying degrees of injury occur to the ALL and PLL. This is an unstable fracture. A relatively high incidence of mortality and morbidity is noted with this injury, particularly neurological sequelae.

5. Other fractures of C2 are odontoid fractures, lateral mass fractures and extension teardrop fractures.

1. The X-ray shows an oblique fracture through the lateral malleolus, which is seen better in the lateral view.

2. Lateral malleolar fracture of the right ankle.

3. Lateral malleolar fracture classification:

    Weber type A (supination adduction injury):

    – transverse avulsion of malleolus sparing tibiofibular ligaments

    – oblique fracture of medial malleolus

    – posterior tibial tip fracture

    Weber type B (supination abduction injury)

    – oblique/spiral fracture of lateral malleolus

    – lateral subluxation of talus

    – partial disruption of tibiofibular ligament, sprain of deltoid ligament, transverse fracture of medial malleolus

    Weber type C (pronation external rotation): fibular fracture, higher than ankle joint, deltoid ligament tear, medial malleolar fracture, tear of tibiofibular ligament, tear of interosseus membrane.

    Dupuytren's fracture: fracture of distal fibula above a disrupted tibiofibular ligament, disruption of deltoid ligament

    LeFort fracture: vertical fracture of anteromedial fracture of distal fibula, avulsion of anterior tibiofibular ligament.

4. Other fractures in the ankle are:

    Tillaux's fracture: avulsion of anterior tibial tubercle at site of attachment of distal anterior tibiofibular ligament

    Masionneuve's fracture: spiral fracture of upper third of fibula, fracture of medial malleolus, with rupture of deep deltoid ligament, tear of distal tibiofibular syndesmosis and interosseus membrane.

5. As in the above case, treatment of a stable, spiral fracture of lateral malleolus is by simple plaster cast. Unstable fractures require close or open reduction and internal fixation.

Case 3.9: Answers

1. The X-ray of the right shoulder joint shows absence of superior part of humeral head and there is increased sclerosis of the bone margin, which is sharp in outline. The humerus has subluxed out of the shoulder joint. Tiny bone fragments are also noted within the joint.

2. Charcot's joint (neuropathic joint).

3. Neuropathic joint is a traumatic arthritis resulting from loss of sensation and proprioception. There are two theories of formation:

    (a) loss of sensation which leads to repetitive trauma and joint destruction

    (b) loss of neural stimuli which leads to loss of sympathetic tone, resulting in vasodilatation and hyperaemia and then in bone resorption.

4. The causes are:

    Congenital: myelomeningocele, congenital insensitivity to pain, Riley–Day syndrome, Charcot–Marie–Tooth disease

    Central neuropathy: brain/cord injury, syringomyelia, syphilis, spinal tumours, infections, cord compression, MS, alcoholism

    Peripheral neuropathy: diabetes mellitus, peripheral nerve injury/tumour, leprosy, polio

    Other: Raynaud's phenomenon, scleroderma, rheumatoid, psoriasis, amyloid, uraemia, pernicious anaemia, pain-relieving drugs, steroids.

5. There are two types: atrophic and hypertrophic:

    Atrophic: most common; osseous resorption, non-weight-bearing joints of upper extremity; usually caused by syringomyelia, peripheral nerve lesion

    Hypertrophic: joint destruction, fragmentation, sclerosis, osteophytes

    Mixed pattern

Musculoskeletal Answers

6. The joints are dislocated and deformed, with degeneration and destruction of articular cortex. Dense subchondral bone is seen as a result of sclerosis and debris as a result of loose bodies. Usually the joints are painless. Joint changes are seen before a neurological deficit manifests. Rapid resorption and fractures are seen. Soft-tissue and vascular calcifications are also seen. Deformities such as licked-candy-stick phalanx and scoliosis may be present.

7. Differential diagnoses for atrophic type: septic arthritis, surgical amputation. Differential diagnoses for hypertrophic type: degenerative joint disease, synovial osteochondromatosis.

8. The causes of neuropathic joint differ, based on the location:

    Shoulder: syringomyelia, cord injury

    Hands and feet: leprosy

    Foot and ankle: diabetes, syphilis

    Spine: spinal injury, syphilis, diabetes, congenital insensitivity to pain, amyloidosis.

Case 3.10: Answers

1. The CT scan shows large, hypodense, rim-enhancing lesions in both psoas muscles, which are enlarged. There are areas of calcification within the left psoas collection

2. Bilateral psoas abscess.

3. The causes of psoas abscess are as follows:

    Primary: immunosuppression, HIV, chronic illness, diabetes, malignancy, drug use

    Secondary: vertebral infections – TB; pyogenic infections

    Bowel infection: Crohn's disease, ulcerative colitis, infective colitis, diverticulitis, appendicitis

    Urinary infection.

4. The most common organisms is *Staph. aureus. Streptococcus pyogenes* and *E. coli* are the other organisms. In secondary psoas abscess, *E. coli* and *Bacteroides* spp. predominate in a mixed culture.

5. Patients present with abdominal pain, back pain, leg pain, flexion deformity and a lump in the groin. On examination, there is fixed flexion deformity of the hip. A lump may be palpable in the inguinal region as a result of extension of abscess to the groin.

6. Ultrasonography shows enlarged psoas and hypoechoic collection in it, with internal echoes. The CT scan with contrast shows a hypodense lesion with rim enhancement. Adjacent bones should be examined for source of infection. The bowel may be inflamed. MRI shows low-signal lesion in T1, high signal in T2 and rim enhancement.

7. Septic arthritis of the hip is a complication. The iliopsoas bursa communicates with the hip joint. Infection can spread to the spine.

8. Intravenous antibiotics are administered after culture of the abscess. Antibiotics are given to cover staphylococci for primary abscess and broad-spectrum antibiotics for an aerobic or anaerobic secondary abscess. Percutaneous drainage is done under CT or ultrasound guidance. Antibiotics are continued until there is no drainage or the fever subsides.

Case 3.11: Answers

1. The X-ray of the left shoulder shows a subtle area of lucency and patchy areas of sclerosis in the head of the left humerus. The joint space is normal.

2. This is MRI of the shoulder, obtained after contrast administration. There is intense, patchy contrast enhancement in the bones and surrounding soft tissues.

3. Acute osteomyelitis.

4. Acute osteomyelitis is an infection of bone, usually caused by *Staphylococcus aureus.*

Children younger than 1 year: group B *Streptococcus* spp., *Staphylococcus aureus, Haemophilus influenzae* and *Escherichia coli*.

Children older than 1 year: *S. aureus, E. coli, H. influenzae, Serratia marcescens*, and *Pseudomonas aeruginosa*.

Older children and adults: group A streptococcus, *H. influenzae*, enterobacteria.

In children, infection is usually acquired through the haematogenous or exogenous route. It is common in long bones, starting in the metaphyseal sinusoidal veins resulting in focal oedema which leads to local tissue necrosis, breakdown of the trabecular bone structure, and removal of bone matrix and calcium. Infection spreads along the Haversian canals, through the marrow cavity, and beneath the periosteal layer of the bone. Subsequent vascular damage causes the ischaemic death of osteocytes, leading to the formation of a sequestrum. Periosteal new-bone formation on top of the sequestrum is known as involucrum. In adults, infection follows open fractures or due to contamination following joint replacement or open reduction of fractures.

5. Clinically there is bone pain, fever, malaise, irritability, restricted limb movement, swelling, tenderness, warmth and regional lymphadenopathy.

6. X-rays are normal in the earlier stages. Subtle soft tissue swelling and displacement of fat planes can be noted. In 10–14 days, a longitudinal lucent destructive lesion with areas of sclerosis and periosteal reaction is seen. Three-phase ^{99m}Tc diphosphonate bone scan (perfusion, blood pool, static) is very sensitive and are positive after 24 hours of onset and show a well-defined focus of tracer uptake in all the phases. It is useful when looking at multifocal sites of osteomyelitis. The uptake on 3-phase bone scans is related to blood flow and osteoblastic activity. ^{111}In- or Tc-labelled leukocytes are very specific in localising infections. Ultrasound can show a hypoechoic collection close to the bone, earlier than X-ray detection. MRI is also a very sensitive tool. Osteomyelitis is seen as low signal in T1 and high signal in T2. MRI is useful in assessing the extent of osteomyelitis and subperisoteal abscess. The inflammatory component enhances on contrast while necrotic pus does not. CT can also detect osteomyelitis earlier than X-ray, but is typically used in chronic osteomyelitis.

7. Differential diagnoses include osteosarcoma, Ewing's sarcoma, lymphoma, sickle cell disease crisis, Gaucher's disease, septic arthritis and juvenile arthritis. Complications are chronic osteomyelitis, metastatic infection, septic arthritis caused by the transphyseal spread of the infection, angular

deformity of bones resulting from arrest of bone growth, pathological fractures, bacteraemia, septicaemia, soft-tissue infection, persistent sinuses and premature epiphyseal fusion.

8. Antibiotics should be started in children after blood culture has been taken. Complete resolution may be expected if antibiotics are started before 48 hours. If diagnosis is made after 48 hours and patient is symptomatic, surgical drainage of pus is indicated.

Case 3.12: Answers

1. The X-ray the right leg shows extensive intramedullary sclerosis, in the distal femoral metaphysis. There is periosteal reaction with Codman's triangle and considerable soft tissue swelling.

2. Osteosarcoma of the right femur.

3. Osteosarcoma is a malignant tumour that arises from undifferentiated mesenchyme, which forms neoplastic immature bone. It has a bimodal age distribution: 10–25 years and > 60 years. Clinical features are sudden onset of pain, swelling, redness, fever, elevation of alkaline phosphatase (ALP) and diabetes mellitus (paraneoplastic syndrome). It is usually seen in the long bones, in the metaphysis.

4. Osteosarcoma is commonly seen in leg bones, with 50–55% seen around the knee joint. It is located within the metaphysis and can extend into other areas. It is very aggressive, with ill-defined tumour margins. The lesion shows extensive areas of new bone formation or lytic areas of moth-eaten or permeative bone destruction. Periosteal reaction produces sunburst, hair-on-end or onion-peel appearance. Codman's triangle and soft tissue mass with new bone formation are seen. A bone scan shows high uptake. A CT scan can demonstrate the new bone formation. MRI shows the extent or marrow involvement, soft tissue involvement, joints and viable tumour for biopsy. Chest X-ray is done for metastasis. Lung metastasis can ossify or cavitate and can produce pneumothorax. Skeletal metastasis is uncommon.

5. Complications are pathological fracture and radiation-induced osteosarcoma, and pneumothorax due to lung metastases.

6. Acute osteomyelitis, sclerosing chronic osteomyelitis and Charcot's joint are the differential diagnoses. Acute osteomyelitis has a similar clinical presentation to osteosarcoma, but extensive new bone formation is not seen.

7. Variants of osteosarcoma:

   Parosteal osteosarcoma: outer layer of periosteum, slow growing, fulminating course once it reaches medulla

   Periosteal osteosarcoma: deep layer of periosteum

   Secondary type: from Paget's disease, irradiation, osteonecrosis, fibrous dysplasia, osteogenesis imperfect, chronic osteomyelitis, retinoblastoma

   Telangiectactic: aneurysmal expansion of bone

   Osteosarcomatosis: multifocal

   Low-grade intraosseous

   High-grade surface

   Extraskeletal osteosarcoma.

8. Metastasis, soft-tissue mass > 20 cm, pathological fractures and skip lesions are bad prognostic indicators. Treatment is by chemotherapy followed by wide surgical resection.

Case 3.13: Answers

1. This is an MRI of the knee, which shows a normal appearing posterior cruciate ligament. However, the anterior cruciate ligament (ACL) is not seen in its normal location.

2. Complete tear of the ACL.

3. ACL injuries occur when landing after a jump. ACL tears occur with or without contact and with the knee in any position from flexed to fully extended. The most common contact mechanism of injury is the valgus/abduction 'clip' injury. These injuries are common in football players and occur with a lateral blow to the partially flexed knee. Hyperextension or varus hyperextension from an anterior blow and pivot shift injury are other

mechanisms. Predisposing factors include joint laxity, large Q angle (angle between a line joining the anterosuperior iliac spine and the midpoint of the patella and a line joining the mid-point of the patella to the tibial tubercle) and narrow intercondylar notch.

4. The ACL originates from the posteromedial aspect of the lateral femoral condyle and courses through the lateral intercondylar notch in an anterior, inferior and medial direction. It inserts on the tibia approximately 2–3 mm posterior to the anterior edge of the tibia, just anterior and lateral to the medial intercondylar eminence (tibial spine).

5. Medial and lateral meniscal injuries, medial and lateral collateral ligament injuries, posterior cruciate ligament injuries, posterolateral corner structure injuries and second fractures are associated. Pain, a snapping or popping sound, giving out of the knee, swelling, loss of knee motion and the ability to continue sport are common symptoms of ACL injury.

6. MRI is useful for confirming the tear and assessing whether it is partial or complete and to find associated injuries that alter the prognosis. The primary signs of an ACL tear are disruption, increased signal intensity in the substance of the ACL on T2-weighted images, abrupt angulation or wavy appearance, and abnormal ACL axis. The axis of the ACL is abnormal if it is more horizontal than a line through the intercondylar roof (Blumensaat's line) on sagittal images.

7. Lachman's test and the anterior drawer test are the most useful in diagnosis of ACL injuries. Slocum's test and the pivot shift test are other tests.

8. In non-athletes, non-surgical treatment with rehabilitation physiotherapy is appropriate. Surgical reconstruction is essential in athletes for restoration of function and prevents long-term complications. Patellar tendon, hamstring tendon, quadriceps tendon and Achilles' tendon are some of the tendon grafts used for ACL reconstruction. Intensive physiotherapy is required to restore hamstring proprioception.

Case 3.14: Answers

1. The first X-ray shows hallux valgus, vascular calcification and subtle increased density in the second metatarsal bone. In the second X-ray, there has been marked resorption of the heads of the second to fifth metatarsals and mild resorption of the first metatarsal. There are multiple loose bodies seen within the metatarsophalangeal (MTP) joints.

2. Diabetic foot.

3. Of people with diabetes 25% develop foot problems. Diabetic foot is a combination of peripheral arterial disease, neuropathy (**sensory** – loss of pain and protective reflexes; **autonomic** – decreased sweat, thick skin, increased vascularity resulting from sympathetic imbalance; **motor** – altered weight distribution causes ulcers at pressure points).

4. Gas in the soft tissue, ulcer, sinus tracts, fractures, cellulitis, abscess, osteomyelitis, neuropathic joints, septic arthritis and gangrene are pathological changes. Deformities and neuropathic changes are seen in the midfoot.

5. Radiographic change in diabetic feet are due to a combination of neuropathy and infection. On X-ray, vascular calcification is seen. Antibiotic impregnated pellets can also be visualised. Ulcer is noted as a soft tissue defect. Gas may be seen in soft tissue. There is increased risk of fractures due to stress and altered biomechanics. Fracture may be in advanced stage by the time of diagnosis. MRI shows soft tissue and bone marrow oedema, with low signal in T1 and high signal in T2, with no contrast enhancement. In a chronic neuropathic joint, toes, midfoot and ankle are affected. Mid-tarsal joints are the most commonly affected joints. Changes can be hypertrophic or atrophic. In the hypertrophic type there is bone destruction, fragmentation, loose bodies, disorganisation, debris and effusion. High uptake is seen on a bone scan. No enhancement is seen in MRI or CT scan, which differentiates it from infection (which shows intense enhancement). Atrophic neuropathic changes may manifest as complete resorption of metatarsal heads with bone tapering (licked candy appearance). Osteomyelitis results from contiguous spread. First and fifth metatarsal heads are most commonly affected. Plain X-ray is positive after 10–21 days. Increased uptake is seen in bone scan, gallium scan and ^{111}In-leukocyte labelled scan. MRI shows low signal in T1, high signal in T2, with contrast enhancement. Cortical erosion and soft tissue oedema are

Musculoskeletal Answers

also seen. Chronic osteomyelitis shows a mixture of bone destruction and remodelling. Septic arthritis is common in MTP and IP joints. Joint effusion, osteopenia, marginal sclerosis, bone erosion and joint space narrowing are seen. Abscess is seen as a focal collection. MRI shows rim enhancement.

6. Imaging is tailored according to the individual patient's symptoms. Clinical assessment and high quality plain films play an important role in diagnosis. Plain film demonstrates osteomyelitis, soft tissue gas, ulcers, neuropathic joints, antibiotic pellets and deformities. Bone scan is not specific and shows increased uptake both in infection and neuropathic joints. ^{111}In-labelled leukocytes show high uptake in infection. CT scan detects soft tissue gas, periosteal reaction and sequestra. MRI is used to assess extent of infection.

Case 3.15: Answers

1. Sagittal T1 and fat-suppressed images show a high signal within the posterior horn of the medial meniscus, which is seen extending to the inferior articular surfaces.

2. Medial meniscus tear.

3. The medial meniscus is crescentic, occupies 50% of the articular contact of medial joint compartment, is C shaped, with the limbs of the C facing centrally, its superior surface is concave and it has a posterior horn body and anterior horn. The attachment of the medial meniscus to the joint capsule is more rigid than the lateral meniscus, making it susceptible to injury. The medial meniscus transmits 40–50% of the axial load of the medial compartment. It is anchored to the tibia via the meniscotibial ligament.

4. Medial meniscal injury is produced by compressive force coupled with rotation of the flexed knee as it starts to move into extension. During internal rotation of the femur on the tibia with knee in flexion, the femur tends to position the medial meniscus posteriorly toward the centre of the knee joint. The posterior part of the meniscus is caught between the femur and tibia, and torn longitudinally when the joint is suddenly extended. Clinically, the knee gives way with clicking, locking and limping. McMurray's test and the Apley–Grinding test are positive.

5. Types of tears:

Longitudinal tears: horizontal cleavage, bucket handle, peripheral

Oblique tears: parrot beak, flap

Transverse/radial tear

Meniscocapsular separation.

6. MRI is the mainstay in the diagnosis of meniscal tears. A normal meniscus is seen as a dark structure on T1- and T2-weighted images. High signal in the meniscus can be seen as a result of degenerative changes or vascularity. A meniscal signal can be classified into three types:

Type I: punctate high signal completely within the meniscus, indicating mild to moderate degenerative process.

Type II: horizontal linear area of increased signal intensity that extends to, but does not involve, the articular surface which indicates severe degenerative process, but not a tear.

Type III: abnormal signal intensity within the meniscus extending to one or both articular surfaces, the hallmark of a meniscal tear.

When torn, the menisci have an abnormal shape. The tear direction can be seen in images as oblique, horizontal or longitudinal. In bucket-handle tear, there is a longitudinal vertical tear with the inner fragment unstable and displaced medially into the joint compartment. Traumatic tears are often vertical longitudinal tears, but degenerative tears are usually horizontal cleavage tears or flaps. Meniscal cysts, adjacent bone marrow changes and degenerative changes may be associated.

7. Differential diagnoses: normal structures mimicking tear on MRI, such as meniscofemoral ligaments, transverse ligament, superior recess on posterior horn of medial meniscus and popliteal hiatus. A healed meniscus with a persistent high signal, degenerative changes and discoid meniscus are other differential diagnoses.

8. The posterior horn is involved in 60%, the body in 18% and the entire meniscus in 22%. Stable tears (partial thickness, oblique tears, 10 mm, stable radial tears < 5 mm) are treated conservatively. Arthroscopic partial meniscectomy is done for complicated tears.

Case 3.16: Answers

1. In the sagittal MRI views of the ankle, normal Achilles' tendon (dark structure posteriorly) is seen in the proximal portion. However, there is no normal tendon, for a distance of 10 cm from the level of calcaneum. The tendon sheath is swollen and filled with haemorrhage, which is of intermediate signal in the T1 and heterogeneous in T2 MRI.

2. Complete tear of Achilles' tendon.

3. Achilles' tendon is formed from tendinous contributions of gastrocnemius and soleus, which coalesce, 15 cm proximal to insertion. The tendon spirals 30–150° until it inserts into the calcaneal tuberosity. The tendon has no proper sheath, only a paratendon.

4. Rupture of Achilles' tendon is commonly located in the tendon substance, about 2.5–5 cm above its insertion to the calcaneus. Poor conditioning, advanced age and over-exertion are risk factors. The common precipitating event is a sudden eccentric force applied to a dorsiflexed foot. Risk factors are recreational athlete, age 30–50, prior injury or rupture, prior tendon steroid injections or fluoroquinolone use, abrupt changes in training, intensity or activity, participation in a new activity, gout, SLE and rheumatoid arthritis.

5. Achilles' tear can be complete or incomplete.

6. Ultrasonography is a simple and dynamic examination. A normal Achilles' tendon is seen as a bright echogenic structure in the posterior aspect of the ankle joint. In tears, there is discontinuity. In a partial tear, there are low echoic areas within the tendon, caused by haemorrhage and debris. In a complete tear, there is no continuity. The gap may be filled with haemorrhage or debris. The ankle is then dorsiflexed, when the gap increases. The exact dimension of the gap is measured in plantar and dorsal flexion and marked on the surface. This might be useful when planning surgical repair. MRI shows a normal tendon as a low-intensity structure. The tear is seen as a defect. The tendon is swollen. Occasionally the gap may be filled with debris. In partial tears, the tendon is thickened and there are areas of abnormal signal intensity within the lesion.

7. The differential diagnosis is tendinosis: the tendon is swollen and shows heterogeneous signal within it.

8. Acute ruptures, large partial ruptures and re-ruptures are indications for surgery. Elderly, inactive patients, with systemic illness, are managed without surgery, with a short leg cast and the ankle in plantar flexion. The repair could be open or percutaneous.

Case 3.17: Answers

1. Ultrasonography shows a cystic, anechoic (dark) lesion in the posterior aspect of the knee joint, which communicates superiorly with the knee joint. MRI demonstrates a cystic lesion, showing high signal on T2-weighted images with fat suppression, in the posterior aspect of the knee joint; this communicates with the knee joint and extends between the medial head of gastrocnemius and semimembranosus.

2. Baker's cyst or popliteal cyst.

3. Baker's cyst is a synovial cyst in the posterior aspect of the knee joint, communicating with the joint capsule. It is caused by synovial effusion into one of the bursae with trapping of the fluid by a one-way valve mechanism. There are two types of valves: the **Bunsen value**, where the expanding cyst compresses the communicating channel, and the **ball type**, which is composed of fibrin and cellular debris plugging the communication channel. The cyst functions as a protective mechanism, reducing destructive pressure of effusion in the joint.

4. The most common location is in the gastrocnemius semimembranosa bursa, which is situated posterior to the medial femoral condyle between the tendons of the medial head of gastrocnemius and semimembranous. This communicates with the joint through a slit-like opening at the posteromedial aspect of the knee capsule just superior to the joint line. Occasionally, fluid collects in the superolateral bursa between the lateral head of gastrocnemius and the distal end of biceps, or in the popliteal bursa beneath the lateral meniscus.

5. Causes include rheumatoid or degenerative arthritis, gout, psoriasis, SLE, pigmented villonodular synovitis or internal derangements of the knee (meniscal/ligament tear), infection, haemophilia, chronic dialysis, hypothyroidism and sarcoidosis.

6. An intact cyst, dissected cyst (cyst extending along fascial planes between gastrocnemius and soleus) and ruptured cyst are the various types of Baker's cyst.

7. An X-ray can show soft-tissue mass, and degenerative changes in the knee joint. Ultrasonography is the most useful imaging technique for evaluation of a popliteal cyst. The cyst is a well-defined anechoic structure with posterior acoustic enhancement, which communicates with the knee. Internal debris can be seen when the cyst is complicated. Colour Doppler ultrasonography is useful in assessing for vascular flow and excluding popliteal artery aneurysm. CT is as good as ultrasonography and useful for finding bony fragments and mass effect, wall thickening and bone erosion. MRI shows the cyst with low signal intensity on T1- and high signal on T2-weighted images. It demonstrates the communication with the joint capsule more easily than other imaging techniques and differentiates it from cystic tumours.

8. Rupture of dissection (pseudothrombophlebitis syndrome), haemorrhage, infection, posterior compartment syndrome and trapped calcified bodies are the primary complications. Compression on the popliteal vein may result in deep vein thrombosis (DVT) and complications related to DVT.

9. Differential diagnoses: meniscal cyst (close to joint line), tibiofibular cyst (close to tibiofibular joint), ganglion cyst (surrounds cruciate ligaments), popliteal artery aneurysm, cystic tumours (neurilemmoma, myxoid liposarcoma) and traumatic tear of gastrocnemius,

10. Conservative treatment is with NSAIDs, ice and assisted weight bearing, and correction of underlying intra-articular disorders. Radioactive synovio-orthosis is used for inflammatory arthritis and haemophilia. The cyst is excised when it is unresponsive to all therapies.

1. The X-ray shows a fracture dislocation through the base of the metatarsals. The lateral border of the first metatarsal is not aligned with the lateral border of the medial cuneiform bone. The medial border of the second metatarsal bone is not aligned with the medial border of the intermediate cuneiform bone. The medial and lateral borders of the third metatarsal are not aligned with the medial and lateral borders of the lateral cuneiform bone. The lateral part of the fifth metatarsal is projecting far beyond the margin of the cuboid bone.

2. Lisfranc's fracture dislocation.

3. Lisfranc's fracture dislocation is the most common dislocation of the foot. Lisfranc's joints are tarsometatarsal joints. Lisfranc's fracture dislocation is caused by falling from a height, falling down stairs or stepping off a curb Mechanisms of injury are rotation around a fixed forefoot (eg falling from a horse with the foot caught in the stirrup) or longitudinal compression of a foot. In this second mechanism, the metatarsal head is fixed, with the weight of the body on the hindfoot against the base of metatarsals along with rotation; these forces result in a distal dorsal dislocation of the metatarsal. It can be seen in parachute jumpers.

4. On the AP view, the lateral border of the first metatarsal should be aligned with the lateral border of the medial cuneiform, and the medial border of the second metatarsal with the medial border of the intermediate cuneiform bone. On the oblique view, the medial and lateral borders of the third metatarsal should be aligned with the medial and lateral borders of the lateral cuneiform bone and the medial border of the fourth metatarsal with the medial border of the cuboid bone. The fourth and fifth metatarsals are aligned with the cuboid bone, but the lateral part of the fifth metatarsal can project beyond the margin of the cuboid bone, up to 3 mm.

5. Lisfranc's dislocation consists of dorsal dislocation of the tarsometatarsal joints:

Homolateral dislocation: lateral dislocation of the first or second to fifth metatarsals.

Divergent dislocation: lateral dislocation of the second to fifth metatarsals and medial dislocation of the first metatarsal.

Lateral displacement is associated with cuboid fractures. Isolated dislocations involve one or two metatarsals displaced from the others. The fracture at the base of the second metatarsal or anterior aspect of the cuboid may be the most obvious indication of Lisfranc's injury.

6. Treatment is by closed reduction with percutaneous pinning or open reduction with internal fixation.

Case 3.19: Answers

1. The right humeral head overlaps the glenoid and is situated medially under the coracoid process

2. Anterior dislocation of the shoulder.

3. Anterior dislocation accounts for 97% of all shoulder dislocations. It is caused by indirect force, such as abduction, extension and posteriorly directed force applied to the arm. The humeral head is driven anteriorly, tearing the shoulder capsule, detaching the labrum from the glenoid and producing a compression fracture of the humeral head. The humeral head lies inferior and medial to the glenoid in the subcoracoid region.

4. The X-ray of the shoulder includes AP, transaxillary and axial views. On an AP view, the anterior dislocated head of the humerus is lodged under the coracoid process. In the normal axillary or the scapular Y view, the humeral head is seen in the glenoid. On the axial view, the golf ball of the humeral head lies within the T of the glenoid. On anterior shoulder dislocation, the humeral head is anterior to the scapula in the axillary view and anterior to the glenoid rim on the axial view.

5. **Posterior dislocation** is produced as a result of direct force, such as seizures and electric shock. On an AP view the humerus may be normal, or it may resemble a light bulb or ice-cream cone, depending on the degree of rotation. The axillary view demonstrates the dislocation better. A Hill–Sachs lesion and Bankart's lesion result from the humerus striking the inferior rim of the glenoid. **Hill–Sachs** defect is seen in the posterolateral aspect of the humeral head. **Bankart's** lesion is seen in the anteroinferior glenoid rim. Both these lesions predispose to recurrent shoulder dislocations and labral injuries.

6. The dislocated shoulder should be reduced as soon as possible and rested in a sling for 10 days. Prolonged immobilisation does not appear to alter the incidence of recurrent dislocation. Complications are mainly due to palsy of axillary and suprascapular nerves (5%) and recurrent dislocation of the shoulder, particularly in the younger age group.

Case 3.20: Answers

1. The X-ray shows a comminuted fracture of the tibial plateau. The CT scan in coronal and sagittal views show a split, comminuted fracture with depression of the lateral tibial plateau.

2 **Schatzker's classification** is commonly used for tibial plateau fractures:

Type I: lateral split

Type II: split with depression

Type III: pure lateral depression

Type IV: pure medial depression

Type V: bicondylar

Type VI: extension to metaphysis.

3. The most common type is type II.

4. The mechanism of injury depends on the type:

Type I: valgus stress in younger patients, with strong bones resistant to depression, often resulting from a bumper injury

Type II: split depression of the lateral tibial plateau, caused by valgus or axial stress; seen in older patients whose osteoporotic bones do not resist depression

Type III: seen in older patients with osteoporosis, after a fall

Type IV: medial fracture; can be a split or split depression type, caused by varus stress

Type V: split of both medial and lateral tibial plateaus; metaphysis is still in continuity with the diaphysis; caused by pure axial stress with severe trauma

Type VI: metaphyseal fracture that separates the articular surface from diaphysis and involves medial, lateral or both articular surfaces; caused by high energy trauma.

5. Associated complications are:

Type I: can be associated with lateral meniscal injury

Type II: associated with meniscal injuries and medial collateral ligament injury

Type III: associated with joint instability if depressed fragments are posterior and lateral

Type IV: associated with avulsion of intercondylar eminence, injury to anterior cruciate ligament/lateral collateral ligament/peroneal nerve/popliteal artery

Type V: associated with neurovascular, ACL and meniscal injuries

Type V: associated with neurovascular injury, compartment injury, meniscal, ACL and collateral ligament injuries.

6. A CT scan with coronal and sagittal reconstructions is vital for assessing the type of fracture and determining the optimal treatment.

7. CT scan is used to assess the degree of displacement, degree of comminution, open/closed status of fracture, and associated soft-tissue/ligamentous/neurovascular injuries.

8. Treatment of tibial plateau fractures

Type I: lateral fixation

Type II: lateral fixation, with elevation of depressed bone fragments and support with a bone graft

Type III: if there is instability, the fractured fragments are elevated and supported with a bone graft and lateral internal fixation

Type IV: medial plate and screws

Types V and VI: medial and lateral internal fixation.

Case 3.21: Answers

1. There is a fracture at the neck of the fifth metacarpal, with deformity due to angulation of the distal fragment.

---

2. Boxers' fracture.

---

3. Boxers' fracture (brawlers' fracture) is a fracture of the neck of the fifth metacarpal bone, caused by a direct blow with a clenched fist.

---

4. Transverse fracture of the distal metacarpal neck, usually in the fifth metacarpal bone. The distal fracture fragment is volarly angulated and may be externally rotated.

---

5. Only the collateral ligaments remain attached to the proximal phalanx and the metacarpal head is freed from any proximal stabilising influence. The metacarpal head tilts volarly, causing the joint to lie in hyperextension and collateral ligaments become lax. If the joint is allowed to remain in hyperextension, collateral ligaments will shorten, leading to limited metacarpophalangeal (MCP) flexion. Clawing results from palmar displacement of the metacarpal head. Closed or open reduction is performed.

Case 3.22: Answers

1. The X-ray shows a fracture in the proximal shaft of the ulna with anterior dislocation of radial head. No fracture of the radius is seen.

---

2. Monteggia's fracture.

---

3. Monteggia's fracture is a fracture of the ulnar shaft with dislocation of the radial head. The mechanism is a direct blow, hyperpronation and hyperextension.

---

4. There are four types (**Bado's classification**):

298 Surgical Radiology: Clinical Cases

Type I: classic Monteggia – anteriorly angulated proximal ulnar fracture, with anterior dislocation of the radial head

Type II: reverse Monteggia – dorsally angulated ulnar fracture with dorsal dislocation of the radial head

Type III: ulnar metaphyseal fracture with anterior dislocation of the radial head

Type IV: fracture of proximal ulna and radius at same level with anterior displacement of the radial head.

For radial dislocation, a line drawn through the radial shaft and head should align with the capitellum in any position if the radial head is in the normal position.

5. Galeazzi's fracture is caused by fall on an outstretched hand with the elbow flexed. There is a radial shaft fracture and dislocation of the distal radioulnar joint.

6. Complications are non-union, limitation of movement and nerve abnormalities (posterior interosseus nerve palsy). In children fracture may be amenable to close reduction but in majority cases and adults, open reduction and fixation of fracture is necessary.

Case 3.23: Answers

1. The X-ray of the pelvis shows a fracture of the left acetabulum. The left femoral head is externally rotated and not contained in the acetabular cavity; it appears smaller than the right femoral head.

2. Left hip dislocation.

3. Hip dislocation can be posterior, anterior or central. **Posterior hip dislocation** is the most common and results from dashboard injury where the flexed knee strikes against the dashboard. It is associated with fractures to the acetabular rim and femoral head. **Anterior hip dislocation** constitutes 5–10% of all hip dislocations; it is uncommon and characterised by anterior obturator dislocation or superoanterior/pubic dislocation. It is associated with fractures of the acetabular rim, greater trochanter, femoral neck and femoral head, which have

characteristic depression on posterosuperior and lateral portions. A central acetabular fracture dislocation is caused by force applied to the lateral side of the trochanter.

4. **Thompson–Epstein** classification is based on radiological findings:

Type 1: with or without minor fracture

Type 2: with large single fracture of the posterior acetabular rim

Type 3: with comminution of rim of acetabulum, with or without major fragments

Type 4: with fracture of the acetabular floor

Type 5: with fracture of the femoral head.

X-rays for hip dislocation include AP, Judet's, and inlet and outlet views. On an AP view, the femoral head appears smaller than normal in posterior dislocation and larger in anterior dislocation. The exact location of the femoral head is identified. Loose fragments can be assessed. A CT scan is helpful for diagnosing loose bodies and fragments that impede closed reduction and evaluating acetabular injuries. Loose bodies, soft-tissue injury and post-reduction widening are best assessed on a CT scan.

5. Complications are sciatic nerve damage, failure to reduce and recurrent dislocation. Treatment is with closed reduction under general anaesthesia. Surgical reduction is done when closed reduction fails or bony fragments or soft tissue in the joint prevents reduction when the joint is unstable.

Case 3.24: Answers

1. The X-ray shows a comminuted fracture in the calcaneum.

2. The CT scan with axial and sagittal reconstruction shows a comminuted fracture of the calcaneum, which extends superiorly to the articular surface of the subtalar joint (talocalcaneal joint).

3. Calcaneal fracture.

4. Calcaneal fracture is the most commonly fractured tarsal bone. It is commonly caused by a fall from heights and axial loading. In adults 75%

fractures are intra-articular, but, in children, most are extra-articular. Intra-articular fractures have a shear line and a compression line. Shear fracture occurs in the sagittal plane and runs through the posterior facet, dividing it into anteromedial and posterolateral fragments. A compression line runs in the coronal plane and extends medially to split the middle facet and the anteromedial fragment. Of the fractures 75% involve the subtalar joint and 10% are bilateral. Extra-articular fractures account for 25% of fractures not involving the posterior facet. Associated fractures are burst fractures of the spine and pylon fractures of the distal tibia.

5. In addition to the AP and lateral views of the foot, an axial view is done for complete evaluation of the calcaneum. On X-ray, a comminuted fracture is visualised, but subtle fractures may not be visible and may be missed. Bohler's angle is produced by intersection of a line drawn from the most cephalic point of the tuberosity to the highest point of the posterior facet with the line from the latter to the most cephalic part of posterior process of calcaneus. Normally it is between 20 and 40°. In calcaneal fracture, the angle is decreased below 20°. The apex of the lateral talar process does not point to the critical angle of Gissane.

6. A CT scan is very useful for accurate characterisation of the fracture. Axial images are acquired and the images are reconstructed in the coronal and sagittal planes. The features are: loss of height of calcaneum, increase in width due to lateral displacement of the tuberosity and disruption of posterior facet of subtalar joint. Tendon entrapment can be assessed.

Sanders' classification has surgical significance and prognostic value:

Type I: non-displaced fracture

Type II: two articular pieces, involve posterior facet

Type III: three part fracture

Type IV: four or more articular fragments.

CT gives an idea of the number of fracture lines that must be reduced. It indicates the size of the sustentacular fragment, since the calcaneus is rebuilt in reference to the sustentacular fragment. CT also shows location and plane of variable fracture lines separating the anterolateral fragment. The precise location of the lateral wall, in relation to lateral malleolus and peroneal tendons, is also appreciated on a CT scan.

7. Type I requires no surgery. Types II and III usually have good results; only 9% of type IV get a good result.

1. AP X-ray shows a transverse fracture of the distal radius. Lateral view shows dorsal displacement of the distal fragment.

2. Colles' fracture

3. Colles' fracture is an extra-articular fracture of the distal radius occurring in elderly individuals. It is caused by a fall onto outstretched hands or forced dorsiflexion of the wrist, when the dorsal surface undergoes compression while the volar surface undergoes tension.

4. The X-ray shows dorsally angulated fracture of the distal radial metaphysis, 2–3 cm proximal to the wrist joint. Ulnar styloid fracture may be associated. The initial fracture line is almost always seen on the volar side. It is associated with a triangular fibrocartilage complex (TFCC) tear.

5. **Smith fracture**: reverse Colles' fracture – distal radius fracture with ventral displacement of the fragment.

    Barton fracture: intra-articular oblique fracture of the ventral/dorsal lip of the distal radius.

    Chaffeurs' fracture (Hutchinson's fracture): triangular fracture of the radial styloid process.

6. Complications are extensor pollicis longus rupture, degenerative arthritis, reflex sympathetic dystrophy, median nerve compression, malunion and distal radioulnar joint injury.

7. Treatment is with closed reduction, percutaneous pinning or open internal reduction. External fixators are rarely necessary. Residual positive ulnar variance >5 mm indicates unsatisfactory outcome. Dorsal angulation or palmar tilt >15° decreases grip strength.

Case 3.26: Answers

1. The X-ray of the right leg shows a well-defined, expansile, multiloculated, lytic lesion arising from the proximal metaphysis of the tibia, causing cortical thinning No periosteal reaction or soft-tissue component is identified. The knee joint appears normal. MRI (T2 weighted) shows high signal intensity lesion in the proximal tibia, suggestive of a fluid containing lesion.

2. Aneurysmal bone cyst

3. An aneurysmal bone cyst is an expansile osteolytic lesion with a thin wall, containing blood-filled cystic cavities. It seen at ages between 5 and 20 years. Pain, swelling and limitation of joint movements are some of the clinical features.

4. Aneurysmal bone cyst can arise secondary to pre-existing bone tumours in 30% of cases, such as chondroblastoma, fibrous dysplasia, giant cell tumour and osteoblastoma.

5. Common locations are in the metaphysis of long tubular bones, and the posterior elements of the spine and pelvis.

6. An aneurysmal bone cyst is usually seen, in the metaphysis, as an expansile, multiloculated (soap bubble), eccentric lesion, with thin intact cortex, resecting epiphyseal plate and no periosteal reaction (unless fractured). Fluid–fluid levels are seen in cystic components. Large lesions can be aggressive similar to lytic metastasis. MRI shows low-to-intermediate signal on T1 and heterogeneous low-to-intermediate signal on T2. High signal on T1 can be seen in acute haemorrhage. A fluid–fluid level is a characteristic finding on MRI and CT. A bone scan shows high uptake in the margin.

7. Fractures can be seen. Periosteal reaction is seen if there is a fracture. Treatment is with surgical resection or curettage. Ethibloc can be injected into the lesion under CT guidance as an alternative to open surgery.

8. Differential diagnoses include **simple bone cyst** (unicameral, located centrally), **giant cell tumour** (seen after epiphyseal fusion,

narrow transition point, may be locally aggressive, may erode into joint), **subarticular geode, Brodie's abscess, benign fibrous histiocytoma, chondroblastoma, haemophilic pseudotumour, expansile neuroblastoma metastasis**. Differential diagnoses of a fluid–fluid level in a bone lesion on MRI include aneurysmal bone cyst, simple bone cyst, chondroblastoma, giant cell tumour, telangiectactic osteosarcoma and fibrous dysplasia.

Case 3.27: Answers

1. The X-ray of the left fibula shows a lytic lesion in the proximal fibula, which is associated with bony destruction, multilamellated periosteal reaction and soft-tissue swelling

2. Ewing's sarcoma of the left fibula

3 Ewing's sarcoma is the second most common primary malignant bone tumour of childhood. It is more common in boys and seen between age 5 and 15. Pain, swelling, tenderness, mass, fever, weight loss and irritability are the common clinical features, and these can mimic a systemic infection

4. It is more common in the lower limbs around the knee in the mid-diaphyseal location. It is also seen in flat bones, especially in older children. Five per cent are seen in vertebrae. In the vertebra, it is seen in posterior elements and occasionally it can be seen purely in extraskeletal soft tissue.

5. The X-ray shows a permeative or moth-eaten pattern of bone destruction with a wide zone of transition, indicating its aggressive nature. It contains both sclerotic and lytic elements. A soft-tissue component is seen and is often very large. It can be seen without visible cortical destruction as a result of the spread through haversian canals. Periosteal reaction is seen and is similar to an onion-skin (lamellated) or spiculated and perpendicular sunburst pattern. Codman's triangle is seen as a result of elevation of the periosteum and central destruction of the periosteal reaction caused by the tumour. A CT scan demonstrates the destructive lesion and soft-tissue component and delineates the accurate extent of the mass. MRI shows low signal on T1 and high signal on T2. Accurate delineation of the intramedullary extent is best seen on T1. After treatment, bone marrow shows low signal resulting from fibrosis. A high signal is seen on a bone scan. Metastasis is seen in 25%. A PET (positron emission tomography) scan is very sensitive in diagnosis and follow-up of the therapeutic response.

6. Differential diagnoses of an aggressive lesion with periosteal reaction and soft-tissue swelling in long bones include acute osteomyelitis, metastatic neuroblastoma, leukaemia, osteosarcoma, fibrosarcoma, lymphoma and eosinophilic granuloma. It might be difficult to differentiate from acute osteomyelitis, which also has Codman's triangle, destruction and soft-tissue swelling. Osteosarcoma has an osseous matrix.

7. Bad prognostic factors are male sex, age > 12 years, anaemia and elevated LDH.

8. As most patients have occult metastatic disease at the time of presentation, treatment consists of neoadjuvant chemotherapy followed by wide or radical excision with or without radiotherapy.

Case 3.28: Answers

1. The X-ray shows multiple, punched-out lytic lesions of varying sizes in the skull. The X-ray of the lumbar spine shows osteopenia and mild compression fractures of several vertebral bodies.

2. Multiple myeloma.

3. Multiple myeloma is the most common primary malignant neoplasm of bone in adults. It is caused by monoclonal neoplastic proliferation of plasma cells, which produces immunoglobulins. These proliferate in the marrow and subsequently spread to the bones, causing destructive bone lesions.

4. Myeloma can be disseminated or focal (< 2%). The disseminated form can be seen anywhere in the axial skeleton and anywhere where there is red marrow, although it is more common in the vertebrae, ribs and skull. Solitary plasmacytoma is seen in the vertebrae, pelvis, skull, sternum and ribs.

5. The clinical features are bone pain, renal insufficiency, proteinuria, hypercalcaemia, Bences Jones proteinuria, normochromic/normocytic anaemia and increased globulin production.

6. Radiological features are:

Diffusely low density bones with coarse trabecular pattern (15%). Punched out lesions with endosteal scalloping and uniform size is a pathognomonic finding. Expansile osteolytic lesions, soft-tissue mass adjacent to the bone lesion and involvement of the mandible are other features. Spine lesions: interspersed on a background of osteopenia, soft-tissue mass, do not involve pedicles first as in metastasis. Sclerosis: can be focal or diffuse, may be seen after chemo- or radiotherapy and may be the main presentation (3%). Often a skeletal survey is performed to detect myelomatous foci in the bones. Bone marrow: isotope bone scan is negative unless the tumour is sclerotic or there is a pathological fracture. MRI can be done to scan all the bones of the axial and appendicular skeleton for myelomatous involvement. MRI is also used to evaluate cord compression.

7. Differential diagnoses:

Diffuse osteopenic form: postmenopausal osteoporosis (it is difficult to exclude myeloma in a patient with diffuse osteoporosis), hyperparathyroidism

Lytic lesions: metastasis (not punched out, spares mandible), amyloidosis, myeloid metaplasia

Expansile lytic lesion such as a solitary plasmacytoma: renal cell carcinoma metastasis, giant cell tumour, hydatid cyst

Sclerotic lesion: lymphoma, osteopoikilosis, mastocytosis, myelosclerosis, osteoblastic metastasis, renal osteodystrophy

Spinal tumour: metastasis (involves posterior elements, large paraspinal mass).

8. **POEMS** syndrome: **p**olyneuropathy, **o**rganomegaly, **e**ndocrine anomalies, **m**yeloma, **s**kin changes.

1. The bone scan shows multiple hot areas in the spine, ribs and peripheral skeleton. Coronal views on the CT scan show multiple destructive lesions in the spine, few of which are seen in the pedicles.

2. Metastatic bone disease.

3. Common primaries causing bony metastases are cancers of the breast, prostate, lung, kidney, uterus, stomach, thyroid, kidney and colon, and lymphoma, neuroblastoma and Ewing's sarcoma.

4. Metastasis can be:

    Lytic: lung, breast, thyroid, kidney, colon, neuroblastoma

    Blastic (Sclerotic): prostate, breast, lymphoma, carcinoid, adenocarcinoma of gastrointestinal tract, TCC of bladder, pancreas, neuroblastoma

    Mixed blastic and lytic: breast, prostate, lymphoma.

    Expansile lesion: kidney, thyroid

    Permeative: Burkitt's lymphoma.

    Sunburst periosteal reaction: prostate, retinoblastoma, neuroblastoma, gastrointestinal tract

    Calcification: breast, osteosarcoma, testes, thyroid, ovary, mucinous adenocarcinoma of the gastrointestinal tract

    Metastasis with soft-tissue mass: thyroid, kidney

    Children: neuroblastoma, retinoblastoma, rhabdomyosarcoma, hepatoma, Ewing's tumour.

5. After diagnosing metastasis, a bone scan is done to identify other locations of metastasis. MRI is also a very sensitive method and can be used to diagnose bony metastases. Differential diagnoses of metastasis are multiple myeloma, osteomyelitis, primary bone tumours, lymphoma, osteopoikilosis, mastocytosis and bone islands.

Case 3.30: Answers

1. This is a cross-table, horizontal-beam, lateral view of the knee joint.

2. There is a fat–fluid level in the suprapatellar pouch of the right knee joint. This is called lipohaemarthrosis

3. Lipohaemarthrosis indicating an underlying intracapsular fracture.

4. The CT scan shows lipohaemoarthrosis. There is a fat–fluid interface, with low-density fat lying superficial to the fluid. There is a comminuted fracture in the tibial plateau.

5. Lipohaemarthrosis is an accumulation of fat and blood in the joint space. When there is an intra-articular fracture, fat and blood from the bone marrow extrude through an osteochondral defect. Fat, being lighter, floats above the blood and joint fluid.

6. The CT shows a fat–fluid level resulting from fat–blood interface, with the darker fat, superficial to the soft tissue density fluid. MRI shows four layers. The first layer is fat, then there is another bright layer due to chemical shift artifact at the junction of fat and blood, followed by two more layers of blood, with the inferior layer more cellular.

7. Lipohaemarthrosis can be seen in other joints such as the shoulder, elbow and hip, but it is most common in the knee joint. The X-ray beam should be tangential to the fat–fluid interface to visualise this.

8. Lipohaemarthrosis in the knee joint is usually caused by a tibial plateau fracture. Even if no fracture is visible in a patient with haemarthrosis, it indicates an occult fracture.

Case 3.31: Answers

1. The X-ray of the pelvis shows expansion, sclerosis and coarsened trabecula on the right side. The X-ray of the skull shows a cotton-wool appearance of the skull, resulting from extensive sclerosis and expansion of the diploic space.

2. Paget's disease of bone.

3. Paget's disease is a multifocal disease of exaggerated bone remodelling. The exact aetiology is not known. Infection by paramyxovirus is one of the proposed aetiologies.

4. There are three phases:

   Osteolytic phase: with intense osteoclastic activity and resorption of bone

   Mixed phase: osteoclastic and osteoblastic activity – lytic and sclerotic lesions are seen

   Late quiescent phase: decreased osteoblastic activity with decreased bone turn over – sclerosis.

   Fourth phase: if malignancy develops.

5. Paget's disease may be asymptomatic. Fatigue, neuropathy, enlarging head circumference, brainstem compression, pain, hearing loss, blindness, facial palsy and hyperthermia are the common clinical features. The serum calcium and phosphorus are normal, but serum alkaline phosphatase is increased and there is increased excretion of hydroxyproline in the urine.

6. The common locations are the pelvis, spine, proximal femur, skull, scapula, distal femur, proximal tibia and proximal humerus. Most cases are polyostotic.

   Skull: early stage is osteoporosis circumscripta – a geographical lytic area in the anterior frontal bone, followed by a cotton-wool appearance of mixed lysis and sclerosis. There is widening of the diploic space, basilar invagination and sclerosis of the skull base.

   Long bones: there is expansion of bones with coarsened trabecula, cortical thickening and cyst-like areas. The appearance is similar to a candle flame or a blade of grass, with a V-shaped defect starting in the epiphysis and advancing to the diaphysis. Deformities are anterior or lateral curvature, such as shepherd's crook deformity of the femur.

Pelvis: protrusio acetabuli.

Spine: **picture frame** – expansion of bone – sclerosis at margins, expansion of bone with coarse trabecula; **ivory vertebra** – completely sclerotic with ossification of the ligaments.

A bone scan shows increased uptake in the active phase and normal in burned-out cases. MRI shows reduction of marrow cavity size, low signal on T1, high signal on T2 in active stages and low signal in burnt-out cases.

7. Differential diagnoses are metastasis, lymphoma, vertebral haemangioma and fibrous dysplasia. In metastasis there is no cortical bone expansion and no coarsening of the trabecula.

8. Complications are: **neoplasia** (1% risk, 20% are multifocal) (osteosarcoma, fibrosarcoma, malignant fibrous histiocytoma, chondrosarcoma) – osteolysis develops in previous Paget's disease, increasing soft-tissue mass and pain; **fractures** (vertebral compression fractures, banana fractures on convex surfaces of long bones); **deformity** (shepherd's crook, lentosis ossia, ivory vertebra); **brain-stem compression** by basilar invagination and hydrocephalus; **spinal stenosis; osteoarthritis; narrowing of neural foramina**; and high-output **cardiac failure**. Treatment is with calcitonin, bisphosphonates or mithramycin.

Case 3.32: Answers

1. The X-ray of the pelvis shows subtle increased density of the right femur, and there is some flattening of the femoral head at the site of the sclerosis.

2. MRI of the pelvis shows a geographical area of low signal in the head of the right femur.

3. Avascular necrosis of the right femoral head (most likely steroid induced).

4. Causes of avascular necrosis of the hip are: idiopathic, Perthes' disease, drugs (steroids), vasculitis (SLE, polyarteritis nodosa, rheumatoid arthritis), renal failure/dialysis, trauma, neoplasm, radiation, thermal injury, Caisson's disease, sickle cell disease and Gaucher's disease.

5. Findings on a plain X-ray are delayed and not sensitive. Sclerosis of the femoral head, crescent sign (subchondral fracture), preservation of joint space and flattened articular surface, which collapses eventually, are the findings. A bone scan is more sensitive than a plain film but less sensitive than MRI. Bone marrow imaging is more sensitive. In the early stages, the lesion is cold because of necrosis. Once revascularisation starts, there is high uptake surrounding the cold area, giving the doughnut sign. CT shows changes similar to a plain film, but is more sensitive. MRI is the most sensitive investigation. The signal changes on MRI, depending on the stage

Michell's classification of MRI pattern within necrotic area

Stage	Representing	T1	T2
A	Normal fatty marrow	High	Intermediate
B	Subacute bleed	High	High
C	Fluid	Low	High
D	Fibrosis	Low	Low

Differential diagnoses are bone marrow oedema (not well defined, no reactive interface), epiphyseal fracture and spondyloarthropathy.

6. The disease is staged based on the radiological appearances. The higher the stage, the worse the prognosis (**Steinberg's classification**).

Stage 0: normal

Stage I: normal X-ray, abnormal bone scan or MRI

Stage IIA: focal sclerosis/osteopenia

Stage IIB: distinct sclerosis/osteoporosis, early crescent sign

Stage IIIA: crescent sign/cyst formation

Stage IIIB: subchondral fracture, altered femoral contour

Stage IV: marked collapse, acetabular involvement

Stage V: joint space narrowing, acetabular degeneration.

7. Complications are secondary osteoarthritis and chondrolysis of the femoral head.

8. Treatment options are core decompression (successful if < 25% of femoral head is involved), osteotomy or arthroplasty/arthrodesis/total hip replacement.

Case 3.33: Answers

1. AP and lateral views of the elbow show complete malalignment of the elbow joint, which is displaced posteriorly and laterally.

2. Posterior dislocation of elbow.

3. Elbow dislocation is the most common dislocation in children and the second most common dislocation in adults after the shoulder; 90% are posterior dislocations. A fall on outstretched hands with slight abduction and flexion results in compressive forces directed to the outstretched hand, the radius and ulna; together with a valgus force at the elbow, this results in posterolateral dislocation, which is usually associated with other fractures. Hyperextension of the elbow is also seen. Anterior dislocation is usually caused by a direct posterior blow to a flexed elbow. Fracture of the olecranon is associated. Divergent dislocation – radius and ulna dislocated in opposite directions – requires a high impact trauma.

4. AP and lateral views are essential for diagnosis. The elbow joint is dislocated anteriorly or posteriorly. CT is used when the full extent of fractures needs to be evaluated. Associated fractures noted are of distal humerus, radial head and coronoid process of ulna.

5. Complications are brachial artery disruption, ulnar nerve/median nerve injury, fractures of radial neck/epicondyles/corocoid process, compartment syndrome, ectopoic calcification and myositis ossificans. Emergency closed reduction is required to prevent neurovascular damage.

Case 3.34: Answers

1. The X-ray of the spine shows narrowing of the disc space at T9/T10 with irregular end-plates. There are paravertebral soft tissue masses on both sides. MRI shows narrowing of the T9–10 disc space with irregular end-plates. There is also protrusion of a soft tissue epidural mass. Axial image demonstrates paravertebral and epidural soft tissue masses.

2. Tuberculous spondylitis.

3. Tuberculous spondylitis is caused by *Mycobacterium tuberculosis*. The infection reaches the vertebrae usually by haematogenous spread via Batson's plexus; it spreads to adjacent vertebrae in the subligamentous space beneath the anterior and posterior longitudinal ligaments. Contiguous spread occurs through the subchondral plate into the disc space.

4. Spinal TB is common in the lower thoracic and upper lumbar vertebrae, with L1 being the most common vertebra. In the vertebra, it starts in the anterior aspect of the body adjacent to the superior or inferior endplate, from where it spreads to the other parts.

5. Clinically TB of the spine presents with backache, stiffness and tenderness or with deformity in advanced stage.

6. The characteristic features of tuberculous spondylitis are narrowing of the disc space and irregular endplates. Collapse of a vertebral body leads to gibbus, kyphotic deformity and vertebra plana. Paravertebral extension causes widening of the paravertebral soft-tissue opacity. Calcification can be seen. The bone density is decreased in chronic cases, and ivory vertebra is seen during the healing phase. A CT scan shows a destructive, stippled bone pattern in the vertebra, with calcified paravertebral soft tissue. MRI is very sensitive and accurate in characterising and evaluating the disease extent. The lesion is low on T1 and high on T2. An abscess can be seen in the epidural or paravertebral space, which shows rim enhancement and calcification.

7. The differential diagnoses are: **pyogenic spondylitis** (rapid destruction, no calcification of abscess rim, posterior elements not involved, little new bone formation), **tumour** (multiple lesions, non-contiguous, no disc destruction, no soft-tissue abscess), **brucellosis** (minimal paraspinal mass, lower lumbar spine, gas within disc) and **sarcoidosis**.

Case 3.35: Answers

1. The X-ray of the face shows depression and irregularity of the floor of the left orbit. Coronal CT scan shows fracture of the inferior wall of the left orbit. Inferior rectus muscle is seen herniating through the defect into the left maxillary sinus.

2. Blow-out fracture of the left orbit.

3. Blow-out fracture of an orbit is an isolated fracture of the orbital floor or, less commonly, the medial wall with an intact rim, caused by increased intraorbital pressure. A sudden direct blow to the globe, by a closed fist or a ball, results in increased intraorbital pressure that is transmitted to the weak orbital floor. Clinical findings are pain, decreased visual acuity, vertical/oblique diplopia (especially in upgaze), enophthamos, soft-tissue oedema, haematoma and facial anaesthesia (infraorbital nerve distribution). It is associated with similar fracture to the medial orbital wall in 20–50%. Globe rupture is associated in up to 30%.

4. Radiological findings are soft-tissue mass extending into the maxillary sinus through the orbital floor as a result of herniation of orbital fat or muscle. Complete opacification of the maxillary sinus is seen as a result of a haematoma or oedema. Displacement of a bone fragment into a maxillary sinus (trap door sign), orbital emphysema, depression of the orbital floor and opacification of adjacent ethmoidal air cells are seen. A CT scan with coronal and sagittal reconstruction is mandatory before treatment. It shows a fracture line or depression in the orbital floor. Herniation of orbital fat can be visualised.

5. The most important clinical information in relation to the treatment is the herniation of inferior rectus.

6. Complications are entrapment of the inferior rectus muscle, which results in vertical diplopia, limiting upgaze. Enophthalmos results from herniation of the orbital contents into the maxillary sinus, which is worsened by a fracture of the medial wall, when the contents herniate into the ethmoidal sinus. The risk is higher when > 50% of the floor is involved. Orbital oedema at the time of injury may mask the enophthalmos. Injury to the infraorbital nerve causes hypoaesthesia of the cheek and upper gum.

7. Blow-out fractures are managed by surgery and there is a 2-week window before fibrosis, contracture and entrapment set in. Surgery is usually performed after dissipation of oedema and haemorrhage, which helps in assessing extraocular muscle function and enophthalmos. Diplopia presenting 10–14 days after trauma, diplopia in children (incarceration of muscle in trapdoor fractures causes early and permanent damage), enophthalmos > 2 mm for 10–14 days after trauma and fracture involving a third or more of orbital floor require surgery. Tense inferior rectus incarceration requires emergency surgery. Early repair is also indicated when diplopia is present within 30° of primary gaze with a positive forced duction test and CT confirmation of fracture.

Case 3.36: Answers

1. On the AP view of the wrist, the lunate has a triangular shape. In the lateral view, the capitate and other bones are aligned with the distal radius. However, the lunate is displaced to the volar aspect, with its distal articular surface facing forward.

2. Lunate dislocation.

3. Carpal dislocations result from hyperdorsiflexion. Severe ligament injury is necessary to tear the distal row from the lunate to produce perilunate dislocation. Lunate dislocations are the most severe of the carpal instabilities and are very commonly associated with a trans-scaphoid fracture.

4. Radiological appearances:

    Normal appearance: normal gap between scaphoid and lunate on AP view: < 3 mm. On the AP view, lunate is normally quadrilateral. On the lateral view, the distal radius, lunate and capitate form a single straight line.

    Scapholunate angle: angle between the scaphoid long axis and a line through the lunate; normal 30–60°.

    Capitolunate angle: angle between lines drawn along the scaphoid and capitate; normal < 20°.

    The continuum of perilunate injuries ranges from dissociation to dislocation. There are four successive stages progressing from the radial to the ulnar side. Lunate dislocation is the final stage in this continuum and is caused by rupture of the dorsal radiocarpal ligament. The lunate dislocates in a volar direction and rotates forwards on a lateral view. The concave distal surface of the lunate comes to face anteriorly. Other carpal bones including the capitate are normally aligned and posterior to the lunate on the lateral view. The capitate drops into the space vacated by the lunate. It involves all the intercarpal joints and results in disruption of most of the major carpal ligaments.

5. Other ligamental instabilities:

    VISI (volar intercalated segmental instability): the lunate is tilted in a volar direction. This decreases the scapholunate angle and increases the capitolunate angle.

    DISI (dorsal intercalated segmental instability): the lunate is tilted dorsally. The scapholunate and capitolunate angles are increased.

6. Complications are carpal instability, vascular complications, degeneration and chronic wrist pain. Surgical treatment options are closed reduction and casting/percutaneous pin fixation or open reduction, open ligamentous repair with internal fixation or percutaneous pin fixation.

Case 3.37: Answers

1. The anterior humeral line is seen intersecting anterior to the posterior third of the capitellum. The radiocapitellar line is not intersecting the centre of the capitellum. A fracture line is seen in the distal humerus.

2. Supracondylar fracture of the humerus.

3. A fall onto outstretched hands with a hyperextended elbow, or a fall onto a flexed elbow resulting in vertical stress, is the mechanism for supracondylar fracture. This is the most common elbow fracture in children aged < 10 years. There are two broad types: extension (95%) and flexion:

Type I: undisplaced

Type II: displaced with intact cortex

Type III: complete displacement.

4, A proper AP view of the elbow should be performed with the forearm in supination and the elbow in extension. Assess for the ossification centres. Look for the following things on the lateral view:

Anterior fat pad displacement: anterior fat pad can be seen as a lucent area in the anterior aspect of the distal humerus, even in normal individuals. It is displaced anteriorly and superiorly when there is elbow effusion.

Posterior fat pad: this is over the olecranon fossa and not normally seen. Visualisation of posterior fat pad indicates haemarthrosis secondary to intra-articular fracture.

Anterior humeral line: this line is drawn along the anterior surface of the distal humerus and in normal individuals intersects the middle third of the capitellum. In supracondylar fracture with posterior displacement of the fragments, the line intersects the anterior third of the capitellum or passes completely anterior to it.

Radiocapitellar line: line drawn along the central axis of the radius should intersect the centre of the capitellum. If this line does not transect the middle of the capitellum, it indicates radial neck fracture or radial head dislocation.

Fracture lines: transverse fracture lines can be seen. The distal fragment is posteriorly displaced.

5. Suspected supracondylar fractures are initially splinted at 20° of elbow flexion pending evaluation. Closed reduction under anaesthesia is the definitive treatment. Percutaneous pin fixation is indicated for type II fractures and most type III fractures. Open reduction is indicated when closed reduction fails to achieve adequate alignment or with vascular injuries. Complications are malunion with restriction of function, injury to the brachial artery, neurological injury (radial nerve or less frequently median nerve) and Volkmann's ischaemic contracture causing flexion contracture of wrist and fingers.

Case 3.38: Answers

1. AP and oblique X-rays of the hand show an oblique lucency running through the metaphysis of the proximal phalanx of the 5th finger, extending into the growth plate, resulting in a triangular fragment.

2. Salter–Harris type II fracture of the phalanx. This is the most common type of Salter–Harris fracture, accounting for 75% of cases.

3. The cartilaginous growth plate of a paediatric skeleton separates the metaphysis and epiphysis. The germinal layer for the growth plate is contiguous with the epiphysis and supplied by epiphyseal vessels. Injuries to the growth plate heal rapidly except when the epiphyseal blood supply or germinal layer has been damaged. Of the layers of the growth plate, the resting cartilage, proliferating cartilage and one provisional calcification have a strong matrix, which resists shearing force. The zone of hypertrophying cartilage is the weakest zone and vulnerable to shearing injuries. The cartilaginous growth plate is weaker in children than the capsule and ligaments, so any force that produces sprain or dislocation in adults causes growth plate injury in children.

4. **Salter–Harris classification of epiphyseal injuries**:

   Type 1: slip of epiphysis, periosteum remains intact

   Type 2: fracture line through the physis and metaphysis, separating a triangular metaphyseal fragment

   Type 3: fracture in the epiphysis extending to the physis

   Type 4: fracture involving the metaphysis, physis and epiphysis

   Type 5: crush injury of the physis

   Rang–Ogden's additions:

   Type 6: injury to perichondrial structures

   Type 7: isolated injury to the epiphyseal plate

Type 8: isolated injury to the metaphysis, with potential injury related to endochondral ossification

Type 9: periosteal injury interfering with membranous growth.

5. Type 2 epiphyseal injuries need closed reduction and immobilisation to avoid damage to the cartilage, which might hinder growth or produce deformity, depending on the extent of involvement. Damage to either the epiphyseal or the metaphyseal vascular supply disrupts bone growth. The damage to the cartilage layer may not, however, be significant if the surfaces are reapposed and vascular supply is not permanently interrupted.

Case 3.39: Answers

1. There is a fracture dislocation at the base of the first metacarpal bone. A small fragment of the first metacarpal is articulating posteromedially, with the trapezium.

2. Bennett's fracture.

3. Bennett's fracture is the most frequent of all thumb fractures. It is a fracture dislocation at the base of the thumb's carpometacarpal (CMC) joint. It is caused by an axial blow direct against the partially flexed metacarpal.

4. The X-ray shows an oblique intra-articular metacarpal fracture, which remains attached to the palmar beak ligament. There is a triangular fragment at the ulnar base of the metacarpal. A triangular fragment remains attached to trapezium with proximal displacement of the metacarpal. Note the size of the volar lip fragment and the amount of displacement of the shaft.

5. Rolando's fracture is a three-part fracture at the base of the metacarpal. In addition to volar lip fracture (as seen in Bennett's fracture), there is also a large dorsal fragment resulting in a Y- or T-shaped intra-articular fracture. It is a comminuted intra-articular fracture at a base-of-thumb metacarpal, even if a Y or T shape is not present. Rolando's fracture is uncommon but has a worse prognosis than Bennett's fracture

6. Reduction, percutaneous pin fixation and open reduction are the treatment options, with immobilisation for 5 weeks. Complications include malunion, restriction of function and osteoarthritis of the first CMC joint.

Case 3.40: Answers

1. MRI shows a complete detachment of the supraspinatus tendon from the site of insertion into the greater tuberosity of the humerus. Note that there is no tendon crossing the humeral head to reach the greater tuberosity. In normal patients the supraspinatus tendon is located here.

2. Complete supraspinatus tear.

3. The rotator cuff is made up of tendons from four muscles: supraspintaus, infraspinatus, teres minor and subscapularis. The tendons blend 15 cm from their lateral margins, before they insert into the greater tuberosity.

4. Theories of formation of cuff tear are: extrinsic compression of cuff (by anterior acromion, coracoacromial ligament and acromioclavicular joint), intrinsic tendon degeneration (zone of hypovascularity in supraspinatus tendon 1 cm from insertion into greater tuberosity is called the critical zone; articular surfaces have less blood supply than bursal surfaces), muscle imbalance and scapular dyskinesis.

5. The most common location of the degenerative tear is in the supraspinatus tendon, 1 cm from its insertion site – the critical zone, which is hypovascular.

6. Classic presentation is chronic ache in the lateral aspect of the shoulder, aggravated by attempts to abduct the arm, especially in the 60–120° range of abduction and forward flexion. There is weakness during abduction or forward flexion. Neer and Hawkins tests are positive.

7. MRI is the technique of choice for detecting cuff tears. T2-weighted images are obtained in the coronal oblique, sagittal oblique and axial planes Tear can be full thickness or partial thickness. In a full-thickness tear, the entire craniocaudal thickness of the cuff is torn and there is free communication between the joint and subacromial bursa. In a partial-thickness tear only a portion of the thickness of the tendon is torn. This can be on the articular surface or the bursal surface or in the tendon substance. This is seen as a high signal intensity area in the articular or bursal surface of the tendon. Complete tears extend the whole AP distance. Incomplete tears are still attached in some parts. When there is a full-thickness tear, the exact size of the tear should be measured and atrophy of the surrounding muscles assessed. Most of the tears occur in the critical zone. In young patients, an avulsion-type partial-thickness tear can occur adjacent to the greater tuberosity. Osteophytes, hooked acromion and os acromiale are seen. Differential diagnoses are tendinopathy, degeneration and cuff strain.

8. High-resolution ultrasonography is a cheaper, dynamic and effective examination. Ultrasonography is as good as MRI in diagnosis of cuff tears. Normal tendons are bright structures. Tears are dark, with irregular ends of tendons. MR arthrography, which is performed by injecting contrast into the joint prior to MRI, is very effective for diagnosing small tears, because it distends the joint. If there is a full-thickness tear, contrast extends through the defect into the subacromial bursa.

9. Treatment options are physical therapy and anti-inflammatory drugs, but definitive treatment depends on the presence and severity of symptoms. In absence of impingement, small tears are treated conservatively. Symptomatic tears with impingement require decompression surgery. Large tears require closure of tear with or without decompression.

Case 3.41: Answers

1. On the AP view, the lunate has a triangular shape. The lateral view shows normal alignment of the lunate with the radius, but the capitate and other carpal bones have been dislocated dorsally.

2. Perilunate dislocation.

3. Carpal dislocations result from hyperdorsiflexion. Severe ligament injury is necessary to tear the distal row from the lunate to produce perilunate dislocation. Perilunate dislocations are usually secondary to a fall onto an

outstretched, hyperextended hand. It is very commonly associated with scaphoid fracture and sometimes with a ulnar styloid fracture.

4. Radiological appearances:

Normal appearance: normal gap between scaphoid and lunate in AP view − < 3 mm

On the lateral view, the distal radius, lunate and capitate form a single straight line

Scapholunate angle: angle between the scaphoid long axis and a line through the lunate; normal 30−60°

Capitolunate angle: angle between lines along the scaphoid and capitate; normal < 20°.

The continuum of perilunate injuries ranges from dissociation to dislocation and depends on the severity of force. There are four successive sages progressing from the radial to the ulnar side:

Stage 1: scapholunate dissociation − rupture of the scapholunate ligament: Terry Thomas sign positive (> 3 mm scapholunate distance). On a PA view a ring sign is seen, as a result of rotatory subluxation of scaphoid

Stage 2: perilunate dislocation − rupture of the capitolunate ligament. The capitate is dislocated dorsally. On the lateral view the lunate is normally sited and aligned with the distal radius. The capitate, along with the other carpal bones, is dislocated dorsally. It may be accompanied by trans-scaphoid, triquestrum, capitate or radial styloid fracture.

Stage 3: midcarpal dislocation − rupture of the triquetrolunate ligament. The capitate and carpus are dislocated dorsally.

Stage 4: lunate dislocation − rupture of the dorsal radiocarpal ligament. Lunate dislocates in a volar direction in the lateral view. Other carpal bones including the capitate are normally aligned.

5. Other ligamental instabilities (this is discussed in the answer to question 5 of Case 3.36):

VISI: the lunate is tilted in a volar direction. This decreases the scapholunate angle and increases the capitolunate angle.

DISI: the lunate is tilted dorsally. The scapholunate and capitolunate angles are increased.

6. Complications are an unstable wrist and secondary degeneration. Surgical treatment options are closed reduction and casting/percutaneous pin fixation or open reduction, open ligamentous repair with internal fixation.

Case 3.42: Answers

1. The X-ray shows a lucent line through the scaphoid bone, without displacement of the bony fragments.

2. Scaphoid fracture.

3. Scaphoid is the most common carpal bone to be fractured and fracture is caused by a fall onto a dorsiflexed outstretched hand. Differential diagnoses are distal radius fracture, trans-scaphoid perilunate dislocation and scaphoid impaction syndrome. Clinically there is tenderness over the anatomical snuffbox, with tenderness on palpation over the scaphoid tuberosity, limitation of wrist flexion and extension, tenderness with axial compression of the thumb towards the snuffbox, tenderness as the patient supinates the forearm against resistance, and pain on radial and ulnar deviation and forced dorsiflexion.

4. Scaphoid fracture is seen in plain X-rays, but is often not detectable in the initial X-ray. Scaphoid views are taken when there is clinical suspicion. AP with 30° supination and ulnar deviation, a pronated oblique view, a lateral view, and a PA of the wrist are done as part of the scaphoid series. Absent or abnormal scaphoid fat stripe is a good indicator of fracture.

5. The initial X-ray is negative in up to 65% of cases. If the initial X-ray is negative the patient is put in a cast and a repeat X-ray done in 2 weeks' time. If there is still no fracture, but clinical suspicion is high, MRI of the wrist is done. On MRI, high signal in the bone marrow indicates bone marrow oedema and might be a result of microfracture of the scaphoid bone. Hence, MRI is the most sensitive method for diagnosing a scaphoid fracture. Alternative methods are CT of the wrist or a nuclear medicine bone scan. A CT scan is also useful for determining stability, if there is > 1 mm step-off, > 60° of scapholunate angulation or > 15° of lunocapitate angulation, PA angulation > 35°, or lateral interscaphoid angulation > 25°, or if there is instability.

6. **Fracture displacement** > 1mm indicates a bad prognosis. Location of fracture in the proximal third indicates high risk of non-union because the blood supply is derived from the distal part. **Orientation of fracture**: vertical oblique fractures are unstable. Good prognosis is seen with a distal fracture, no displacement and no ligamentous injury.

7. Complications are non-union, avascular necrosis of the proximal fragment and scapholunate advanced collapse (SLAC).

8. Non-displaced fractures are treated by casting or percutaneous fixation. Displaced fractures require fixation with a screw. Plaster immobilisation is required for at least 8 weeks. Delayed union or non-union requires bone graft and internal fixation.

Case 3.43: Answers

1. MRI of the right arm shows a round, soft tissue mass arising from deep inside the muscle and extending anteriorly. After contrast, there is very intense enhancement of this mass, with central areas of necrosis.

2. Soft-tissue sarcoma.

3. Malignant fibrous histiocytoma, fibrosarcoma, liposarcoma, leiomyosarcoma, rhabdomyosarcoma, neurofibrosarcoma, synovial sarcoma, alveolar soft-tissue sarcoma and epithelioid sarcoma are the histological types of sarcoma.

4. Pain, swelling, tenderness and neurovascular compression are the most common symptoms.

5. X-rays show large soft-tissue masses. Calcification is seen in haemangiomas and synovial sarcomas. Excessive fat in the tumour can produce lucencies. Ultrasonography visualises a solid mass, which shows intense vascularity on Doppler examination. A CT scan can show the bony involvement. MRI is the test of choice for diagnosis and staging. The whole tumour and any needle tracks are included in the scan. T1- and T2-weighted images with STIR are obtained in multiple planes before and after contrast. The tumour enhances intensely and

heterogeneously. MRI can identify the tumour, characterise it to a certain extent (presence of fat indicates liposarcoma, and serpiginous vascular lesions haemangiopericytoma). Most of these tumours are large and heterogeneous, with areas of haemorrhage and necrosis and intense contrast enhancement. MRI is used to assess the compartments involved, which is useful for treatment planning. Invasion of bone, bone marrow and neurovascular structures is noted. A chest CT scan is essential to rule out pulmonary metastasis. A bone scan shows high uptake. Ultrasound-guided biopsy is useful for determining the diagnosis.

6. Imaging enables diagnosis. An X-ray shows calcification, phleboliths, lucencies and secondary bone changes. Ultrasonography is useful in superficial tumours, haemangiomas and tumour vascularity. A biopsy for tissue diagnosis is obtained, under ultrasound guidance. MRI is the best imaging modality because the soft-tissue contrast is superior and multiplanar views are acquired. The most common soft-tissue tumour is lipoma, which is easily identified on any imaging modality. Any other solid tumour is suspicious for soft-tissue sarcoma and should be considered a sarcoma unless proved otherwise.

7. Resection of the tumour with adjuvant chemotherapy. Soft tissue sarcomas respond poorly to radiotherapy.

8. MRI is useful in follow-up surveillance after resection. Tumour recurrence is differentiated from postoperative changes using dynamic MRI.

Case 3.44: Answers

1. MRI shows a large mass arising from the vertebral body at the level of C7, which extends into the spinal canal and causes compression of the spinal cord. This is seen well on the axial view, which shows the soft-tissue mass narrowing the spinal canal.

2. Spinal cord compression by metastasis.

3. Causes of spinal cord compression:

    Congenital (os odontoideum, hemivertebra, diastomatomyelia,

    Trauma (haematoma, fracture fragment), discal herniation, infection with abscess formation (TB, pyogenic, fungal), tumours (secondary – metastasis, lymphoma; primary – any primary bone tumour such as haemangioma, aneurysmal bone cyst, osteochondroma, osteoblastoma, extradural tumours such as meningioma, neurofibroma, leptomeningeal metastasis), vascular (AV malformation, hematoma)

Arthritis (rheumatoid arthritis, ankylosing spondylitis, synovial cysts of facet joint, diffuse idiopathic skeletal hyperostosis, calcium pyrophosphate deposition disease, ossified posterior longitudinal ligament/ligamentum flavum, gout, Paget's disease), **spinal stenosis**, **severe scoliosis**, **mucopolysaccharidoses** and **achondroplasia**.

4. Clinical features depend on the extent and rate of development of cord compression. Motor symptoms are fatigue and gait disturbance. Cervical spinal lesions produce quadriplegia, thoracic spinal lesions produces paraplegia, and lumbar spinal lesions affects L4, L5 and the sacral nerve roots. Sensory symptoms are sensory loss and paraesthesiae. Light touch and proprioception are reduced. Tendon reflexes are: increased below level, absent at level and normal above level. Reflex changes may not correlate with the sensory level. Sphincter disturbances are late features of cervical and thoracic cord compression. Cauda equina compression produces loss of perianal sensation, root pain in both legs and painless urinary retention Spinal pain is present in most surgically treatable causes. Extreme tenderness suggests an epidural abscess. Low-grade background pain suggests a tumour or osteomyelitis.

5. MRI confirms the diagnosis of compression, identifies the cause of compression, finds the level(s) of compression and enables treatment planning. In some patients non-neoplastic findings are discovered. Compression can occur at multiple levels. On MRI a malignant tumour is seen with collapse of vertebrae and high signal on T2 and STIR sequences. There is a soft-tissue mass, extending into the paraspinal space, and more importantly into the spinal canal, causing compression of the spinal cord or conus medullaris. When the compression is mild, there might be some cerebrospinal fluid (CSF) space left between the mass and spinal cord. Thecal sac compression without spinal cord compression may cause neurological abnormalities via a vascular mechanism. When the CSF space is completely obliterated, it indicates severe compression. Usually the sensory levels found in clinical examination do not correlate well with MRI, and they can be below or above the clinical level. MRI enables planning for radiotherapy. High signal inside the cord indicates cord oedema.

6. Acute cord compression is a surgical emergency. Spinal decompression and stabilisation of the spine are required. Malignant cord compressions are treated with radiation.

Case 3.45: Answers

1. The X-ray shows a rib arising from the seventh cervical vertebra on both sides.

2. Cervical rib with thoracic outlet syndrome.

3. Cervical rib can be complete or incomplete type, bony or fibrous type. It can be unilateral or bilateral.

4. In the X-ray, the rib is seen arising from the seventh cervical vertebra. Differential diagnosis includes a hypertrophied transverse process of the C7 vertebra or a hypoplastic first thoracic rib. The rib may fuse with the first rib anteriorly and the adjacent transverse process is angulated inferiorly. It can be associated with Klippel–Feil syndrome. Other investigations such as venogram, arteriogram or duplex ultrasound may be required to assess for vascular compression.

5. Cervical rib is seen in 0.2–2.0% of the population. Usually cervical ribs are asymptomatic, but they can produce thoracic outlet syndrome due to elevation of the floor or scalene triangle with decrease of costoclavicular space. Some 10–20% of those with thoracic outlet syndrome have a cervical rib; 5–10% of those with complete cervical rib have symptoms. Thoracic outlet syndrome presents with neurological, venous or arterial symptoms. Neurological symptoms involve the nerve roots C8, T1 or the upper three nerve roots, C5, C6, C7. Pain is present in the medial aspect of the arm, forearm, ring and small digits, paraesthesias, loss of dexterity, cold intolerance and headache. Claudication with arm activity is the vascular complication. Elevated arm stress test is the most reliable test. The patient sits with arms abducted 90° from the thorax, and the elbows are flexed 90°. Then the patient opens and closes the hands for 3 minutes. Those with the syndrome have reproduction of symptoms in these 3 minutes. Tenderness, sensory loss, weakness, oedema, cyanosis, pallor, pulselessness and low blood pressure are other clinical features. Cervical ribs are found in most cases with arterial symptoms. Occasionally thrombus from post-stenotic dilatation of the brachial artery may cause embolic episodes distally in the hands and fingers.

6. The cervical rib is resected if is found to be the cause of thoracic outlet syndrome.

Case 3.46: Answers

1. Sagittal MRI of the left side of lumbar spine shows a dark structure protruding posteriorly from the disc space at L5–S1 level and compressing the nerve roots. Axial view at the level of the L5–S1 disc shows a dark structure protruding posterolaterally on the left side and compressing the transiting S1 nerve root.

2. Disc protrusion with nerve root compression.

3. Disc disease is due to degenerative changes in the spine. Dehydration of the nucleus pulposus leads to narrowing of disc space, vacuum disc, and disc calcification and bone sclerosis. Displacement of the nucleus pulposus in an anterior and anterolateral direction results in traction on osseus attachment of the annulus fibrosis, producing end-plate osteophytes. Tear of the annulus posteriorly allows the nucleus pulposus to herniate within the spinal canal and cause nerve root compression.

4. Prolapse of disc material can compress the nerves in the central canal, exit foramen or lateral recess (transiting nerve roots). In the lumbar level it is most common at L4–5 > L5–S1. In the cervical spine, it is most common at C6–7. In the thoracic spine, it is more common in T11–12.

5. Types of degenerative discal disease:

   Disc bulge: lengthening of annular fibres; concentric smooth circumferential expansion of disc

   Disc protrusion: weakening/tear of outer fibres of annulus fibrosis resulting in broad-based protrusion of disc material limited by posterior longitudinal ligament

   Disc extrusion: tear of outer fibres of annulus fibrosis, with a narrow, focal extension of disc material through the defect, and only a narrow isthmus connecting to the parent disc; intact or ruptured posterior longitudinal ligament; the fragment may extend at the same level or above it

   Disc sequestration: the disc loses its communication from the parent fragment and can be located many segments away from the parent disc.

6. The disc is a hypovascular fibrous structure. On MRI, it is seen as a hypointense, dark area on T1 and T2. The disc bulge can be posterolateral, posterocentral, bilateral or lateral. A large central bulge narrows the spinal canal and causes spinal stenosis. A posterolateral protrusion can compress the transiting root at the lateral recess or the exiting root at the intervertebral foramen. A diffuse bulge is seen as a diffuse extension of the disc behind the posterior border of the vertebra. Normally it is concave, but in a diffuse bulge it looks convex. Presence of osteophytes in the spinal canal and exiting foramen will increase the nerve root compression.

7. In the upper cervical level, the nerve root exits above the corresponding vertebra, eg the C4 nerve root exits above the C4 vertebra, ie at the C3–4 level. The C7 root passes at C6–7 level. The C8 root exits below C7 at the C7–T1 level. All the nerve roots from this level exit below the corresponding vertebra, so the L3 nerve root exits at the L3–4 level. The transiting roots are seen in the lateral recess at the same level.

8. In the lumbar spine, nerve root compression is a common complication, causing back pain and sciatica, followed by altered sensation and muscle weakness. Serious neurological symptoms such as deranged bladder emptying and gross neurological deficits in lower limbs require urgent surgery.

Case 3.47: Answers

1. The X-ray of the left leg shows a well-defined, expansile, multiloculated, lytic lesion arising from the proximal metaphysis of the tibia, extending to the subarticular surface and causing cortical thinning. No periosteal reaction or soft-tissue component is identified. The knee joint appears normal.

2. Giant cell tumour.

3. Clinical symptoms are localised swelling and pain. The patient seeks medical attention following trauma, which accentuates the symptoms. Typically it is seen in the mature skeleton, but is occasionally seen in younger patients. It is more common around the knee.

4. Giant cell tumor of the bone is a relatively uncommon, usually benign tumour that is characterised by the presence of multinucleated giant cells. The basic proliferating cell is the background mononuclear stromal cell, in which the characteristic osteoclast-like giant cells are uniformly distributed. Giant cell tumors have an indolent course, but they can recur locally in as many as 50% of cases. Metastasis to the lungs may occur. The tumors are malignant in 5–10% of patients. Malignant giant cell tumors of the bone usually result from secondary malignant transformation after radiation treatment.

5. Most giant cell tumours (60%) occur in the long bones, and almost all are located at the articular end of the bone. Metaphyseal involvement may occur in skeletally immature patients. Common sites include the proximal tibia, distal femur, distal radius and proximal humerus, although giant cell tumours have also been reported to occur in the pubic bone, calcaneus and feet, and occasionally in vertebrae.

6. Typical giant cell tumours are expansile, bubbly, multiloculated, osteolytic, lucent lesions without sclerotic margins or periosteal reaction. Most tumours are eccentric and subarticular and have a narrow transition zone with a sclerotic margin. The tumour originates in the metaphysis and epiphyseal involvement is caused by skeletal maturity. On MRI, on a T1-weighted image, the lesion is homogeneous or heterogeneous, and of low signal intensity except in cases of haemorrhage. On T2-weighted images, heterogeneous low-to-intermediate signal intensity is noted. Cystic areas are seen as high signal on T2. Haemosiderin appears dark in both sequences. Fluid–fluid levels are present inside the lesion in MRI, due to haemorrhage.

7. Fractures can be seen. Periosteal reaction is seen if there is a fracture. Although they are benign tumours, metastasis to the lung is seen in 3% of cases. Spontaneous malignant transformation is not uncommon and is defined as a sarcoma associated with a benign typical giant cell tumour. There is a strong association between radiotherapy and malignant transformation of giant cell tumours. Treatment options include curettage, curettage and bone grafting, curettage and PMMA cement insertion, cryotherapy, chemical adjuvant therapy, primary resection, radiotherapy and embolisation of feeding vessels.

8. Differential diagnoses include: **simple bone cyst** (unicameral, located centrally), **aneurysmal bone cyst** (seen before epiphyseal fusion, can extend to subarticular region), **subarticular geode, Brodie's abscess, benign fibrous histiocytoma, chondroblastoma** (epicentre in epiphysis, chondroid calcification), **haemophilic pseudotumour, expansile neuroblastoma metastasis**. Differential diagnoses of a fluid–fluid level in bone lesions on MRI include **aneurysmal bone cyst, simple bone cyst, chondroblastoma, giant cell tumour, telangiectactic osteosarcoma** and **fibrous dysplasia**.

4
NEURORADIOLOGY
QUESTIONS

Case 4.1

A 61-year-old woman presents with loss of consciousness, headache and weakness in her right leg, after a minor road traffic accident several weeks ago. On examination, her GCS is 7. Her pupil is dilated on the left side. There is reduced power on her right side with increased reflexes.

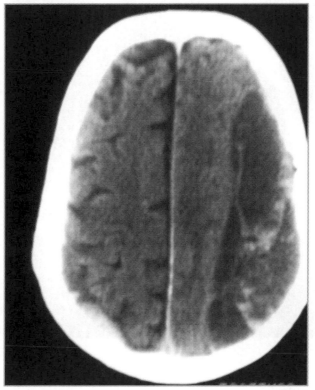

Fig 4.1

1. What are the findings on the CT scan?
2. What is the diagnosis?
3. What is the mechanism?
4. What is the usual location?
5. What are the radiological features?
6. What is the prognosis?
7. What is the differential diagnosis?
8. What are the complications?

Answers *on pages 363–393*

A 34-year-old woman presents at hospital with sudden onset of a severe headache and photophobia. On examination, she is afebrile and has neck stiffness with decreased power in all four limbs.

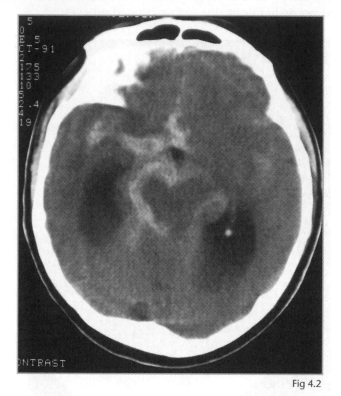

Fig 4.2

1. What does the CT scan show?

2. What are the diagnosis and the causes?

3. What complication has developed in this patient and what other complications are encountered in this condition?

4. If the CT scan is normal, are further investigations required?

5. Are further radiological investigations required with this CT appearance?

6. What is the classic presentation of this condition?

7. What conditions are associated with this pattern?

8. How is this condition managed?

9. What is the rate of recurrence of this condition?

10. What is the role of radiology in treatment of this condition?

Answers on pages 363–393

Case 4.3

A 56-year-old woman presents with sudden onset of weakness in the left arm and leg. On examination, she is fully conscious, but she has a power of 0/5 in her left arm and leg with exaggerated deep tendon reflexes and a brisk plantar response.

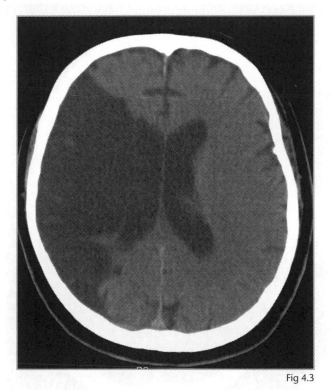

Fig 4.3

1. What do you observe on the CT scan of the brain?
2. What is the diagnosis?
3. What are the causes of this disease?
4. What is the common location?
5. What are the tests that are used for early diagnosis?
6. What are the earliest signs on CT?
7. What are the findings in established disease?
8. What are the changes after the acute stage?
9. What are the contraindications for thrombolysis?

Answers *on pages 363–393*

A 52-year-old woman presents with weakness in her right arm. On examination, the power is 3/5 in the right arm with exaggeration of deep reflexes.

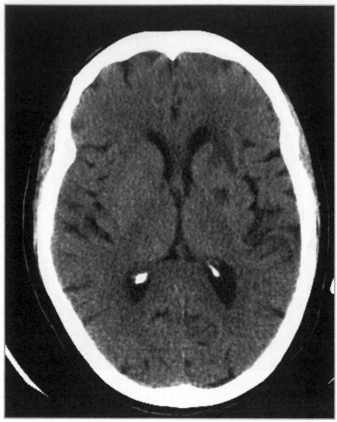

Fig 4.4

1. What do you see on the CT scan?
2. What is the diagnosis?
3. What are the causes?
4. What is the most common location?
5. What are the clinical syndromes?
6. What are the findings on CT and MRI?
7. What is the differential diagnosis?

Answers on pages 363–393

A 29-year-old man presents with severe headache, intermittent seizures, and weakness of his right arm and leg. On examination, there is no neck stiffness, but there is reduced power in the right arm and leg (3/5).

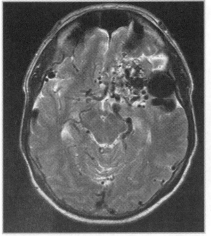

Fig 4.5a

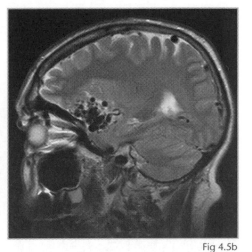

Fig 4.5b

1. What do you see on MRI?
2. What is the diagnosis?
3. What are the causes?
4. What are the types and the vascular supply?
5. What are the common locations?
6. What are the imaging findings?
7. What is the role of radiology in treatment?
8. What are the complications and prognosis?

Answers on pages 363–393

A 31-year-old man presents with weakness in his arms and legs and reduced vision. On examination the power and tone of his limbs are decreased and there are exaggerated reflexes. The visual acuity is reduced.

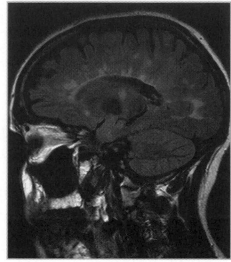
Fig 4.6a

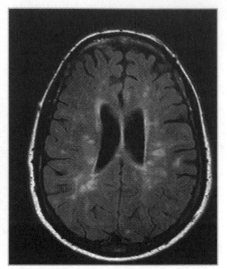
Fig 4.6b

1. What are the findings on MRI of the brain?
2. What is the diagnosis?
3. What are the various types of the disease?
4. What are the clinical features?
5. What are the radiological features?
6. What are the other investigations that are required for confirmation of the diagnosis?
7. What is the radiological differential diagnosis?
8. What is the management?

Answers *on pages 363–393*

Case 4.7

A 35-year-old woman presented with severe headache and photophobia.

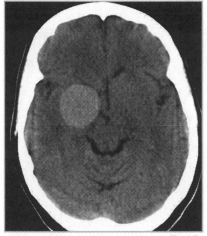

Fig 4.7a

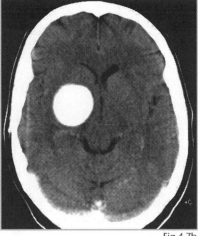

Fig 4.7b

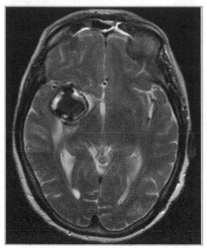

Fig 4.7c

1. What do you see on this CT scan and on MRI?

2. What is the diagnosis?

3. What are the causes?

4. What are the risk factors?

5. What are the common locations?

6. What are the imaging findings?

7. What are the new techniques and the role of radiology in treatment?

8. What are the complications and the prognosis?

Answers on pages 363–393

A 45-year-old woman presents with headache, seizures, nausea, progressive dementia and some limb stiffness, over a period of several months. A CT scan was performed.

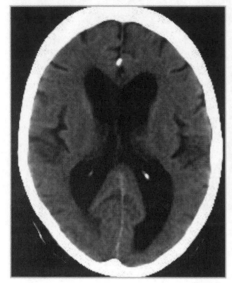

Fig 4.8a

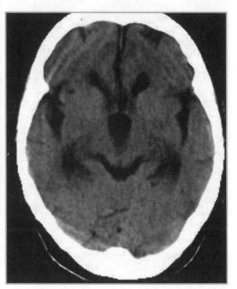

Fig 4.8b

1. What are the findings on the CT scan?
2. What is the diagnosis?
3. What are the types of this disease?
4. What is the normal route of flow?
5. What are the radiological findings?
6. What is the differential diagnosis?

Answers on pages 363–393

Case 4.9

A 47-year-old woman presents with left-sided deafness and tinnitus.
Examination reveals left sensorineural deafness and normal hearing on the
right side.

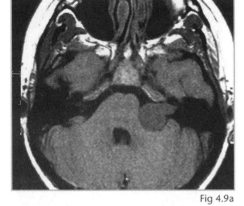

Fig 4.9a

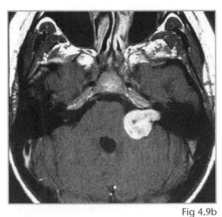

Fig 4.9b

1. What are the findings on MRI?
2. What is the diagnosis?
3. What is the origin of this lesion?
4. What are the pathological and clinical features?
5. What are the radiological features?
6. What are the other types of the disease?
7. What are the associations?
8. What is the differential diagnosis?

Answers on pages 363–393

Case 4.10

A 12-year-old girl presents with severe right orbital pain and swelling. On examination, her right eye is swollen, red and tender, with proptosis. Lateral eye movement is limited.

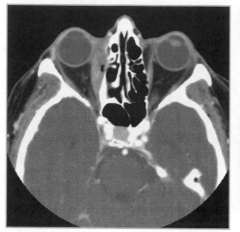
Fig 4.10a

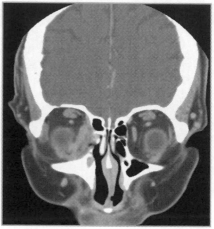
Fig 4.10b

1. What are the findings on the CT scan?
2. What is the diagnosis?
3. What are the causative agents?
4. What is the mode of spread?
5. What is the common location?
6. What are the radiological features and the role of imaging?
7. What is the differential diagnosis?
8. What is the treatment?

Answers on pages 363–393

Case 4.11

A 35-year-old man presents with proptosis and swelling in his right eye and limitation of lateral gaze. On examination, there is right-sided proptosis with no pulsations.

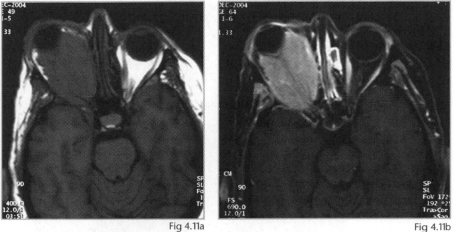

Fig 4.11a   Fig 4.11b

1. What do you find on MRI?

2. What is the diagnosis?

3. What are the pathology and the causes?

4. What are the associations?

5. What is the location?

6. What are the radiological features?

7. What is the differential diagnosis of intraorbital lesions?

8. What is the treatment?

Answers on pages 363–393

A 28-year-old man presents with headache, nasal stuffiness and post-nasal drip. On examination, there is tenderness over the sinuses and nasal blockage.

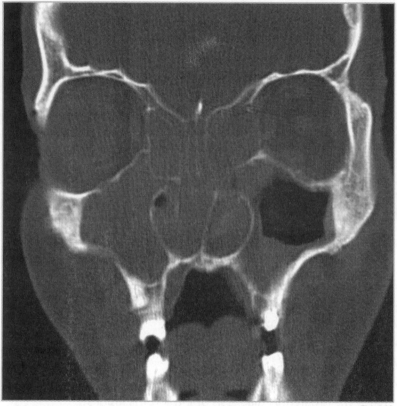

Fig 4.12

1. What are the findings on the CT scan?
2. What is the diagnosis?
3. What are the causes and the types?
4. What is the relevant anatomy?
5. What are the radiological findings?
6. What are the important things to be noted on the CT scan? What is the differential diagnosis?
7. What are the complications?
8. What is the treatment?

Answers *on pages 363–393*

A 27-year-old man presents with headache, drowsiness and history of loss of consciousness following a fight. On examination he is disoriented and does not respond to verbal stimuli. His BP is normal, pulse rate is 60 and respiratory rate is 24/minute. The left pupil is dilated and there is weakness in the right lower extremity.

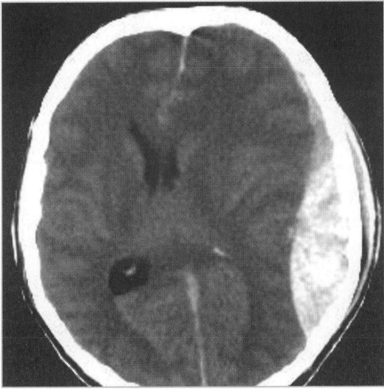

Fig 4.13

1. What are the findings on the CT scan?
2. What is the diagnosis?
3. What is the mechanism?
4. What are the clinical features?
5. What are the radiological features?
6. What are the complications and the treatment of this condition?

Answers on pages 363–393

Neuroradiology Questions

A 9-year-old boy presented with nystagmus, seizures and headache.
Clinical examination showed truncal ataxia, dysdiadochokinesia and poor
coordination. Power was reduced and reflexes were exaggerated.

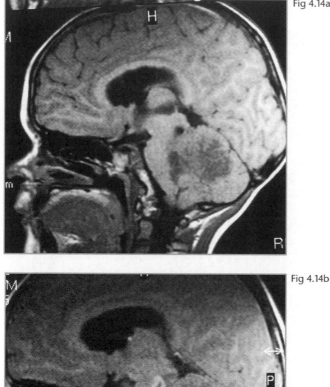

Fig 4.14a

Fig 4.14b

1. What do you observe on MRI of the brain?
2. What is the diagnosis?
3. What are the clinical features?
4. What are the radiological findings?
5. What is the differential diagnosis?

Answers on pages 363–393

Case 4.15

A 37-year-old man presents with recurrent intermittent pain and swelling of the right side of his face.

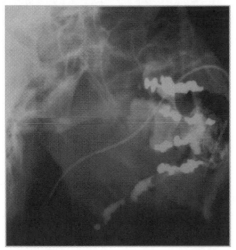

Fig 4.15a

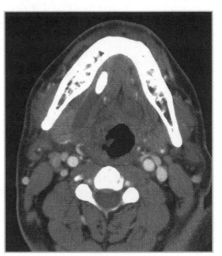

Fig 4.15b

1. What is the first investigation and what do you observe?
2. What do you observe on the CT scan of the face?
3. What is the diagnosis?
4. What is the composition?
5. What are the common locations?
6. What are the radiological features?
7. What are the complications?
8. What is the treatment?

Answers on pages 363–393

Case 4.16

A 26-year-old man was involved in a road traffic accident and is brought unconscious to A&E. Clinical examination revealed a GCS of 4.

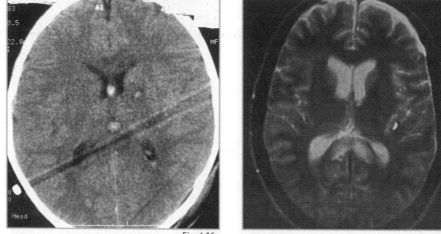

Fig 4.16a   Fig 4.16b

1. What are the findings on the CT scan or on MRI?
2. What is the diagnosis?
3. What is the mechanism?
4. What is the usual location?
5. What are the radiological features?
6. What is the prognosis?

Answers on pages 363–393

Case 4.17

A 4-year-old girl presented with nystagmus, syncopal episodes and weakness of her upper limbs. On examination, there was decreased power in the upper extremities. Reflexes were exaggerated.

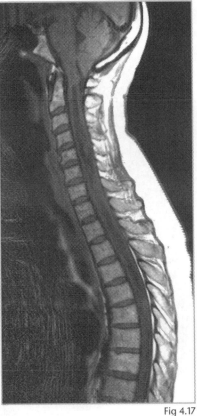

Fig 4.17

1. What are the findings on MRI?
2. What is the diagnosis?
3. What are the types of this disease?
4. What are the radiological features?
5. What are the clinical features and treatment of this condition?

Answers on pages 363–393

A 51-year-old presents with a history of loss of consciousness and headache, after a high-velocity motor vehicle accident. On examination, the GCS is 13–15. There is bruise over the right frontal region.

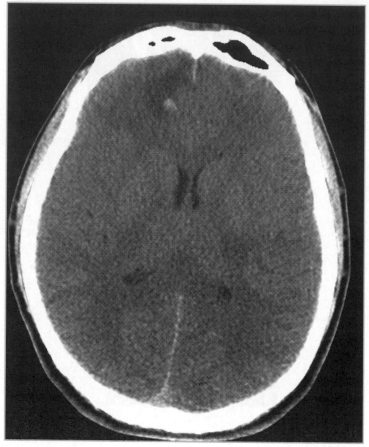

Fig 4.18

1. What are the findings on the CT scan?
2. What is the diagnosis?
3. What is the mechanism?
4. What are the types?
5. What are the usual locations?
6. What are the radiological features?
7. What are the complications?

Answers on pages 363–393

Case 4.19

A 47-year-old patient was brought to A&E unconscious after he was found unconscious in his bed. On examination, his GCS was 4.

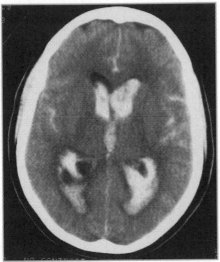

Fig 4.19a

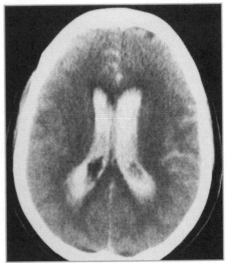

Fig 4.19b

1. What are the findings on the CT scan?
2. What is the diagnosis?
3. What are the causes?
4. What are the radiological findings?
5. What are the complications?
6. What is the treatment?

Answers *on pages 363–393*

A 65-year-old presents with headache, seizures and right-sided hemipariesis. Clinical examination showed poor motor function and increased reflexes on the left side.

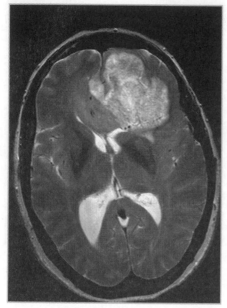

Fig 4.20a

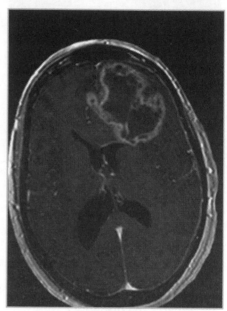

Fig 4.20b

1. What are the findings on MRI?
2. What is the diagnosis?
3. What are the common locations?
4. What are the associations of this disease?
5. What are the radiological features?
6. What are the other types of this disease?
7. How does this disease spread?
8. What is the differential diagnosis of MRI features of the above lesion?

Answers on pages 363–393

Case 4.21

A 37-year-old woman presents with headache, weight gain and visual difficulties. Clinical examination showed bitemporal hemianopia with normal power and reflexes. MRI was done for diagnosis. There was a sudden deterioration in her consciousness level on the second day of admission and a second MRI was done.

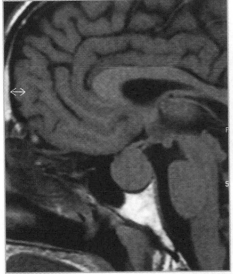
Fig 4.21a

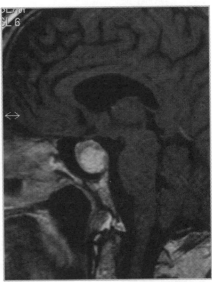
Fig 4.21b

1. What are the findings on this MR scan?
2. What is the diagnosis? What complication do you see on the second MR scan?
3. What are the types of this disease?
4. How is it classified?
5. What are the radiological findings?
6. What is the important information to be obtained from MRI?
7. What are the complications and the treatment?
8. What is the differential diagnosis?

Answers on pages 363–393

A 35-year-old woman presented with right-sided neck pain, a lump and hypertension. On examination, a firm lump is palpated in the right side of neck, which does not move with swallowing.

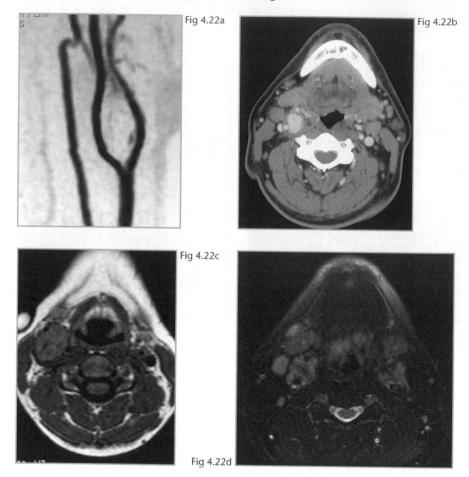

Fig 4.22a

Fig 4.22b

Fig 4.22c

Fig 4.22d

1. What do you see on the angiogram, and on CT and MRI?
2. What is the diagnosis?
3. What is the cell of origin of this lesion?
4. What are the anatomy and the function of this organ?
5. What are the common locations?
6. What are the radiological features?
7. What are the differential diagnoses?
8. What is the clinical course and treatment of this lesion?

Answers on pages 363–393

Case 4.23

A 23-year-old woman with relevant family history presents with headache, gait disturbance and nystagmus. On examination, the cerebellar signs are positive.

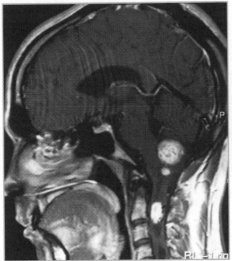

Fig 4.23a

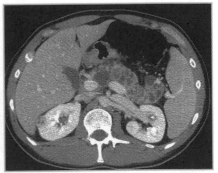

Fig 4.23b

1. What do you observe on MRI?
2. What is the diagnosis?
3. What is the underlying associated condition?
4. What do you observe on the CT scan of the abdomen?
5. What are the radiological features?
6. What are the findings on the associated syndrome?
7. What is the differential diagnosis?

Answers on pages 363–393

A 38-year-old patient presents with back pain and paraesthesiae along the chest wall. On examination, there is tenderness in the lower dorsal spine. Multiple nodules are seen on the skin.

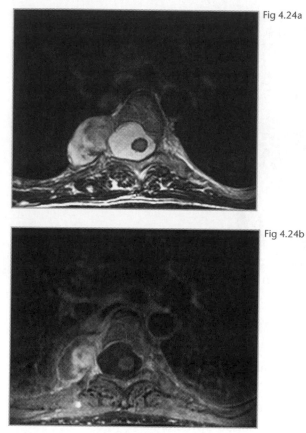

Fig 4.24a

Fig 4.24b

1. What are the findings on MRI?
2. What is the diagnosis?
3. What is the pathology of the lesion?
4. What are the most common locations?
5. What is the most common association?
6. What are the radiological features?
7. What are the complications?
8. What is the differential diagnosis?

Answers *on pages 363–393*

Case 4.25

An 11-year-old girl presents with paraesthesiae in the upper limbs. On examination, there is loss of pain and temperature sensation in the upper limbs, and muscle weakness.

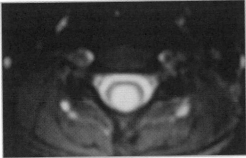

Fig 4.25a

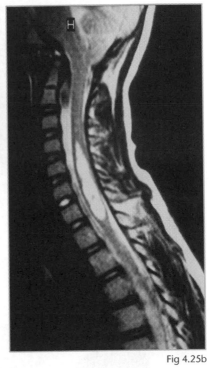

Fig 4.25b

1. What are the findings on MRI?
2. What is the diagnosis?
3. What is the aetiopathology of this disease?
4. What are the clinical presentations?
5. What are the radiological features?
6. What is the differential diagnosis?
7. What are the treatment options?

A 21 year old presents after a road traffic accident with loss of consciousness, headache and vomiting. On examination, there is weakness in the left arm and leg.

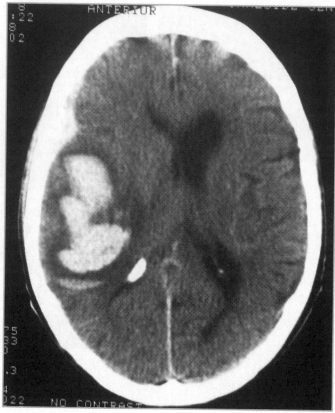

ANTERIOR

NO CONTRAST

Fig 4.26

1. What are the findings on the CT scan?

2. What is the diagnosis?

3. What is the mechanism?

4. What is the usual location?

5. What are the radiological features?

6. What are the other non-traumatic causes of this appearance?

7. What are the complications and the treatment?

Answers on pages 363–393

Case 4.27

A 36 year old presents with headache and seizures. Clinical examination is unremarkable. Power, tone and reflexes are normal.

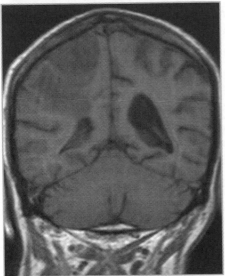

Fig 4.27a

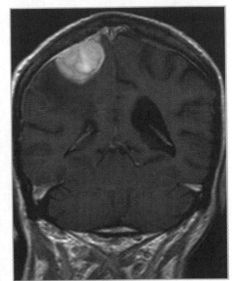

Fig 4.27b

1. What are the findings on MRI?
2. What is the diagnosis?
3. What is the cell of origin?
4. What are the common locations?
5. What are the associations?
6. What are the types?
7. What are the radiological appearances?
8. What is the vascular supply?
9. What are the differential diagnoses?
10. What is the treatment?

Answers *on pages 363–393*

A 38-year-old woman presented with pain in the right cheek and swelling.

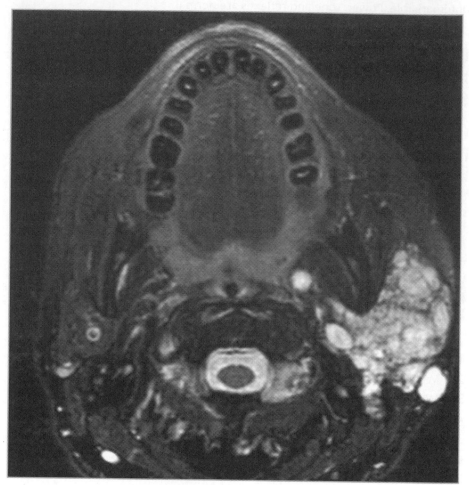

Fig 4.28

1. What are the findings on MRI?
2. What is the diagnosis?
3. What is the pathophysiology?
4. What are the radiological features?
5. What are the important points to be considered in imaging?
6. What are the complications and the treatment?
7. What is the differential diagnosis?

Answers on pages 363–393

Case 4.1: Answers

1. The cranial CT scan shows a crescenteric hypodense collection in the left convexity with areas of high density within it.

2. Acute-on-chronic subdural haematoma.

3. Subdural haematoma is a collection of blood in the potential space between the dura mater and the leptomeninges. It is caused by trauma, resulting in differential movement of the brain and adherent cortical veins in relation to the skull, which tears the bridging subdural veins that run from the cortical veins to the dural sinuses.

4. The haematoma is located in the subdural space. It extends across the suture lines, limited only by the interhemispherical fissure and tentorium. It is most commonly seen in the convexity, with extension to the interhemispherical fissure, along the tentorial margins, inferior temporal and occipital lobe. It does not cross the midline and is bilateral in 10–15%. Interhemispherical subdural haematoma is a feature of non-accidental injury (NAI) in children.

5. CT is the investigation of choice. A CT scan shows a crescenteric collection in the subdural space (extradural haematoma is biconvex). The haematoma is hyperdense in the acute stage and gradually becomes isodense over 1–2 weeks and hypodense within 3–4 weeks. Acute-on-chronic subdural haematoma presents with areas of high density within a predominant hypodense collection. The haematoma results in loss of the grey–white matter interface, with effacement of the sulci, compression of the ventricle and midline shift to the opposite side. The most difficult cases are isodense subdural haematomas in the acute stage, which might be a result of low haemoglobin or CSF dilution from an arachnoid tear. In these cases, the haematoma has the same density as that of the brain parenchyma. The CT scan should be carefully examined for haematoma, changing the window settings. There is thickening of the skull with effacement of sulci. Sulci not traced to the brain surface indicate a mass effect Ventricular compression displacing the grey–white matter interface and midline shift are also seen. No contrast enhancement is seen in the haematoma. Interhemispherical subdural haematoma has a crescenteric shape with a flat medial border and might be difficult to differentiate from an interhemispherical subarachnoid haemorrhage.

6. Subdural haematoma has a high mortality as a result of associated brain injury, mass effect, rapid rate of accumulation and complications.

7. Differential diagnosis: extradural haematoma – lentiform, crosses suture.

8. Complications are herniation, death, AV fistula and underlying brain injury.

Case 4.2: Answers

1. A non-contrast CT scan shows bright density within the basal cisterns and sulci. The bright density is blood. In addition, the lateral ventricles appear dilated.

2. The patient has a subarachnoid haemorrhage. The most common cause is rupture of an aneurysm. Other causes are AVMs, hypertension and cryptogenic.

3. She has developed acute hydrocephalus, which is caused by decreased drainage of cerebrospinal fluid. Complications of subarachnoid haemorrhage are rebleeding, vasospasm (seen in 70–90%, leading to stroke in 50%) and mortality (10% die before reaching hospital). Other complications that may develop are electrolyte disturbances, arrhythmias, neurogenic pulmonary oedema and hypoxia.

4. If the CT scan is normal in a patient with strong clinical suspicion, a lumbar puncture is done to exclude subarachnoid haemorrhage. The presence of blood and xanthochromia confirms the diagnosis.

5. If the CT scan shows bleeding as in this case, conventional angiography is required to determine the presence of an aneurysm. This is being replaced by CT angiography, which identifies an aneurysm and determines whether intervention is appropriate.

6. Headache of sudden onset is the classic presentation. Other presentations are meningism (photophobia, vomiting, neck stiffness), third nerve palsy, fits, altered consciousness and focal neurological deficits.

7. Marfan syndrome, Ehlers–Danlos syndrome, polycystic kidney disease, coarctation of aorta and AVMs are associated conditions.

8. Calcium channel blockers are used to reduce vasospasm. Surgical clipping or endovascular coiling is done to treat the aneurysms. AVMs are managed by embolisation with coils. Cerebral oedema is managed by steroids. Hydrocephalus requires shunting.

9. If untreated, the risk of rebleeding is 10–20% in the first 2 weeks and 50% in the first 6 months. The mortality rate from rebleeding is 70–90%.

10. Radiology not only is used in diagnosis, but plays a major role in treatment. GDC (Gugleimi detachable coils) are used to embolise the aneurysms, using selective catheterisation of the involved arteries.

Case 4.3: Answers

1. The CT scan shows a large area of low density in almost the entire right cerebral hemisphere. There is minimal compression of the right lateral ventricle, but there is no midline shift to the left side.

2. Large infarct in the right cerebral hemisphere, in the right middle cerebral arterial (MCA) territory.

3. Infarct results from a thrombotic or embolic occlusion of a large artery, small vessel occlusion, coagulopathies, cardiac causes, vasculitis and non-arteriosclerotic causes.

4. Cerebral hemispheres are the most common location, with the MCA territory being the most commonly affected.

5. Routine CT is not positive until 12–24 hours. MRI is positive within a few minutes of onset of the stroke. Early diagnosis is useful if intra-arterial thrombolysis is contemplated. The MRI protocol consists of T1- and T2-weighted images, susceptibility imaging (for haemorrhage), diffusion and perfusion imaging.

6. Earliest signs on CT are: dense MCA sign (bright middle cerebral artery as a result of hyperdense thrombus), insular ribbon sign (hypodense external capsule not distinguishable from insular cortex), loss of differentiation between grey and white matter, low-density basal ganglia and subtle sulcal effacement.

7. CT shows obvious changes from 24 hours. Hypodense wedge-shaped lesion results from cytotoxic oedema. Mass effect is seen in the acute stage, with sulcal effacement and herniation. Enhancement of the cerebral gyri may be seen at between 7 and 30 days. MRI shows low signal on T1 and high signal on T2, with blurring of the grey–white matter junction, meningeal enhancement, enhancement of cortical arteries and gyriform enhancement.

8. Haemorrhagic conversion occurs after 2–4 days, as a result of leakage of blood from ischaemically damaged capillaries following reperfusion. Eventually the infarct liquefies and leaves an area of encephalomalacia and brain atrophy with gliosis. Calcification can be seen in children.

9. The presence of haemorrhage and a massive infarct involving more than two-thirds of a cerebral hemisphere are contraindications for thrombolysis.

Case 4.4: Answers

1. CT shows a well-defined small hypodensity in the lentiform nucleus of basal ganglia on the left side.

2. Lacunar infarct.

3. Lacunar infarcts are small infarcts < 15 mm, caused by fibrinoid degeneration and occlusion of small penetrating vessels, which are the lenticulostriate, thalamoperforating, pontine perforating and recurrent artery of Heubner. It is seen in patients with diabetes or hypertension.

4. The upper two-thirds of the putamen, caudate nucleus, thalamus, pons and internal capsule are the common locations.

5. Pure motor syndrome, pure sensory syndrome, ataxia, dysarthria, clumsy hand syndrome and abnormal movements are the various types of lacunar infarct syndromes.

6. CT shows well-defined hypodense lesions, < 15 mm, in the basal ganglia and thalamus. The lesions show higher signal than CSF as a result of gliosis. MRI shows low signal on T1 and high signal on T2.

7 Differential diagnoses of T2 bright lesions: MS, ischaemic changes, vasculitis, infection (TB, cysticercosis).

Case 4.5: Answers

Neuroradiology Answers

1. MRI (axial and sagittal views) shows tortuous, vascular structures in the left temporal lobe, extending to the parietal lobe

2. Cerebral AVM.

3. AVM is a malformation that consists of a nidus of abnormal, dilated, tortuous arteries and veins with no intervening normal brain parenchyma. The affected arteries have thin walls with gliotic parenchyma in vessels. AVMs are congenital malformations. They may be associated with other syndromes such as Wyburn–Mason and Sturge–Weber syndromes.

4. An AVM can be a pial or dural AVM. Other malformations are cavernous angiomas, capillary telangiectasia and cortical venous anomalies. Most AVMs are supplied by pial branches of the internal carotid artery. Occasionally dural branches of the external carotid artery may supply an AVM.

5. The majority are located in a supratentorial location, particularly in the parietal and frontal lobes. An infratentorial location is seen in 10%.

6. A non-contrast CT scan shows an irregular hyperdense lesion with large feeding arteries and draining veins. Calcifications can be seen. Haemorrhage can occasionally be seen. Usually there is no oedema or mass

effect, but when there is haemorrhage, mass effect is noted. On contrast CT scans, there is dense, serpigineous enhancement of the tortuous vessels. If the AVM is thrombosed, there is no contrast enhancement. MR shows a flow void in non-contrast scans and serpigineous contrast enhancement. Angiogram shows dilated efferent and afferent vessels with AV shunting.

7. Transcatheter embolisation can be performed under image guidance.

8. Complications are haemorrhage, infarction and atrophy. AVMs are seen by the end or the fourth decade, and present with headaches, seizures, mental deterioration and neurological deficit. Risk of rebleeding is 2–3% per year. The mortality rate is 10%.

Case 4.6: Answers

1. T2-weighted MRI of the brain shows elongated, oval, hyperintense lesions extending perpendicularly from the corpus callosum. The second axial image shows multiple, hyperintense, bright lesions in the periventricular white matter.

2. Multiple sclerosis (MS).

3. MS is the most widespread acquired demyelinating disease. The aetiology is uncertain and is probably an autoimmune response against myelin triggered by a previous virus infection or exogenous agent acting on inherited susceptibility. There are many types, including classic Charcot's, neuromyelitis optica (Devic syndrome), Balo's concentric sclerosis and Schilder's diffuse sclerosis. The classic form has four subtypes: relapsing–remitting, chronic progressive, secondary progressive and benign.

4. Most patients present in the third or fourth decade; 15% are seen before age 20 and 10% after age 50. Females are more commonly affected. Clinical symptoms are visual disturbance (optic neuritis), weakness, numbness, tingling and gait disturbance, loss of sphincter control, blindness, paralysis and dementia.

5. MR has the highest sensitivity in the diagnosis of MS (85%), even better than evoked potentials and CSF oligoclonal bands. Sagittal FLAIR (**fl**uid

attenuation inversion recovery) sequences are the most sensitive. This sequence suppresses the fluid signal from the CSF, which appears dark, and any subtle high signal in the subcallosal region will be seen as a bright lesion. Most plaques are iso- or hypointense on T1-weighted images and hyperintense on T2-weighted images. They are typically ovoid, from medial to lateral, and are mainly close to the periventricular white matter. They extend perpendicularly from the surface of the corpus callosum (Dawson's fingers caused by perivenular demyelination). Other appearances are small subcortical punctuate lesions, tumour-like plaques involving a large part of centrum semiovale, and confluent periventricular and peritrigonal plaques. Plaques can enhance in the acute stage.

6. CSF analysis for oligoclonal bands is the other test that could be performed to confirm the diagnosis.

7. Other diseases that produce white matter hyperintensities are degeneration, vasculitis, metastasis, infection and haemorrhage. Oval hyperintensities in the periventricular white matter, caused by perivenous demyelination, are specific for MS and not seen in any of these other conditions.

8. Immunomodulators such as interferon- 1a and - 1b, glatiramer acetate and nalalizumab, corticosteroids and immunosuppressants such as cyclophosphamide, methotrexate, mitoxantrone and azathioprine are used for treatment.

Case 4.7: Answers

1. The CT scan shows a hyperdense lesion in the non-contrast scan, which enhances intensely after contrast, located in the right parietal region. T2-weighted MRI shows a heterogeneous lesion, predominantly low signal intensity in the right parietal region.

2. Cerebral aneurysm.

3. Most of the aneurysms are congenital berry aneurysms. The rest of the aneurysms are atherosclerotic, mycotic, traumatic, neoplastic, as a result of collagen vascular disease or fibromuscular disease.

4. Risk factors are family history, age > 50, female, Marfan syndrome, Ehlers–Danlos syndrome, pseudoxanthoma elasticum, neurofibromatosis type 1, polycystic kidney disease and AVM. Multiple aneurysms are seen in fibromuscular hyperplasia, coarctation, Ehlers–Danlos syndrome, AVM, SLE, polycystic kidney disease and coarctation

5. The most common location of cerebral aneurysm is the circle of Willis, especially at the bifurcations. The most common location is the anterior communicating artery, the posterior communicating artery and the middle cerebral artery (MCA) bifurcation.

6. Aneurysms present with subarachnoid haemorrhage, which is seen as bright blood in the sulci, cisterns and fissures. An aneurysm can be calcified or non-calcified. In the non-contrast scan, it is hyperdense (especially if there is thrombus) or hypodense. Contrast enhancement is homogeneous when there is no thrombus and circumferential if there is central thrombosis. The MRI signal depends on thrombus and flow. There might be a signal void if there is fast flow and a mixed signal if there is mixed thrombosis. CT/MRA shows aneurysm in the same way as proper angiography. When an aneurysm ruptures, intracerebral haematoma occurs. The underlying aneurysm can be diagnosed based on the location of the haematoma:

Interhemispherical fissure: anterior communicating artery (AcoA)

Sylvian fissure: middle cerebral artery

Prepontine cistern: basilar artery

Foreman magnum: posterior inferior cerebellar artery (PICA)

Corpus callosum: pericallosal artery.

7. Previously all suspected aneurysms were diagnosed with cerebral angiography. Currently, all patients with suspected aneurysm, based on the presence of subarachnoid haemorrhage, undergo CT angiography or MRA, which gives information about the location, number, size, neck and sac of aneurysm. If the patient is fit for intervention, coil occlusion of the aneurysm is done by interventional neuroradiologists. Surgical clipping of aneurysms is performed only when coil occlusion cannot be done.

8. A total of 10% die within 24 hours due to haemorrhage, brain herniation, infarction and brainstem haemorrhage. Complete recovery is seen in 5%. Rebleeding is seen in 5% in the first 24 hours and 10–20% in the first 2 weeks, and 50% in 6 months. Risk of death from surgery is 50% for ruptured and 1–3% for unruptured aneurysms.

Case 4.8: Answers

1. The CT scan shows dilated lateral and third ventricles, but a normal fourth ventricle.

2. Hydrocephalus.

3. Hydrocephalus is a disturbance of formation, flow or absorption of CSF, which leads to an increase in volume occupied by this fluid in the central nervous system (CNS). Based on time of onset, hydrocephalus can be **acute**, **subacute** or **chronic**.

   Communicating hydrocephalus: communication between ventricles and subarachnoid space seen (overproduction of CSF/defective absorption/venous insufficiency)

   Non-communicating hydrocephalus: no communication between ventricles and subarachnoid space (obstruction at any level in the ventricles or outlets to subarachnoid space)

   Benign external hydrocephalus (self-limiting absorption deficiency of infancy and childhood, with large subarachnoid spaces and intracranial pressure)

   Hydrocepalus *ex vacuo*: as a result of brain atrophy

   Arrested hydrocephalus: stabilisation of ventricular enlargement, secondary to compensatory mechanisms.

4. Normally CSF is produced in choroid plexus, flows through lateral ventricle →→ foramen of Monro →→ third ventricle →→ cerebral aqueduct of Sylvius →→ fourth ventricle →→ foramen of Luschka and Magendie → → subarachnoid space →→ arachnoid granulations →→ dural sinus →→ cerebral veins.

5. In hydrocephalus, the ventricles are dilated and there is effacement of sulci. Diagnostic criteria for hydrocephalus: visualisation of temporal horns > 2 mm, ratio between width of frontal horns and internal diameter of skull > 0.5, ratio of largest width of frontal horns to maximal biparietal diameter > 0.3, periventricular hypodensities, ballooning of frontal and third horns, and upward bowing of corpus callosum. Transependymal seepage of CSF results in periventricular hypodensities. In chronic hydrocephalus, temporal horns are less prominent, the head is large and the corpus callosum is atrophied, the sella turcica may be eroded and the third ventricle herniates into the sella turcica.

6. Most common differential diagnosis is atrophy with dilatation of the ventricles. In atrophy, the temporal horn is not prominent and CSF spaces are very prominent.

Case 4.9: Answers

1. MRI shows a well-defined, cone-shaped mass arising in the left cerebellopontine angle (CPA). The mass is seen extending into the internal acoustic meatus. The mass is isointense on a non-contrast scan and shows intense contrast enhancement after administration of gadolinium.

2. Left-sided acoustic neuroma.

3. Acoustic neuroma arises from the vestibular division of the eighth cranial nerve. In 15% it arises from the cochlea; 85% of these lesions arise from inside the internal auditory canal and extend to the CPA.

4. The tumour is a schwannoma with cellular dense regions (Antoni A) and loose areas with widely separated cells in reticulated matrix (Antoni B). Clinically it presents with slowly progressive sensorineural deafness, tinnitus, pain, diminished corneal reflex, unsteadiness, vertigo, ataxia and dizziness.

5. The CT scan shows a round, isodense mass arising from the internal auditory canal and extending into the CPA. There is a funnel-shaped component extending into the internal auditory canal. The CPA cistern is widened. Hydrocephalus can be seen. The mass is isodense on non-contrast with areas of cyst formation and necrosis, and no calcification. There is homogeneous enhancement. MRI shows iso- or hypointense signal on T1 and hyperintense signal on T2, and an intense enhancing homogeneous mass with contrast. An acoustic neuroma is usually diagnosed by high-resolution axial MRI. Images are taken in axial and coronal planes, without contrast. Normally there is high signal around nerve VIII roots. Absence of this high signal indicates a neuroma. Large tumours do not require further evaluation. If there is a small suspicious lesion, contrast is administered for optimal evaluation.

6. Intracanalicular neuroma. This type of acoustic neuroma is confined to the internal auditory canal, and is best diagnosed by contrast-enhanced MRI.

7. Acoustic neuroma is associated with neurofibromatosis type 2, although most of the neuromas are sporadic.

8. Differential diagnoses: meningiomas (broad based, no intracanalicular extension, dural tail), aneurysm, epidermoid cyst (high signal on T1, increased diffusion signal), arachnoid cyst (same signal as CSF in all sequences), ependymoma, trigeminal neuroma and metastasis.

Case 4.10: Answers

1. The CT scan shows a hypodense, ill-defined lesion in the right extraconal space close to the medial wall of the orbit. There is a locule of gas within this lesion. The coronal scan with contrast shows no rim enhancement.

2. Orbital cellulitis.

3. Orbital cellulitis is an acute bacterial infection, caused by infection with staphylococci, streptococci or pneumococci.

4. Usually the infection spreads from adjacent sinuses or eyelids. The infection can extend into the intracranial space.

5. The most common location is the extraconal space in the medial wall of the orbit. Patients present with proptosis and pain.

6. CT scan is the diagnostic procedure of choice. It shows proptosis, enlarged extraocular muscles, increased soft-tissue stranding in retro-orbital fat and obliteration of fat planes. Ill-defined stranding is also seen in the medial wall in the extraconal space. The ethmoidal and maxillary sinuses may be opaque. On MRI, it is hypointense on T1 and high on T2, with contrast enhancement. The main aim of imaging is to confirm the clinical diagnosis, define the extent of disease and rule out abscess formation.

7. Differential diagnoses: **abscess** – seen in the medial wall, and should be differentiated from cellulitis, because management is different; seen in the subperiosteal region, and there is displacement of the periosteum medially, giving a convex appearance with contrast enhancement; **preseptal cellulitis** – in the eyelid. Other lesions such as lymphoma, haematoma, dermoid cyst, lacrimal cyst, lymphangioma, haemangioma and hydatid should also be differentiated.

8. Orbital cellulitis is treated with intravenous antibiotics and steroids. An abscess requires surgical drainage.

Case 4.11: Answers

1. T1-weighted images of the orbits show a homogeneous mass in the right orbit, surrounding the optic nerve. There is also proptosis. There is no destruction of the underlying bone and intense enhancement after contrast administration. The left eye is normal.

2. Optic nerve sheath meningioma.

3. Optic nerve sheath meningioma accounts for 10% of orbital neoplasms and is commonly seen in middle-aged or elderly women. It arises from arachnoid rests on the meningeal surface of optic nerves in the orbit or middle cranial fossa.

4. It is associated with neurofibromatosis. Clinically it presents with progressive loss of visual acuity over months and proptosis.

5. It is located in the intraconal space surrounding the optic nerve.

6. An X-ray shows an enlarged optic nerve canal. Ultrasonography shows a hypoechoic tumour with an irregular border. CT and MRI are the most useful in diagnosis. On CT the mass is seen as a tubular/fusiform mass around the optic nerve. Calcification is frequently seen. Dense linear bands or ring-like enhancement is seen as a result of tumour around a non-enhancing optic nerve. MRI shows an extrinsic mass surrounding the optic nerve, which is hypointense to fat on a T1-weighted image, and enhances with gadolinium.

7. Orbital lesions are classified based on their location within the orbit:

Intraconal (inside the muscle cone): haemangioma, optic glioma, meningioma, metastasis, retinoblastoma, melanoma, pseudutomour, Graves' disease, cellulitis

Extraconal: dermoid, teratoma, haemangioma, lymphangioma, neurofibroma, pseudotumour, histiocytosis, lymphoma, leukaemia, metastasis, rhabdomyoscarcoma

Superolateral quadrant: lacrimal gland tumour, metastasis, lymphoma, pseudotumour, sarcoid, metastasis, Wegener's granulomatosis, mucocele of ethmoidal and frontal sinuses.

8. Treatment is with surgical resection.

Case 4.12: Answers

1. The CT scan shows complete opacification of the right maxillary sinus with mucosal thickening of the osteomeatal complex. There is lesser degree of mucosal thickening in the left maxillary sinus, with narrowing of the osteomeatal complex. Mucosal thickening of nasal cavity and ethmoidal sinuses is present. There is no bone destruction.

2. Pansinusitis.

3. Sinusitis is mucosal congestion as a result of infection, which causes apposition of mucosal surfaces and results in retention of secretions with bacterial superinfection. Sinusitis can be acute or chronic. Causes are bacterial (streptococci, *Haemophilus* spp., β_1-haemolytic streptococci, staphylococci, fusobacteria), allergic, fungal (*Aspergillus* spp., mucormycosis, *Candida* spp.). There are four basic patterns:

Infundibular: obstruction of inferior infundibulum above maxillary ostium; isolated maxillary sinus

Osteomeatal: mucosal thickening in middle meatus, osteomeatal complex, maxillary sinus, anterior ethmoidal cells, frontal sinus

Sphenoethmoidal recess: sphenoid and posterior ethmoid

Sinonasal polyposis: replacement of sinus space with polyps.

4. There are four sinuses: maxillary, ethmoidal, frontal and sphenoidal. The middle meatus drains frontal, maxillary and anterior ethmoidal sinuses. A sphenoethmoidal recess drains the posterior ethmoidal and sphenoidal sinuses. The osteomeatal complex is the control point for drainage from the frontal, anterior ethmoidal and maxillary sinus. Its medial wall is formed by the uncinate process, the suprolateral wall by the inferior orbital wall. The infundibulum leads to the hiatus semilunaris. Through the nasofrontal duct, the frontal sinus drains directly into the frontal recess of the middle meatus, but in 15% a nasofrontal duct drains the frontal sinus into the ethmoid infundibulum.

5. Plain X-ray shows opacification of paranasal sinuses or air fluid levels. A coronal CT scan is performed for evaluation of sinus disease. In sinusitis, the sinuses are opacified due to mucosal thickening. In allergic sinusitis, the mucosal thickening is lobular, with little fluid collection. In infective sinusitis, air–fluid levels are seen in the sinuses or complete opacification of sinuses may be seen. MRI shows mucosal thickening, with low signal intensity in T1 and high signal in T2 sequences.

6. Features to be noted are: the pattern of sinus disease; patency of the osteomeatal complex; infundibula, anatomical variants such as concho bullosa; septal deviation; paradoxical middle turbinate; reversed uncinate process; inferiorly migrated ethmoidal bullae; location of carotid artery close to the clinoid; Onodi's cells (most posterior ethmoidal cells, surrounding optic canal and nerve); and Haller's cells (posterior ethmoidal cells invading the medial floor of orbit, can obstruct ostia). Differential diagnosis is haematoma and tumour.

7. Complications are mucus retention cyst, mucocele, extension through the neurovascular foramen, orbital cellulites, septic thrombophlebitis, an intracranial extension to produce meningitis, epidural abscess, subdural empyema, venous sinus thrombosis and cerebral abscess.

8. Acute sinusitis needs antibiotics for several weeks. Nasal decongestants may help in drainage. Antral lavage may help in drainage and obtain samples for bacteriology. Recurrent sinusitis is treated with FESS (functional endoscopic sinus surgery), which enlarges the infundibulum and maxillary ostia, amputates the uncinate process and creates a common channel for anterior ethmoidal cells.

Case 4.13: Answers

1. The CT scan shows a well-defined, lentiform, bright haematoma in the left parieto-occipital region. There is oedema in the underlying brain and compression of the left lateral ventricle, with subfalcine herniation to the right side.

2. Acute left-sided extradural haematoma.

3. Extradural haematoma is an accumulation of haematoma between the dura mater and the inner table of the skull. Direct trauma results in laceration of arteries, usually the middle meningeal artery. Occasionally meningeal veins, dural venous sinuses or diploic veins are lacerated. It is more common in younger age groups.

4. Patients present early after injury, with loss of consciousness. There might be a lucid interval, where the patient is normal, and then he or she deteriorates. Focal neurological signs, such as hemipariesis and seizures, might develop. Venous bleed is slow and presents late.

5. The CT scan is the main test used for diagnosis. Acute haematoma is hyperdense, subacute is isodense and chronic is hypodense. If there is hypodense swirl within the hematoma, it indicates active bleeding. The most common location is the temporopariteal region. It is usually associated with skull fractures (85%). The haematoma is in the extradural compartment and has a lentiform shape (subdural hematoma is crescenteric). The venous sinuses are separated from the skull. The haematoma produces a mass effect with effacement of the underlying gyri and sulci and midline shift with displacement of ventricles and herniation. MRI shows signal intensity depending on the stage of haematoma. It shows displacement of venous sinuses away from the inner table.

6. Emergency surgical decompression is indicated and the haematoma is evacuated. Following surgery, the patient is ventilated in ICU. Intracranial pressure (ICP) is maintained below 25 mmHg and cerebral perfusion pressure (CPP) above 70 mmHg. Complications include cerebral oedema, cerebral ischaemia, infection, epilepsy and residual neurological deficit.

1. MRI done in the sagittal plane shows a well-defined hypointense mass in the cerebellar hemisphere. The second post-contrast MR scan shows cystic lesion with peripheral solid enhancement. There is mild anterior compression of the fourth ventricle.

2. Cerebellar pilocytic astrocytoma.

3. Pilocytic astrocytoma is the second most common posterior fossa tumour in children. It is more common in children and there is no specific age distribution. It usually originates in midline with extension to the cerebellar hemispheres. The vermis, tonsils and brain stem are also affected. It is a benign tumour. Malignant transformation is very rare. It presents with truncal ataxia and dysdiadochokinesia.

4. The lesion is usually cystic with a mural nodule. Astrocytomas in the cerebellar hemispheres are usually cystic. Some lesions are solid with a cystic necrotic centre and others are purely solid. Calcification is seen in 20%. CT shows a cyst with CSF value and contrast enhancement of the wall. In MRI, it is hypo intense on T1 and hyper in T2.

5. Differential diagnoses: **haemangioblastoma** (< 5 cm, vascular nodule), **arachnoid cyst**, **trapped fourth ventricle**, **megacisterna magna**, **Dandy–Walker cyst**. Differential diagnoses of solid astrocytoma: **medulloblastoma** (hyperdense mass, non-calcified) and **ependyoma** (fourth ventricle, 50% calcification).

Case 4.15: Answers

1. The first investigation is a submandibular sialogram. This procedure is performed by cannulating the submandibular duct under the tongue and injecting small amounts of radio-opaque contrast material. There is a large filling defect seen in the distal aspect of the submandibular duct, with proximal dilatation.

2. The second CT scan of the face shows a large ovoid radiodensity in the distal part of the right submandibular duct, with proximal dilatation of the submandibular duct.

3. Submandibular calculus with ductal dilatation.

4. Submandibular calculi are classified as rock like, granular and globular. The core has a circular or polygonal structures forming a honeycomb pattern, surrounded by small projections distributed radially.

5. 80% of salivary calculi are found in the submandibular duct. The predisposing factors are – an alkaline pH that precipitates salts, thicker and more mucous saliva, higher concentration of hydroxyapatite and phosphatase, narrower Wharton's duct orifice (compared with lumen of duct) and uphill course of salivary flow in Wharton's duct (when patient is in upright position). Poor-fitting dentures, dehydration, recurrent infection and trauma are added risk factors. Clinically submandibular calculus produces intermittent swelling of salivary gland associated with meals and lasting for 2–3 hours.

6. An X-ray shows the calculus in 50%. Radiolucent calculi are best seen on a sialogram, where it is seen as a filling defect with proximal dilatation of the duct. A CT scan can show incidental calculus; 25% of cases have multiple stones. An MR sialogram is a non-invasive alternative to conventional sialography. Heavily T2-weighed sequences are taken and hence the ducts are seen as bright structures and calculus is seen as a dark area (area of signal void).

7. Complications are obstruction, strictures, sialadenitis and submandibular abscess.

8. Treatment consists of removing the calculus, if possible, or excising the submandibular gland, in particular for multiple and recurrent calculi formation and presence of calculi within the intraglandular duct system.

Neuroradiology Answers

Case 4.16: Answers

1. The CT scan shows high density, fresh hemorrhages in the white matter of the right occipital region and the left internal capsule. MRI shows high signal areas in the posterior area of corpus callosum and in the region of left lentiform nucleus and external capsule.

2. Diffuse axonal injury.

3. Diffuse axonal injury is a shearing injury caused by high-velocity trauma, resulting in an acceleration/deceleration force. The cortex and deep structures move at different speeds, causing shearing stress of the axons and small white matter vessels. The damage to nerves results in wällerian degeneration and the damage to vessels causes petechial haemorrhages

4. The grey–white matter junction in the cerebral hemispheres, internal capsule, external capsule, basal ganglia, corona radiata, cerebellar peduncles, corpus callosum and posterolateral aspect of the brain stem are the common locations of diffuse axonal injury. There is sparing of the cortex.

5. A CT scan shows small high-density haemorrhages. If the diffuse axonal injury is non-haemorrhagic, a CT scan is normal. MRI shows low signal intensity on T1 and high intensity on T2.

6. Diffuse axonal injury indicates severe head injury and the prognosis is poor. Brain atrophy is seen with enlargement of the sulci and ventricles.

Case 4.17: Answers

1. Sagittal views of the brain stem and cervical spine show herniation of the cerebral tonsil below the level of the foramen magnum. There is also an abnormal, long segment of low signal intensity in the cervical and thoracic spinal cord.

2. Arnold–Chiari I malformation associated with syringohydromyelia of the cervical and upper thoracic cord.

3. Arnold–Chiari malformation is a congenital malformation resulting from defective neural tube closure. There are four types:

I: Downward herniation of the cerebellar tonsils below the level of foramen magnum(>5 mm)

II: Caudal herniation of tonsils and vermis, small posterior fossa, towering cerebellum, beaked tectum

III: Chiari II findings + encephalocele (hydrocephalus is almost always present)

IV: Severe cerebellar hypoplasia.

4. In the normal sagittal pictures of the craniocervical junction, the cerebellar tonsils are above the level of the foramen magnum. If they extend below the foramen magnum, they do not extend > 5 mm. Any descent > 5 mm is considered to be tonsillar herniation and is a feature of Arnold–Chiari I malformation. The fourth ventricle can be elongated, but remains in a normal position. It is associated with syringomyelia in 50% of cases. Syringomyelia is seen as a low signal intensity lesion on T1- and high signal intensity on T2-weighted images.

5. Arnold–Chiari I malformation is associated with intermittent compression of the brain stem, which manifests as nerve palsies, atypical facial pain, respiratory depression and long tract signs. Associated features are syringomyelia (50%), hydrocephalus (25%), basilar invagination (30%), Klippel–Feil anomaly (10%) and atlanto-occipital fusion (5%). Treatment of Arnold–Chiari I is by surgical bone decompression of the craniocervical junction.

Case 4.18: Answers

1. The CT scan shows a hypodense lesion in the anterior aspect of the inferior frontal cortex. There is hyperdense, haemorrhage in the posterior aspect of this lesion.

2. Cerebral cortical contusion.

3. Cerebral cortical contusion is caused by trauma, where capillary disruption leads to extravasation of blood, plasma and red blood cells (RBCs). It results from linear acceleration–deceleration forces/penetrating trauma. Pathologically it is made up of petechial haemorrhage, followed by liquefaction, oedema and necrosis. Patients present with confusion, seizures and focal neurological deficits.

4. There are two types of cerebral injuries: coup and contre coup. Coup contusions are seen on the site of impact. Contre-coup contusions are seen opposite to the impact. The contusion can he haemorrhagic or non-haemorrhagic.

5. Common sites are the orbitofrontal, inferior frontal and rectal gyri above the cribriform plate, planum sphenoidale, lesser wing and temporal lobe.

6. The CT scan shows a heterogeneous lesion, which is of low density with an admixture of high-density haemorrhage. The haemorrhage becomes isodense after 2–3 weeks and then hypodense. Contrast enhancement can be seen as a result of leaking new capillaries. MRI shows non-haemorrhagic contusions as low signal on T1 and high signal on T2. Haemorrhagic contusions show hypointense and hyperintense T2 changes initially, but later they become hyperintense on T1 and T2 as a result of methaemoglobin, and then they show low signal on T2 as a result of haemosiderin.

7. Complications of contusions are haematoma, encephalomalacia, porencephaly and hydrocephalus.

Case 4.19: Answers

1. There is high-density blood filling all the ventricles, and also the subarachnoid space.

2. Intraventricular haemorrhage.

3. Intraventricular haemorrhage usually extends from a subarachnoid bleed. The causes are rupture of an aneurysm or an AVM, spontaneous intracerebral haemorrhage, ventricular angiomas, bleeding tumours, blunt head trauma and ventriculitis.

4. The CT scan shows high-density blood in the ventricles. MRI shows signal changes depending on the age of the haemorrhage.

5. If the patient survives the acute episode, hydrocephalus is the main complication. The ventricles are dilated and there may be periventricular hypodensity due to transependymaloedema. Other complications depend on the aetiology of haemorrhage.

6. Intraventricular haemorrhage as such is not a bad prognostic indicator. It usually resolves on its own. The primary condition, eg an aneurysm or AVM, should be treated. If hydrocephalus develops, external ventricular drainage is done with an intraventricular catheter. Drainage is done even when the haemorrhage is near the outlet orifices and hydrocephalus is imminent. The drainage should be slow when there is an unruptured aneurysm. The sudden lowering of CSF pressure might cause a big difference in transmural pressure, which results in rupture of the aneurysm. Thrombolytics can be introduced through the catheter to relieve obstruction.

Case 4.20: Answers

1. MRI shows a large heterogeneously enhancing mass in the left frontal lobe, with large areas of central necrosis and peripherally enhancing wall. There is also perilesional oedema, with compression of the frontal horn of the left lateral ventricle.

2. Glioblastoma multiforme. This is the most malignant form of all gliomas and is the most common primary brain tumour. The peak age is 65–75 years.

3. The common locations are in the cerebral hemisphere: white matter of centrum semiovale, in the frontal and temporal lobes. Other locations are corpus callosum (butterfly glioma), posterior fossa and extra-axial locations.

4. It is associated with neurofibromatosis 1, Turcot syndrome and Fanconi syndrome.

5. The CT shows a heterogeneous mass with areas of haemorrhage, necrosis and cyst formation. The margins are not well-defined and there is significant mass effect with oedema, compression of ventricles and midline shift to the opposite side. There is diffuse heterogeneous enhancement and occasionally it may show a rim enhancement, like an abscess. MRI shows an ill-defined lesion, hypointense in T1 and heterogeneously hyperintense in T2, with surrounding oedema. There is significant contrast enhancement of the solid portions. Increased uptake is seen in the PET scan.

6. The variants are: multifocal, GBM – due to spread of primary GBM; gliomatosis cerebri – diffuse infiltrative tumour; gliosarcoma; giant cell glioblastoma and an inherited tumour.

7. The tumour spreads by direct extension along the white matter, through the subependymal route or via the CSF, or by haematogenous spread.

8. Differential diagnoses for rim-enhancing lesion: abscess, lymphoma, metastasis, haematoma, resolving infarct and tumefactive demyelination.

Case 4.21: Answers

1. In the first picture, a sagittal view of MRI of pituitary fossa shows a homogeneous intrasellar mass, which is extending to the suprasellar region.

2. Pituitary macroadenoma. In the second film, a high signal is seen within the enlarged pituitary, indicating development of haemorrhage into the macroadenoma.

3. Pituitary adenoma is a benign tumour arising from the anterior lobe of the pituitary gland. It can be a macroadenoma, > 10 mm, or a microadenoma, < 10 mm.

4. Pituitary adenomas are classified based on the hormones that they secrete. Prolactinoma, corticotrophic adenoma, somatotrophic adenoma, gonadotrophic cell adenoma, thyrotroph cell adenoma, plurihormonal adenoma, non-functioning null cell adenoma and oncocytoma are the various types. Prolactinoma is the most common type, is large and presents with infertility, amenorrhoea, galactorrhoea, elevated prolactin levels, headache and impotence.

5. Macroadenomas are larger than 10 mm, seen in the sella and extend into the suprasellar region. In CT/MRI, there is an isodense/intense tumour, which enhances homogeneously on contrast. When there is haemorrhage in the tumour, high signal is seen in T1 and T2. Calcification can be seen. Microadenomas are small and in MRI, they may be seen as a small hypointense lesion within the bright signal of the pituitary gland. After contrast, the normal pituitary gland enhances, but the adenoma is seen as a non-enhancing area. Subtle signs of small microadenoma are: height of the gland >10 mm, convexity of the gland, depression of the floor, erosion of the sella, deviation of the pituitary stalk and asymmetry of the gland.

6. Important factors to be assessed in macroadenoma are: extension to the suprasellar and parasellar regions, and compression of the optic chiasmas, ventricles and carotid artery.

7. Necrosis, obstructive hydrocephalus, pituitary apoplexy and encasement of carotid artery are the complications. Prolactinomas can be treated with dopaminergic agonists. Transphenoidal surgery and radiation are used in most tumours.

8. Differential diagnoses are meningioma, metastasis, aneurysm, craniopharyngioma, Rathke's cleft cyst, epidermoid and histiocytosis.

Case 4.22: Answers

1. The angiogram shows splaying of the carotid bifurcation by a soft tissue tumour that is arising at the carotid bifurcation. The CT scan shows a well-defined, round, intensely enhancing tumour in the right carotid space. MRI shows a bright, enhancing tumour in the carotid space, with signal voids within it due to vascularity.

2. Carotid body tumour.

3. Carotid body tumour arises from non-chromaffin tissue, which is an APUD (**a**mine **p**recursor **u**ptake **d**ecarboxylation) system. In the neck it is situated in the carotid body.

4. A carotid body is a $5 \times 3 \times 2$ mm structure situated at the bifurcation of the common carotid artery into the external and internal carotid arteries. It is a chemoreceptor that detects changes in the arterial partial pressures of O_2 and CO_2 and the pH, and regulates pulmonary ventilation through afferent input by the glossopharyngeal nerve to the medullary reticular fibres.

5. A carotid body tumour is made up of nests of epithelioid cells with granular eosinophilic cytoplasm, separated by trabeculated, vascularised, connective tissue. Chromaffin-positive granules are seen. It is a type of paraganglioma. Paraganglia are seen adjacent to the nerves and vessels. In the head and neck, they are seen in the carotid body, jugular foramen, path of the vagus nerve and middle ear.

6. Carotid body tumour is situated in or outside the adventitial layer of the common carotid artery at the level of the bifurcation in the posteromedial wall. It is bilateral in 5%. Ultrasonography shows a well-defined mass in the carotid bifurcation, which is hypoechoic, with internal flow as a result of vascularity. The CT scan shows a well-defined, enhancing mass, splaying the bifurcation. Contrast enhancement is homogeneous. MRI shows a low signal on T1 and high signal on T2. Signal voids (absence of any MRI signal) are seen as a result of vascular channels.

7. The most common differential diagnosis is a schwannoma arising from the vagus nerve or sympathetic nerves. These tumours do not splay the bifurcation, but displace it. Internally they are not homogeneous. They have an extensive cystic component, due to myxomatous stroma, and they show heterogeneous enhancement on contrast. Other differential diagnoses are lymph nodal masses (lymphoma, infection including TB and metastasis).

8. The carotid body tumours grow at the rate of 5 mm/year. Malignant transformation is seen in 6%. Treatment is with surgical resection. Transarterial chemoembolisastion reduces tumour vascularity and makes surgery easier.

1. This is a contrast-enhanced MRI of the brain obtained in the sagittal plane. The MRI shows multiple enhancing masses, in the inferior cerebellum and upper cervical cord.

2. Haemangioblastoma of the cerebellum and upper cervical cord.

3. Von Hippel–Lindau syndrome.

4. The CT scan of the abdomen shows multiple, hypodense cysts in the pancreas. There is a small solid mass on the cortex of the anterior aspect of the right kidney.

5. Haemangioblastoma is a benign tumour of vascular origin. It is commonly seen in the cerebellar hemispheres. It can also be seen in the spinal cord, cerebral hemispheres or brain stem. The lesion can be solid, cystic with mural nodule or cystic. CT shows a well-defined cyst or a cyst with an enhancing nodule or a solid enhancing lesion. MRI shows a cyst with a low signal on T1 and high signal on T2, and a solid nodule within, which shows intense enhancement. Flow voids are seen in the solid component. Haemorrhage is high signal in both sequences. Oedema is seen around the tumour. Angiography shows a vascular nidus in the cyst and draining veins.

6. Haemangioblastomas are associated with von Hippel–Lindau syndrome, which is characterised by cerebellar and spinal cord haemangioblastomas, cysts of the pancreas and kidneys, endolymphatic sac tumour, rhabdomyoma of the heart, renal carcinoma, phaeochromocytoma, cystadenoma of the epididymis, islet cell tumour, liver adenoma and paraganglioma. Renal cell carcinomas in von Hippel–Lindau syndrome occur at a younger age, are frequently multiple and are bilateral compared with renal carcinomas in those without the syndrome.

7. Differential diagnoses: **pilocytic astrocytoma** (cerebellar hemisphere, large cyst > 5 cm, thick wall, mural nodule not as vascular), **medulloblastoma** (solid, vermis), **arachnoid cyst** (no mural nodule) and **metastasis** (more oedema, primary tumour may be known).

1. MRI of the chest shows a large mass in the right paravertebral region, which extends into the spinal canal, causing widening of the intervertebral foramen. There is widening of the spinal canal. There is mild enhancement of the paravertebral mass in the post-contrast scan.

2. Spinal neurofibroma.

3. Neurofibroma is a nerve sheath tumour, which is made up of neuronal elements containing Schwann cells, nerve fibres, fibroblasts and collagen. It is commonly seen at age 20–30 years.

4. In the spine, it is commonly seen in the intradural extramedullary location. It is more common at the cervical and thoracic levels. Other locations are in the peripheral nerves.

5. Neurofibroma is associated with neurofibromatosis type 1. It is a dignostic feature of NF-1.

6. An X-ray shows neurofibromas as paraspinal masses when they are large. In the chest, the ribs are dysplastic and ribbon shaped. MRI shows a well-defined mass with a dumb-bell configuration, which widens the intervertebral foramen with scalloping or erosion of the pedicles. On MRI the lesion is a homogeneous mass, isointense to muscle on T1 and hyperintense on T2. The target sign is characterised by a low signal centre on T2 as a result of collagen and condensed Schwann cells. There is no significant contrast enhancement. CT shows a homogeneous, hypodense, dumb-bell lesion that does not show contrast enhancement. Occasionally soft-tissue nodules are seen in the subcutaneous plane.

7. Cord compression can be seen in large tumours. Malignant transformation is rare.

8. The most common differential diagnoses are meningioma (not dumb-bell, hyperdense, contrast enhancement), metastasis, dermoid, lipoma, ependymoma and neurenteric cyst.

Case 4.25: Answers

1. An axial T2-weighted image shows a bright, fluid-containing space in the centre of the cervical spinal cord. The sagittal view of MRI shows a long cavity, which has high signal intensity on T2-weighted images, extending through the cervical and upper thoracic levels.

2. Syringomyelia.

3. Syringomyelia is a cavity in the spinal cord that may communicate with the central canal, not lined by ependymal tissue. It is caused by interrupted flow of CSF through the perivascular space of cord between the subarachnoid space and the central canal. The causes are trauma, postinflammatory, tumours, vascular insufficiency and idiopathic. Hydromyelia is dilatation of the central canal of the spinal cord. This is associated with a Chiari malformation, Dandy–Walker syndrome, spinal dysraphism, myelocele, scoliosis, diastomatomyelia, Klippel–Feil syndrome, segmentation defects and tethered cord.

4. Loss of pain and temperature, trophic changes in skin, muscle weakness, spasticity, hyperreflexia and abnormal plantar reflexes are seen. It is usually seen in the cervical cord, and can extend to the thoracic level or brain stem.

5. MRI is the imaging procedure of choice. It shows a longitudinal CSF-filled cavity, low signal on T1 and high signal on T2. Usually the wall is smooth, but it may be beaded with metameric haustrations in syringomyelia secondary to tumour. Traumatic syringomyelia has septations, irregular borders and arachnoid loculations. CT shows low-density areas, with no contrast enhancement. The cord is enlarged.

6. Differential diagnoses for other cystic lesions in the spinal cord are cystic tumours such as ganglioglioma, astrocytoma, ependymoma and haemangioblastoma. Other intramedullary lesions are MS, transverse myelitis, sarcoidosis, lipoma, epidermoid cyst, dermoid cyst, teratoma, oligodendroglioma, AVM and metastasis.

7. A variety of surgical treatments is available for syringomyelia, including suboccipital and cervical decompression, laminectomy with syringotomy, shunts (VP shunt, lumboperitoneal shunt, syringo-subarachnoid/syringoperitoneal shunt), fourth ventriculostomy, terminal ventriculostomy, percutaneous needling and neuroendoscopic surgery.

Neuroradiology Answers

Case 4.26: Answers

1. The CT scan shows a very dense lesion seen in the right parietal lobe, with compression of the right lateral ventricle and midline shift to the left side. There is subfalcine herniation, and minimal vasogenic oedema surrounding the lesion, which is seen as a low-density area.

2. Acute cerebral intraparenchymal haematoma.

3. Intraparenchymal haematomas are caused by shear strain injury via a blunt or penetrating trauma, with blood separating the neurons.

4. The most common location for traumatic intracerebral haematoma is low frontal and anterior temporal white matter or the basal ganglia. Hypertensive haematomas are common in basal ganglia, external capsule, thalamus, brain stem, cerebellum and cerebral hemisphere.

5. In a non-contrast CT scan, haematoma is seen as a high-density lesion (50–70 HU), with irregular margins, surrounded by a hypodense oedema. The density of the haematoma increases in the first few days as a result of haemoglobin and clot retraction. Layering may be seen. The density of the haematoma increases in the first week, after which the density decreases, starting from the periphery to the centre and becomes isodense. Contrast study is not advisable because it might increase intracerebral pressure. There might be rim enhancement in the second week as a result of a break in the blood–brain barrier. The MRI appearance of haematoma depends on the stage of haematoma and the type of haemoglobin:

Stage	Time (days)	Haemoglobin	T1	T2
Hyperacute	< 24 h	Oxyhaemoglobin	Iso-	Hyper-
Acute	1–3	Deoxyhaemoglobin	Hypo-	Hypo-
Subacute early	4–7	Methaemoglobin intracellular	Hyper-	Hypo-
Subacute chronic	8–14	Methaemoglobin extracellular	Hyper-	Hyper-
Chronic	> 14	Haemosiderin	Hypo-	Hypo-

6. Common causes of haematoma are chronic hypertension, rupture of an aneurysm or AVM, haemorrhagic infarction, amyloid angiopathy, coagulopathy, haemorrhagic tumour (metastasis from choriocarcinoma, melanoma, renal cancer, thyroid cancer), glioblastoma multiforme, ependymoma, venous infarction, eclampsia, septic embolism and vasculitis.

7. Complications are – compression of brain with herniations, extension of bleeding into ventricles, porencephaly, gliosis and atrophy. Large intraparenchymal haematomas with rising intracranial pressure require urgent surgical evacuation. Intracranial pressure is continually monitored in ICU.

Case 4.27: Answers

1. MRI shows a well-defined, broad-based lesion in the frontoparietal region, with minimal surrounding oedema. Post-contrast MRI shows intense enhancement.

2. Meningioma.

3. Meningioma is the most common benign tumour in the brain. It is derived from arachnoid cap cells, which are meningothelial cells that penetrate the dura.

4. The most common locations are the convexity, parasagittal region, sphenoidal ridge and olfactory groove. It can be seen in the ventricles and other sites in the brain. Ectopic meningiomas can be seen outside the brain.

5. Meningiomas are seen in middle- and old-aged people, more common in women. It is associated with neurofibromatosis type 2, in which meningiomas can be multiple. There is association with basal cell naevus syndrome.

6. The histological types are fibroblastic, transitional, meningothelial and angioblastic. The last two are aggressive. It is multicentric in 2–10%. Meningiomas can be discrete globular masses or seen en plaque, which is associated with just hyperostosis. Other variants are cystic meningiomas and lipoblastic meningiomas.

7. On plain films of the skull, calcification, hyperostosis and prominent vascular grooves are seen. A CT scan shows a well-defined extra-axial mass, which is located outside the brain parenchyma. Meningiomas have a broad base, displace the grey–white matter interface inside and have a cleft between the mass and brain (CSF vascular cleft). The mass is hyper- or isodense, with calcifications and hyperostosis of adjacent bone. After contrast, there is intense enhancement of the mass, with a dural tail of enhancement. There is minimal oedema. MRI shows a similar appearance with low signal on T1. The signal on T2 is lower in fibrous types and higher in more aggressive types, and there is intense contrast enhancement with dural tail.

8. Meningioma, being an extra-axial mass, is supplied by branches of the external carotid artery. The most common supply is from the middle meningeal artery. On angiography, the tumour fills early with contrast and there is a persistent blush. There may be a spokewheel configuration.

9. Differential diagnoses of meningiomas are glioma (intra-axial tumours), melanoma, metastasis, lymphoma and haemangiopericytoma,

10. Asymptomatic small meningiomas are followed up. Large meningiomas are surgically resected.

Case 4.28: Answers

1. This is T2-weighted MRI of the neck. The left parotid gland is normal, but the right parotid gland is abnormal. There is a mass replacing almost the entire parotid gland, which is very bright on T2-weighted images.

2. Pleomorphic adenoma of the left parotid gland.

3. Pleomorphic adenoma is the most common benign tumour of the parotid gland and the third most common parotid tumour in children after **haemangioma** and lymphangioma. Some 80% occur in the superficial lobe and 80% are benign. The tumour is a combination of epithelial and myoepithelial cells and presents as a slow-growing, painless lump in the cheek in the parotid region.

4. Ultrasonography shows a soft-tissue mass, hypo- or isoechoic, with well-defined smooth margins. Calcification can be seen. On a CT scan, the parotid gland has a low density as a result of the fat in the gland. The mass is seen as a soft-tissue density lesion inside the parotid gland. The margins are well defined and there is mild homogeneous contrast enhancement. If the tumour is large, there might be areas of haemorrhage, necrosis in the centre of the lesion. In MRI, the tumour has low signal intensity on T1 and high intensity on T2. Contrast enhancement is seen. There is no invasion of lymph nodes or adjacent structures.

5. The important factors are margins (benign tumours have well-defined margins), involvement of deep part of the parotid gland, involvement of facial nerve (facial nerve and vascular invasion indicates malignancy) and lymphadenopathy.

6. Complications are facial nerve involvement and malignancy. Treatment is facial nerve-sparing parotidectomy.

7. Haemangioma, schwannoma, mucoepidermoid carcinoma and adenoid cystic carcinoma are other tumours in the parotid gland.

5
PAEDIATRIC
RADIOLOGY
QUESTIONS

Case 5.1

A 10-day-old neonate presents with respiratory distress and cyanosis. Resonant note was heard on percussion of the left side of the chest. Decreased breath sounds and abnormal splashing sounds were heard on auscultation of the left side.

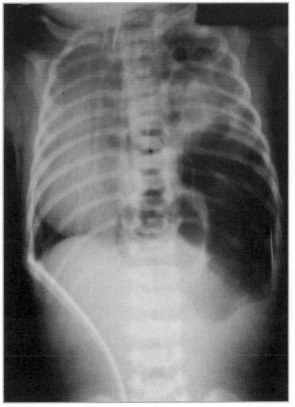

Fig 5.1

1. What do you see on the chest X-ray?
2. What is the diagnosis?
3. What are the types of this disease?
4. What are the radiological findings?
5. What are the prognostic factors?
6. What are the complications?
7. What is the differential diagnosis for this appearance?
8. What is the treatment?

Answers on pages 411–427

Case 5.2

A preterm neonate, born at 30 weeks, with birthweight of 1000 g, developed severe abdominal distension, bilious vomiting and blood in the stools. Clinically she was febrile, with distended abdomen and there were no bowel sounds.

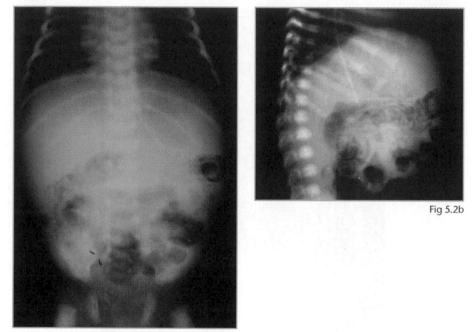

Fig 5.2b

Fig 5.2a

1. What do you observe on the X-ray of the abdomen?
2. What is the diagnosis?
3. What are the predisposing factors for this condition?
4. What is the most common location?
5. What are the clinical features?
6. What are the radiological features of this condition?
7. What are the complications?
8. What is the treatment?

Answers on pages 411–427

Case 5.3

A 4-month-old baby with chronic constipation, abdominal distension, vomiting and failure to thrive was seen in the clinic. Clinical examination revealed gross abdominal distension.

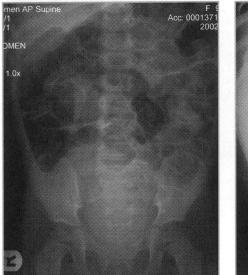

Fig 5.3a

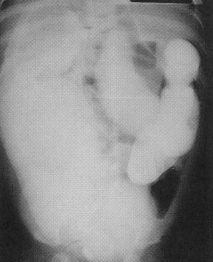

Fig 5.3b

1. What do you see on the plain X-ray?
2. What do you observe on the second examination and what does it show?
3. What is the diagnosis?
4. What are the aetiology and the pathology?
5. What are the clinical features?
6. What are the radiological procedures and findings?
7. What is the diagnostic approach to this patient?
8. What is the treatment?

Answers on pages 411–427

Case 5.4

A 3-week-old boy delivered normally at full term presents with recurrent episodes of bilious vomiting and abdominal distension.

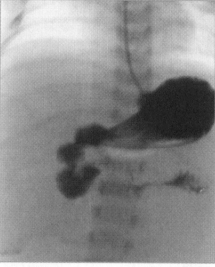

Fig 5.4a

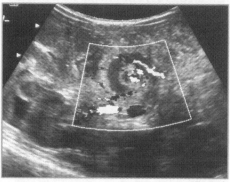

Fig 5.4b

1. What do you see on the plain film of the abdomen?
2. What do you see on Doppler ultrasonography of abdomen?
3. What is the diagnosis?
4. What is the development of this condition?
5. What are the radiological features?
6. What are the complications and the treatment?

Answers *on pages 411–427*

Case 5.5

A 6-week-old boy, delivered at term, presents with projectile vomiting and feeding difficulties. On examination, there is a palpable mass in the upper quadrant of the abdomen.

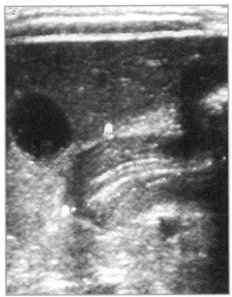

Fig 5.5a

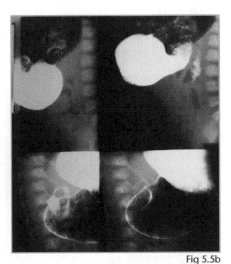

Fig 5.5b

1. What do you observe on this ultrasound examination?
2. What do you observe on the contrast study?
3. What is the diagnosis?
4. What are the aetiology and the clinical features of this disease?
5. What are the ultrasound features?
6. What are the features noted in a contrast study?
7. What is the differential diagnosis?
8. What is the treatment?

Answers on pages 411–427

Case 5.6

A 4-year-old girl presents with recurrent urinary infections, left-sided abdominal pain and oliguria. On examination there is a large cystic mass on the right side of her abdomen in the renal angle. There is renal angle tenderness.

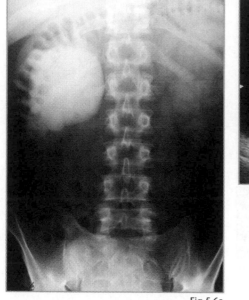

Fig 5.6a

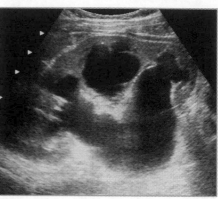

Fig 5.6b

1. What do you observe on IVU?
2. What do you observe on renal ultrasonography?
3. What is the diagnosis?
4. What is the aetiology?
5. What are the clinical features?
6. What are the radiological features?
7. What is the earliest test to diagnose this condition?
8. What is the treatment?

Answers *on pages 411–427*

An 18-month-old boy presents with a history of recurrent UTIs, failure to thrive and dribbling of urine. On examination the abdomen was distended and bladder palpable. A voiding cystourethrogram (VCUG) was performed.

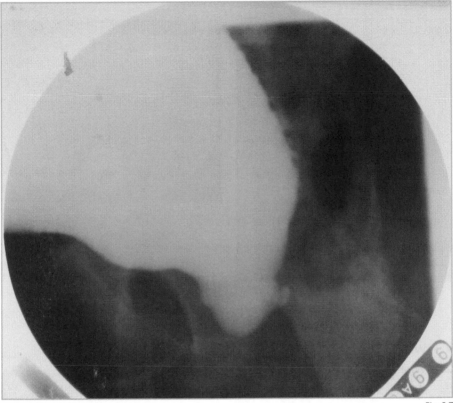

Fig 5.7

1. What are the findings in VCUG?
2. What is the diagnosis?
3. What are the clinical features?
4. What are the types of this disorder?
5. What are the radiological findings?
6. What are the complications?
7. What are the findings of this disease before birth?
8. What is the differential diagnosis?

Answers on pages 411–427

A 5-year-old boy presents with abdominal pain, distension and headache. On examination, there is a large, firm, tender mass in the right side of the abdomen.

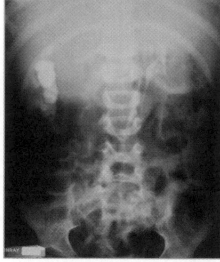

Fig 5.8a

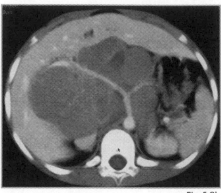

Fig 5.8b

1. What do you see on IVU?
2. What do you observe on the CT scan of the abdomen?
3. What is the diagnosis?
4. What are the pathology and the common locations?
5. What are the clinical features?
6. What are the radiological features and the differential diagnosis?
7. What are the prognostic factors?
8. What is the further management of this patient?

Answers *on pages 411–427*

Case 5.9

A 2-year-old boy presents with failure to thrive, irritability and bowed legs. On examination there are bilateral knock-knees and an abnormal skull.

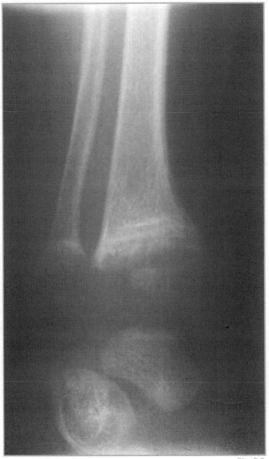

Fig 5.9

1. What are the findings on the ankle X-ray?
2. What is the diagnosis?
3. What is the pathophysiology of this disease?
4. What are the causative factors?
5. What are the radiological and clinical features?
6. What is the differential diagnosis?

Answers on pages 411–427

A 2-year-old boy is brought to A&E with a history of falls from bed. On examination there are bruises on his arms and legs in varying stages of development.

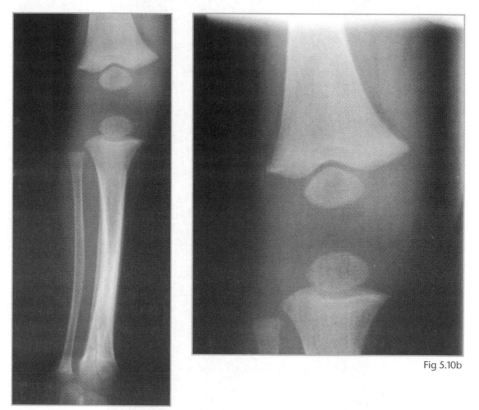

Fig 5.10a

Fig 5.10b

1. What do you observe on the plain X-ray?
2. What is the diagnosis?
3. What is the differential diagnosis for this radiological appearance?
4. What the clinical features of this disease?
5. What are the most suspicious findings?

Answers on pages 411–427

Case 5.11

A 16-month-old baby presents with diarrhoea, rectal bleeding and an incessant cry. An X-ray and ultrasonography of the abdomen were performed.

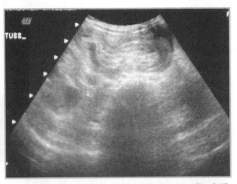

Fig 5.11b

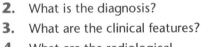

Fig 5.11a

1. What do you observe on the plain X-ray and on ultrasonography?

2. What is the diagnosis?

3. What are the clinical features?

4. What are the radiological features?

5. What do you see on the third picture and what is the management of this patient?

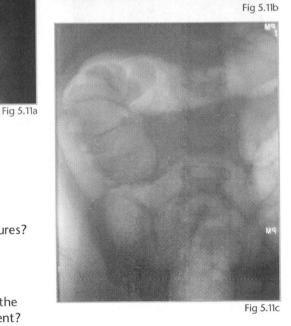

Fig 5.11c

Answers *on pages 411–427*

Paediatric Questions

A 3-year-old boy presents with severe abdominal pain. A plain X-ray, and ultrasound and CT scans were performed.

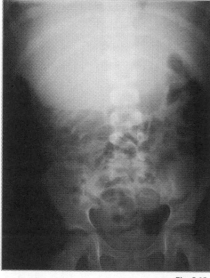

Fig 5.12a

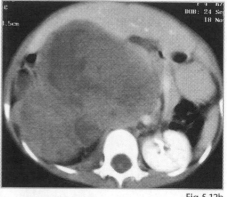

Fig 5.12b

1. What do you see on the plain X-ray and the CT scan?
2. What is the diagnosis?
3. What are the clinical features and associations?
4. What are the radiological features?
5. What is the differential diagnosis in this age group?
6. How will you manage this patient?

Answers on pages 411–427

Case 5.13

A 4-year-old boy falls from a swing and presents to A&E with a painful, swollen left wrist. On examination there is tenderness, and swelling of the left wrist, which has restricted motion.

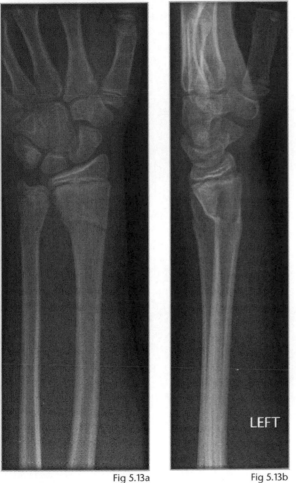

Fig 5.13a   Fig 5.13b

LEFT

1. What are the findings on this X-ray?
2. What is the diagnosis?
3. What is the mechanism of injury?
4. What are the things to look for on the X-ray to confirm the diagnosis?
5. What is the treatment of this condition?

Answers on pages 411–427

A 7-year-old boy twisted his ankle.

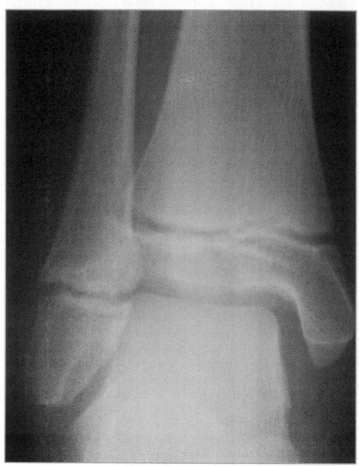

Fig 5.14

1. What are the findings on this X-ray?
2. What is the diagnosis?
3. What is the mechanism of injury?
4. What are the different types of this injury?
5. What is the treatment?

Answers on pages 411–427

Paediatric Questions

Case 5.1: Answers

1. The X-ray shows multiple lucencies in the left thoracic cavity with shift of the mediastinum to the right side. There is paucity of bowel loops in the abdomen.

2. Congenital diaphragmatic hernia.

3. **Bochdalek's hernia** (90%): defect in the pleuroperitoneal canal, seen posteriorly, more frequent on the left side (75%), contains stomach/colon/small intestine/spleen/pancreas/kidneys. The herniated bowel loop frequently malrotates.

    Morgagni's hernia (10%): anterior and more often on the right side, at costophrenic angle, contains omentum or colon, associated with accompanying anomalies.

    Eventration: due to absence of muscle in the dome of diaphragm. Associated with trisomies 13, 18, congenital infections (cytomegalovirus, rubella), arthrogryposis congenita multiplex and pulmonary hypoplasia. Rarely, congenital **hiatus herniation** of the stomach can be seen. There is an association with De Lange syndrome and familial cases have been reported. Children present with respiratory distress.

4. On an X-ray, the lungs are multicystic and the hemidiaphragm is not visualised. Mediastinal shift is seen to the opposite side. There is a paucity of bowel loops in abdomen. The stomach is more centrally placed than normal. Diagnosis becomes difficult when there is no gas in the bowel loops or when there is herniation of liver or solid viscera, in which case there will be homogeneous opacification that needs to be differentiated from fluid or mass. Herniation of bowel loops can be confirmed by contrast examination, which opacifies the bowel loops in the chest. The mortality rate is 60% and higher when associated with other abnormalities, such as neural tube defects and pulmonary hypoplasia.

5. Poor outcome is seen when the stomach herniates (indicates herniation at earlier stage of gestation and hence more pulmonary hypoplasia) or when the hernia is associated with pneumothorax or when it is right-sided. Aerated ipsilateral lung and aerated contralateral lung >50% are favourable features.

6. Complications are pulmonary hypoplasia, gastric volvulus, midgut malrotation and volvulus, gastric or intestinal perforations, hypoplastic left ventricle, pleural effusion and ipsilateral renal hypertrophy.

7. Differential diagnoses for this appearance are: **congenital lobar emphysema** (hyperexpansion of single lobe, attenuated vascular markings), **cystic adenomatoid malformation, congenital diaphragmatic hernia** (bowel loops can be traced going into abdomen), **pneumothorax** (no vascular markings seen), **Swyer–James syndrome** (secondary to viral infection, small hyperlucent lung, pruning of peripheral pulmonary vasculature) and **inhaled foreign body** (change in appearance in expiration and inspiration).

8. Treatment is by surgery. Fetal surgery can be performed to reduce the development of pulmonary hypoplasia, which has a bad prognosis. Emergency postnatal surgical reduction can be performed. Surgery can also be performed with a delay of 24 hours to 10 days, during which time the baby is stabilised and a nasogastric tube is used for decompression of the bowel. Some surgeons prefer to operate on these neonates when normal pulmonary artery pressure is maintained for at least 24–48 hours, based on echocardiography. Postoperative pneumothorax is common.

Case 5.2: Answers

1. The X-ray of the abdomen shows distended loops of small and large bowel. There are subtle areas of gas collection in the wall of the small bowel. Gas is also seen in the peritoneum, which is best seen in the lateral view.

2. Necrotising enterocolitis.

3. Necrotising enterocolitis is the most common gastrointestinal emergency in neonates. It is an ischaemic bowel disease secondary to hypoxia, perinatal stress, infection (no single causative organism) and congenital heart disease. It is common in preterm infants (abnormal intestinal flora, ischaemia and mucosal immaturity), those with Hirschsprung's disease, bowel obstruction resulting from small bowel atresia, pyloric stenosis, meconium ileus and meconium plug syndrome.

4. It is most commonly seen in the terminal ileum, followed by the caecum and right colon. It develops in the first 2–3 days after birth. Pathologically there is widespread transmural necrosis and acute inflammation with mucosal ulceration.

5. Neonates present with gross abdominal distension, bilious emesis, delayed gastric emptying feeding intolerance, decreased bowel sounds, explosive diarrhoea, blood-streaked stools, apnoea, lethargy, shock and generalised sepsis. Elevated WBC count, anaemia, thrombocytosis, metabolic acidosis and hyponatraemia are worrisome features.

6. An X-ray shows dilated small and large bowel loops, with or without air–fluid levels, especially in the right lower quadrant. The bowel gas pattern is disarrayed rather than the normal polygonal pattern. Bowel wall thickening with thumbprinting is also seen. The bowel loops are fixed and do not show any change on sequential films. Pneumatosis intestinalis is a characteristic finding and is characterised by curvilinear (serosal) or bubbly (mucosal) gas collection (hydrogen bubbles produced by bacterial fermentation of intestinal contents). The bowel appears bubbly as a result of gas in the wall, faecal matter that is a mix of blood, sloughed colonic mucosa, intraluminal gas and faecal material. Gas is seen in the branches of the mesenteric vessels and portal vein. Gas in the portal vein does not necessarily imply a grave outcome. Pneumoperitoneum is seen as a result of bowel perforation and warrants surgery. Barium enema is contraindicated in these patients. Absence of bowel gas indicates distension with fluid and is also worrisome. When ascites develops as a result of perforation, the bowel loops float in the centre of the abdomen. Ultrasonography can find the portal gas, any local abscess formation and other abnormalities.

7. Complications are inflammatory stricture and bowel perforation, which is seen in 30% of patients. Short gut syndrome results from removal of long segments of bowel, causing malabsorption. Of patients 75% survive, of whom 50% develop complications.

8. Treatment of necrotising enterocolitis depends on the degree of bowel involvement and the severity of its presentation. Parenteral nutrition and fluid support are initiated. Broad-spectrum antibiotics are given after blood culture. Surgery is indicated when there is bowel perforation

Case 5.3: Answers

1. The plain X-ray shows dilated loops of small bowel and large bowel with air–fluid levels, indicating distal obstruction in the large bowel. There is no gas in the rectum and no pneumoperitoneum.

2. This is an enema of the large bowel performed with water-soluble contrast. A rectal tube is inserted and a radio-opaque contrast introduced to distend the rectum. The study shows a transition point from a normal calibre bowel to grossly dilated proximal bowel.

3. Hirschsprung's disease.

4. Hirschsprung's disease is characterised by the absence of myenteric (Auerbach) and submucosal (Meissner) ganglion cells in the distal alimentary tract as a result of failure of neural crest cells to populate the embryonic colon at around 5–12 weeks of gestation. Hirschsprung's disease can be classified as classic (75%), where the rectosigmoid is involved, long segment (20%) or total colonic (3–12%).

5. Neonates present with failure to pass meconium, abdominal distension and vomiting. Older children present with constipation, abdominal distension, vomiting and failure to thrive. Associated conditions are Down syndrome, multiple endocrine neoplasia and Waardenburg syndrome.

6. The X-ray shows features of bowel obstruction with no gas in the rectum, implying a low large bowel obstruction. Another feature is presence of mixed barium stool pattern in delayed X-rays. An enema with water-soluble contrast agent with a 5 Fr catheter under screening control will often demonstrate a narrow segment of aganglionosis and proximal dilated normal colon with faecal loading. The presence of a transitional zone at the junction of normal and abnormal innervation is a highly reliable sign, but not always seen. Other findings are: irregular bowel contractions in the aganglionic segment, thick nodular mucosa proximal to the transition point and delayed evacuation of contrast.

7. Contrast study has a false-negative rate of 24%. Rectal manometry shows an absence of normal relaxation of the internal sphincter, with a reduction in the intraluminal pressure in the anal canal when the rectum is distended with a balloon. Rectal biopsy (suction or full thickness) has a 100%

negative predictive value. If ganglion cells are present, then Hirschsprung's disease is excluded. Other findings are hypertrophy and hyperplasia of nerve fibres, and an increase in acetylcholinesterase-positive nerve fibres in the lamina propria and muscularis mucosa.

8. Treatment depends on the patient's age and the extent of involvement. The aganglionic bowel is removed or bypassed, with anastomosis of normally innervated intestine to the distal rectum. This can be performed by means of a preliminary colostomy followed by a definitive pull-through procedure or an immediate definitive procedure. Presence of normal ganglion cells in confirmed with frozen section during surgery.

Case 5.4: Answers

1. The barium meal shows a distended stomach. The duodenojejunal flexure is situated in the right side of the lumbar vertebrae.

2. Doppler ultrasonography of the abdomen shows a whirlpool appearance of twisted mesentery. The superior mesenteric artery is situated to the right of the superior mesenteric vein.

3. Intestinal malrotation.

4. Normal intestinal rotation takes place around the superior mesenteric artery (SMA) as axis. The proximal duodenojejunal loops and distal colic loops make a total 270° in rotation during normal development. Both loops start in a vertical plane parallel to the SMA and end in a horizontal plane.

    Stage I (5–10 weeks): the bowel herniates into the base of the umbilical cord. The duodenojejunal loop begins superior to the SMA at 90° and rotates 180° in a counterclockwise direction. At 180° the loop is to the right of the SMA and by 270° it is beneath the SMA. The caecal loop begins beneath the SMA at 270°, rotates 90° counterclockwise and ends at the left at 0°. Both loops maintain these positions until the bowel returns to the abdominal cavity. The midgut lengthens along the SMA and a broad pedicle is formed at the mesentery base.

    Stage II (week 10): bowel returns to abdominal cavity. The duodenojejunal loop rotates 90° to end at the left of the SMA. The caecal loop turns 180° more to place it to the right of the SMA at 180°.

Stage III (11 weeks till term): the descent of the caecum to the right lower quadrant and mesentery fixation.

Arrest in development of stage I causes non-rotation (duodenojejunal junction not inferior and left of the SMA, caecum not in the right lower quadrant, narrow base of mesentery, midgut volvulus).

Incomplete rotation: stage II arrest – peritoneal bands, midgut volvulus depending on rotation before arrest, internal herniations.

Incomplete fixation: no mesenteric fixation, resulting in hernial pouches formation, volvulus if the caecum remains unfixed.

5.   A plain X-ray shows a double-bubble appearance. A barium meal is the mainstay in the diagnosis of malrotation. Small volumes of barium are fed and rapid fluoroscopic images taken. The duodenum and jejunum are located to the right of the spine. The duodenojejunal junction (ligament of Trietz), which is normally located to the left of the spine at the level of T12, is located on the right side. Colonic loops are seen on the left side of abdomen. A corkscrew appearance indicates midgut volvulus. Doppler ultrasonography is used to confirm the diagnosis of malrotation. In normal Doppler ultrasonography, the superior mesenteric vein (SMV) is located to the right of the SMA, but this is reversed in malrotation. Another sign is the whirlpool sign, which is a result of twisted mesentery at the base of the bowel.

6.   Volvulus (a result of clockwise rotation of the midgut), obstruction, ischaemia, perforation, Ladd's bands and internal herniation are the complications. Surgery is done when there is malrotation with volvulus or obstruction.

Case 5.5: Answers

1.   This is an ultrasound of the upper abdomen. The pylorus is visualised here. It is very thick and shows the target sign. The pyloric channel, which is the hyperechoic area in the centre is very long. The redundant pyloric channel is protruding into the gastric antrum.

2.   Contrast study shows a narrow, long, tapered pylorus and proximally distended stomach filled with contrast. There is no flow of contrast distally and a shoulder indentation is noted on the gastric antrum.

3. Congenital hypertrophic pyloric stenosis.

4. Hypertrophic pyloric stenosis is idiopathic hypertrophy of the circular muscle fibres of the pylorus, extending into the gastric antrum. It is seen between 2 and 8 weeks and is more common in first-born boys. Etiology is multifactorial. The baby has projectile vomiting and there might be a palpable olive-shaped mass in the epigastric region.

5. Ultrasound is the mainstay in the diagnosis of pyloric stensis. Ultrasound is done after feeding.

   a. **Target sign** – refers to thickened hypoechoic pylorus with central hyperechoic mucosa

   b. **Pyloric wall thickness** > 3mm. **Pyloric transverse diameter** > 13mm with channel closed

   c. **Elongated pyloric channel** > 17mm

   d. **Pyloric volume** > 1.4cc

   e. **Pyloric length (mm) + 3.64 x muscle thickness (mm)** > 25

   f. **Cervix sign** – indentation of muscle mass on fluid filled antrum

   g. **Antral nipple sign** – redundant pyloric channel protruding into antrum

   h. **Increased peristaltic waves**

   i. **Delayed gastric emptying** of fluid into duodenum.

6. Contrast study shows:

   1. **String sign** – contrast flowing through a small streak through pyloric channel

   2. **Double track sign** – crowding of mucosal folds in pyloric channel

   3. **Diamond sign** – irregular tent like clefts in mid portion of pyloric canal

   4. **Teat sign** – outpouching along lesser curvature

   5. **Beaking** – mass impression on antrum

   6. **Mushroom sign** – indentation of base of bulb.

7. Differential diagnoses: **infantile pylorospasm** (has similar features of pyloric stenosis, with thick muscle, antral narrowing and elongation of pylorus, but it undergoes spontaneous resolution or responds to metoclopromide); **gastritis/milk allergy** (circumferential thickening of antral mucosa); **gastric diaphragm** and **duodenal obstruction from mid-gut volvulus** (whirpool sign – twisted mesentery, reversal of SMA and SMV).

8. Once the diagnosis has been confirmed, the metabolic abnormality, such as hypochloraemic metabolic alkalosis, is corrected. Heller's myotomy is performed. The pylorus muscle is incised longitudinally, leaving an intact mucosa of the pylorus.

Case 5.6: Answers

1. IVU shows gross enlargement of the right renal pelvis and right collecting system. The ureter is not visualised.

2. Ultrasound of the right kidney shows grossly dilated pelvicalyceal system of the right kidney. There is also blunting of the fornices.

3. Obstruction of the pelviureteric junction (PUJ), causing hydronephrotic changes of the right kidney.

4. PUJ obstruction is the most common cause of obstruction in children. Causes:

Primary obstruction:

   – **intrinsic**: functional, excessive collagen, abnormal muscle orientation, abnormal conduction, high ureteral insertion, mucosal folds

   – **extrinsic**: aberrant vessels, kinks, angulations, bands, cysts, aneurysm

Secondary obstruction: stones, ischaemia, infection, trauma, iatrogenic.

5. It is more common in boys, on the left side, and presents with abdominal mass, pain, haematuria and a urinary tract infection (UTI).

6. Ultrasound shows a large dilated anechoic renal pelvis, with no dilatation of the ureter. Dilated collecting system is seen. IVU can show a non-functioning kidney. There might be delayed excretion of contrast. There is dilated renal pelvis without dilated ureters. Abrupt narrowing is seen at the PUJ.

7. PUJ obstruction can be diagnosed antenatally. If the renal pelvis is > 10 mm in the AP direction, it is considered enlarged. A follow-up postnatal ultrasound scan should be done. If there is persistent dilatation, follow-up ultrasonography and VCUG are done to exclude vesicoureteral reflux (VUR). Other tests that may be used for confirmation are diuresis IVU, diuresis renography and Whitaker's pressure–flow urodynamic study.

8. Pyeloplasty is done for surgical correction. The spastic pelviureteric junction is excised and reanastomosed to the pelvis of the kidney.

Case 5.7: Answers

1. Oblique view of VCUG shows grossly distended bladder, with wall trabeculations. The posterior urethra is dilated, with a smooth outline and no contrast is seen in the anterior urethra.

2. Posterior urethral valve, causing chronic bladder obstruction.

3. Posterior urethral valve is seen in boys and usually is seen at first on the antenatal ultrasound, neonatal period or in later childhood. The children present with recurrent UTIs, hesitancy, straining, dribbling, enuresis, palpable kidneys and bladder, failure to thrive or rarely haematuria.

4. Posterior urethral valve is a congenital fold or mucous membrane located in the posterior urethra, which includes the prostatic and membranous portion. There are three types:

    Type I: mucosal folds extend anteriorly and inferiorly from the verumontanum of the urethra and fuse at the lower level

Type II: mucosal folds extend anterosuperiorly from the verumontanum towards the bladder neck

Type III: diaphragm-like membrane, located below the level of the verumontanum.

5. VCUG shows fusiform dilatation and elongation of the posterior urethra, which persists throughout voiding. Occasionally it is seen as a filling defect in the urethra. The distal urethra appears collapsed. The bladder is distended and might show prominent trabeculations or sacculations resulting from obstruction. VUR can be seen. After voiding, a large volume of residual urine is seen in the bladder.

6. Complications are bladder outlet obstruction, VUR, urinary infections renal dysplasia (obstruction during gestation), prune-belly syndrome, neonatal pneumothorax/pneumomediastinum and neonatal urine leak.

7. Posterior urethral valve can be diagnosed on antenatal ultrasound scans, with oligohydramnos, bilateral hydroureteronephrosis, distended urinary bladder, thick-walled bladder, posterior urethral dilatation and dilated utricle in the urethra. Urinary leak and dysplastic kidneys can be seen.

8. Differential diagnoses of distended bladder and bilateral dilated ureters include: posterior urethral valve, congenital urethral stricture, meatal stenosis, vesicoureteral reflux, primary megaureter and megacystis–microcolon–intestinal hypoperistalsis syndrome.

Case 5.8: Answers

1. IVU shows inferior and lateral displacement with moderate hydronephrosis of the right kidney. The left kidney collecting system is normal.

2. The CT scan shows a large mass in the upper retroperitoneum, which completely encases the aorta and coeliac branches, crossing the midline. The mass is overlying the right kidney and is displacing it laterally and posteriorly.

3. Neuroblastoma.

4. Neuroblastoma is the third most common malignancy in children after intracranial tumours and leukaemia. It arises from primitive sympathetic neuroblasts of the neural crest, in either the sympathetic ganglion chain or the adrenal medulla. Although it can occur anywhere along the sympathetic chain from the neck to the pelvis, the most common location is the adrenal gland. Seventy-five per cent of cases are abdominal. Thoracic lesions account for a further 10–15% and pelvic and cervical lesions make up the rest.

5. It is usually seen before the age of 5 years, with most children presenting around age 2. It affects both sexes equally. Unlike Wilms' tumour, the child is usually unwell, with lethargy, anaemia and reduced general status. Sixty per cent of cases present with metastatic disease. Bone pain, limping, ecchymoses, pallor, black eyes, proptosis and facial swelling are signs. Symptoms resulting from renal arterial compression (hypertension), spinal canal invasion and hormonal activity can be encountered such as flushing, sweating, diarrhoea and hypokalemia.

6. Diagnosis is based on imaging and 24-hour urine collection for catecholamines. X-rays can show abdominal mass and skeletal metastasis. Ultrasound is the initial examination, which shows a large adrenal mass, with displacement of the kidneys. It is usually a solid tumour with areas of calcification. Cystic tumours are rare. CT or MRI is required for full assessment. MRI is better for demonstrating intraspinal extension. CT shows calcification. MRI and CT are ideal for demonstrating encasement of coeliac/renal/mesenteric arteries, which is a characteristic feature of neuroblastoma. Bony metastases are seen as hot spots in isotope MDP (methyl diphosphonate) bone scan. Increased uptake is seen in MIBG (^{131}I-labelled meta-iodobenzylguanidine) scan as a result of chromaffin cell activity. Differential diagnoses include Wilms' tumour, lymphoma and sarcoma.

7. The prognosis depends on the staging at presentation and aggressiveness of neoplasm as determined by cytogenetics. Stage IV disease and elevated number of oncogene NMYC within chromosome 2 are associated with poor prognosis. Stage IV neuroblastoma occurs in children less than 12 months of age, with metastasis to bone marrow and not to bone, with good prognosis, with spontaneous remission. Overall survival rate is 30–35%. Infants have a better survival rate of 70%.

8. Children are initially treated with chemotherapy, after biopsy confirmation. This is followed by surgical excision depending on the stage.

1. The X-ray of the ankle shows increased distance between the shaft and epiphyseal centre with cupping and fraying of the metaphysis.

2. Rickets.

3. Rickets is a metabolic abnormality affecting endochondral bone growth, in which the zone of preparatory calcification does not form, with heaping of maturing cartilage cells, and failure of osteoid mineralisation with calcium. The changes are more marked in areas of rapid bone growth.

4. Causes of rickets:

   Primary vitamin D deficiency

   Malabsorption: gastrectomy, enteropathy, enteritis, biliary obstruction, biliary cirrhosis, pancreatitis

   Primary hypophosphataemic vitamin D resistant rickets

   Hypophosphatasia, pseudohypophosphatasia

   Fibrogenesis imperfecta osseum

   Axial osteomalacia

   Hypoparathyroidism, hyperparathyroidism, thyrotoxicosis, Paget's disease, fluoride, neurofibromatosis, osteopetrosis, malignancy, macroglobulinaemia, ureterosigmoidstomy.

5. Radiological features: rickets is commonly seen in the metaphysis of the long bones such as the wrists, ankles and knees. An X-ray shows delayed formation of poorly mineralised epiphysis; the epiphyseal plates are wide and irregular. Increased distance is seen between the end of the shaft and the epiphysis. Cupping and fraying of metaphysis, metaphyseal spurs, coarse trabeculation, periosteal reaction, deformities, such as bowed legs and bowing of the diaphysis, and frontal bossing are other features. Patients suffering from rickets present with irritability, bone pain, tenderness, craniotabes, rachitic rosary, bowed legs, delayed dentition, and swelling of the wrists and ankles.

6. Differential diagnoses: metaphyseal dysplasia and healing scurvy.

1. The plain X-ray shows a spiral fracture in the distal tibial metaphysis, with periosteal thickening.
   There is also a subtle fracture in the medial aspect of the metaphysis of the distal femur (better seen in the magnified view on the second film).

2. Non-accidental injury with corner sign.

3. Metaphyseal irregularity and fracture in children can be seen as a result of trauma, infection, metastatic neuroblastoma, leukaemia, congenital syphilis and scurvy.

4. Non-accidental injury is the third cause of death in children after sudden infant death syndrome and accidents. The children are usually brought to hospital with a history of trauma. Multiple injuries are seen in different stages of healing. Usually they are seen in children aged less than 2 years. The usual sites of fracture are ribs, costochondral junction, acromion, skull, vertebra, tibia and metacarpals. There are multiple fractures in different stages of healing, with exuberant callus formation. Avulsion fracture at ligament insertion is seen without periosteal reaction. The epiphysis is separated, and the metaphysis shows irregularity and fragments. Corner fracture/bucket-handle fracture is a characteristic finding. It is caused by the avulsion of the arcuate metaphyseal fragment overlying the epiphyseal cartilage, resulting from sudden twisting of an extremity. This causes the periosteum to be pulled from the diaphysis, but it remains attached to the metaphysis. A spiral fracture of the diaphysis can be seen. Extensive periosteal reaction may be present.

5. **Fractures pathognomonic of non-accidental injury:**

   – rib fractures, costochondral junction fractures, especially first rib fractures and posterior fractures

   – metaphyseal fractures, bucket-handle type

   – fractures at different stages of healing

   Fractures highly suggestive of non-accidental injury:

   – scapula, outer third of clavicle, vertebral (dorsolumbar, C2–3), digital injuries

   – diaphyseal fractures.

Case 5.11: Answers

1. The plain film shows a claw (meniscus) sign in the middle of the abdomen at the level of L2, with a soft-tissue opacity protruding into a gas shadow of the colon. Ultrasonography shows a pseudokidney sign, with central hyperechogenicity and surrounding hypoechogenicity.

2. Ileocolic intussusception.

3. Intussusception is a common cause of acute abdomen in infancy, and occurs when a segment of bowel, the intussusceptum, telescopes into the bowel distally, the intussuscipiens. It is usually seen between 6 months and 2 years of age. Most are ileoileal or ileo-ileocolic. Most cases are idiopathic and do not have any lead point other than lymphoid hypertrophy (Peyer's patches). About 2% have lead points, which include Meckel's diverticulum, duplication cyst, lymphoma, polyps, Henoch–Schönlein purpura and inspissated mucus in cystic fibrosis. Characteristic features include intermittent colicky abdominal pain with drawing up of legs, vomiting, red-currant-jelly stools and palpable abdominal mass. Drowsiness and lethargy can be seen. Mechanical small bowel obstruction and ischaemia are the complications if untreated

4. Plain X-ray demonstrates a soft-tissue mass in the right upper quadrant, dilated small bowel loops or the classical **claw sign** where the apex of the intussusceptum is outlined by gas in the colon. In ileocaecal intussusception, the caecal gas is absent in the right lower quadrant. Bowel obstruction, perforation and sparse amount of bowel gas are other features. Plain X-ray can be normal. Ultrasound is the most sensitive method in diagnosis. Multiple concentric rings or a pseudokidney or doughnut sign can be seen, due to varying appearances of the telescoping bowel loops. Enlarged Peyer's patches can be seen. Fluid in the intussusceptum indicates vascular compromise.

5. This picture demonstrates air reduction of intussusception. The bowel loops are distended with gas, which has entered the small bowel, indicating successful reduction. Air reduction is attempted for treating intussusception. Surgery is done if three attempts of air reduction fail. The standard treatment is air reduction using oxygen or carbon dioxide. A Foley's catheter is inserted into the rectum and a tight seal is maintained. Air is delivered inside the colon, with a maximum pressure of 120 mmHg. Successful reduction is indicated by air entering the small bowel. Three attempts can be made with three-minute intervals. Contraindications of reduction are: prolonged history >48 hours, signs of peritonism, obstruction and rectal bleeding. Perforation and tension pneumoperitoneum are complications of air reduction. Occasionally, dilute barium can also be used. Surgery is performed for failed reductions. There is 5–10% recurrence after operative or non-operative reduction.

Case 5.12: Answers

1. The plain X-ray shows a large mass in the abdomen, which causes inferior displacement of the bowel loops. The CT scan shows the heterogeneously enhancing mass in the right kidney that causes displacement of the midline major vessels.

2. Wilms' tumour of the right kidney.

3. Wilms' tumour is the most common renal tumour in children (6–10% of all childhood malignancies); 80% occur between 1 and 5 years of age with a peak incidence between 3 and 4 years. The tumour is bilateral in 4–13%, which occurs in a younger age group. Mutations in chromosome 11 are identified. It can be associated with crypto-orchidism, hypospadias, hemihypertrophy, aniridia, Beckwith–Wiedemann syndrome, WAGR syndrome (Wilms' tumour, aniridia, genitourinary anomalies, mental retardation), Bloom syndrome and Drash syndrome. It usually presents as a palpable abdominal mass. Hypertension and microsopic haematuria are other presentations. Gross haematuria is rare and arises from persistent primitive embryonal tissue (mesodermal blastema). The classic Wilms' tumour has a combination of epithelial, stromal and blastema cell lines. The prognosis depends on the cell type and the presence of anaplasia.

4. An X-ray shows a large mass, with displacement of gas-filled bowel loops and effacement of a psoas shadow. Calcification is seen in 9–13%. Ultrasonography shows the mass, which is usually iso- or hyperechoic. Hypoechoic areas are seen as a result of necrosis and occasionally the tumour can be entirely cystic. Vascular invasion can be identified. CT and MRI are better at evaluation of perinephric extension, and the relationship to the great vessels, retroperitoneum and spinal canal. CT shows a heterogeneous, enhancing mass, with occasional specks of calcification, with splaying and displacement of blood vessels. Regional lymphadenopathy can be seen. Metastasis in the lung can be demonstrated on a chest CT.

5. Neuroblastoma is the other most common tumour. It arises from the adrenal gland, causing inferior displacement of the kidney. It crosses the midline and encases the vessels (Wilms' tumour causes displacement of vessels, but not encasement). Bony metastasis is more common than Wilms' tumour.

6. CT-guided biopsy is done for histological confirmation. The tumour is treated by initial resection, followed by chemo- and radiotherapy according to the surgical staging of the tumour and histology. Some centres do biopsy and chemotherapy before surgery, which facilitates later tumour resection and makes inoperable tumours operable.

Case 5.13: Answers

1. AP X-ray shows compression of the distal aspect of the radius and ulna. In the lateral X-ray, there is buckling of the dorsal cortex of the radius, with intact volar cortex. The distal fragment is angulated dorsally. There is also buckling of the distal ulna, but to a lesser extent.

2. Torus fracture of the distal radius and ulna.

3. A fall onto outstretched hands is the common mechanism of a torus fracture of the radius. A torus (protuberance in Latin) fracture is unique to children, because of the weakness of bone's immature mineralisation. When a compressive force is placed on a tubular bone's long axis, the axial stress on the bone causes a buckling reaction, characterised by failure of cortex on the compression side, 2–3 cm proximal to the physis.

4. Torus fractures of the distal metaphysis of the radius and ulna are the most common fractures in the lower forearm in young children. The impact of indirect violence of a fall onto an outstretched hand crumples the dorsal cortex, but the volar cortex remains intact. The distal fragment is angulated dorsally. There is no deformity in torus fracture because the periosteum and cortex are intact on the opposite side of the bone. To summarise, in torus fracture the tension side (anterior) is intact. If the fracture is not on the compression side, the patient has a greenstick fracture, which will result in deformity. In a greenstick fracture, there is failure of the cortex on the tension side (convex side of angulation), with plastic deformation of the cortex on the concave (compression) side. A lateral view of the wrist is important for diagnosis.

5. Treatment consists of a short arm cast for 3 weeks to make the patient comfortable and prevent further injury. As a result of the compressive forces on the radius and the proximity of the radius and ulna, there is often involvement of the ulna, which will result in deformity of the thinner, longer ulna. Treatment is to reverse the torsional mechanism of the injury, ie pronating the fracture with palmar angulation of the bone and supinating the dorsally angulated bone.

Case 5.14: Answers

1. There is a lucent line running in the epiphysis of the distal tibia, which extends to the growth plate

2. Salter–Harris type III fracture of the distal tibia.

3. The cartilaginous growth plate of the paediatric skeleton separates the metaphysis and epiphysis. The germinal layer for the growth plate is contiguous with the epiphysis and supplied by epiphyseal vessels. Injuries to the growth plate heal rapidly except when the epiphyseal blood supply or germinal layer has been damaged. Of the layers of the growth plate, the resting cartilage, proliferating cartilage and one of provisional calcification have a strong matrix that resists shearing force. The zone of hypertrophying cartilage is the weakest zone and vulnerable to shearing injuries. The cartilaginous growth plate is weaker in children than the capsule and ligaments, so any force producing sprain or dislocation in adults causes growth plate injury in children.

4. See answer 4 to Case 3.38 on page 318.

5. A Salter–Harris type III fracture of the ankle requires anatomical reduction, which could be a closed or open reduction, which is then followed by plaster cast immobilisation.

6

CHEST AND CARDIOVASCULAR RADIOLOGY

QUESTIONS

Case 6.1

A 56-year-old presents with difficulty breathing at night and coughing. On examination, the patient has oedema, systolic cardiac murmurs and bilateral crackles in the lungs.

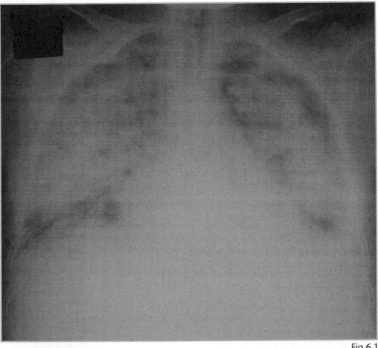

Fig 6.1

1. What do you see on the chest X-ray?
2. What is the diagnosis?
3. What are the causes?
4. What are the radiological findings?
5. What is the reason for this appearance?
6. What are the complications?
7. What is the differential diagnosis?

Answers on pages 451–474

Case 6.2

A 27-year-old man presents with sudden onset of dyspnoea and chest pain. On examination, he is tachycardic, with decreased breath sounds on the right side and a hyperresonant chest on percussion.

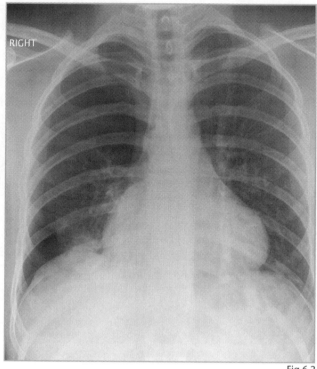

RIGHT

Fig 6.2

1. What are the findings on the chest X-ray?
2. What is the diagnosis?
3. What are the types of this condition?
4. What are the causes?
5. What is the mechanism of spontaneous appearance of this condition?
6. What are the radiological features?
7. What is the indication for treatment?

Answers *on pages 451–474*

Case 6.3

A 43-year-old woman, who underwent pelvic surgery 2 weeks ago, presents with sudden onset of dyspnoea and sharp right-sided chest pain, which increases with deep breathing and coughing. On examination, she is tachycardic. Breath sounds and percussion are normal.

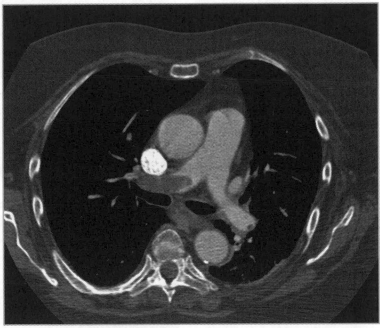

Fig 6.3

1. What is this investigation?
2. What are the findings?
3. What is the diagnosis?
4. What is the imaging protocol for this condition?
5. What are the predisposing factors?
6. What are the clinical features?
7. What is the differential diagnosis?
8. How is this condition managed and what are the complications?

Answers on pages 451–474

A 67-year-old man presents with chest pain and dyspnoea. Clinical examination reveals hypertension and a systolic cardiac murmur. Radiological tests were ordered.

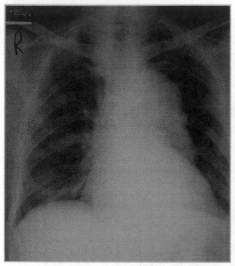

Fig 6.4a

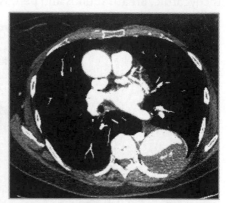

Fig 6.4b

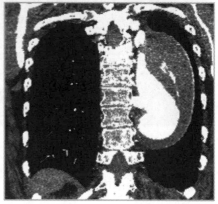

Fig 6.4c

1. What do you see on the chest X-ray and the CT scan?

2. What is the diagnosis?

3. What are the common causes of this condition?

4. What is the classification of this disease?

5. What are the presenting clinical and radiological features?

6. What are the complications?

7. What are the indications for surgery?

8. Which location has the highest morbidity and mortality?

Answers on pages 451–474

A 67-year-old man presented with chest pain, dyspnoea and weight loss. On examination, the patient is anaemic and afebrile. The breath sounds are reduced on the right side and there is a dull note on percussion.

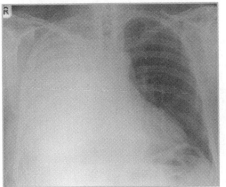

Fig 6.5a

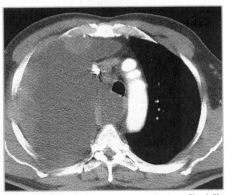

Fig 6.5b

1. What are the findings on the chest X-ray and on CT?
2. What is the diagnosis?
3. What are the predisposing factors?
4. What are the latent period and the histological types?
5. What are the associations?
6. What is the pattern of spread?
7. What are the radiological findings?
8. What is the differential diagnosis?

Case 6.6

A 75-year-old man presents with claudication of the left buttock and both calves. On examination, the pulses are feeble on both sides.

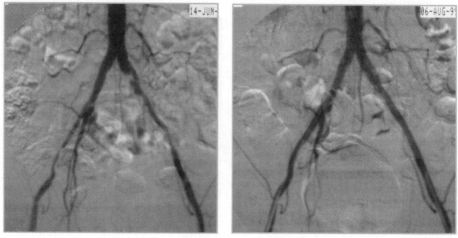

Fig 6.6a   Fig 6.6b

1. What do you see on the first film?
2. What do you see on the second image, obtained after a procedure?
3. What procedure has been done on the patient?
4. What are the causes for the disease?
5. What is the mechanism of this procedure?
6. What are the indications and steps of this procedure?
7. What is the prognosis?
8. What are the complications?

Answers on pages 451–474

A 63-year-old man presented with claudication in his leg. On examination, there is a feeble left femoral pulse and good left popliteal and distal pulses. The patient was investigated with angiography.

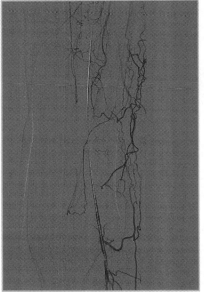

Fig 6.7a

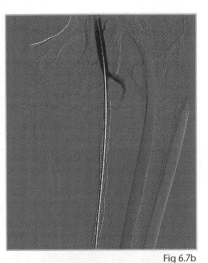

Fig 6.7b

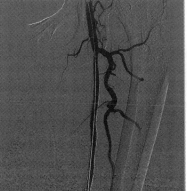

Fig 6.7c

1. What do you observe on the first angiogram?
2. What procedure has been undertaken and what do you observe on the second and third picture?
3. What are the uses of this device?
4. What are the types?
5. What are the other places where it can be used?
6. What are the complications?

Answers on pages 451–474

Case 6.8

A 35-year-old woman presents with severe pain in her left thigh and leg. On examination, her left leg is swollen, tender and oedematous. The pulses are normal.

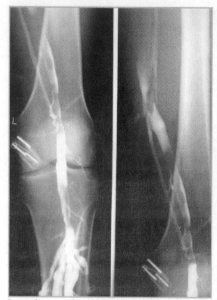

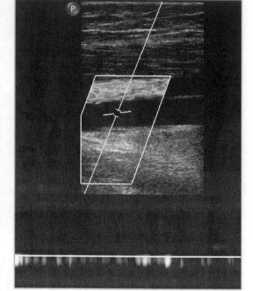

For colour version, see *Colour Images* section from page 475.

Fig 6.8a

Fig 6.8b

1. What is this investigation and what do you find?
2. What is the diagnosis?
3. What are the causes of this disease?
4. What are the common locations?
5. What are the features on Doppler ultrasonography?
6. What are the other investigations that may be of help?
7. What are the complications?
8. What is the management?

Answers *on pages 451–474*

A 49-year-old man presents with intermittent left arm pain, which is worse after exercise, dizziness and vertigo. On examination, the pulse in the left arm is feeble compared to the right side.

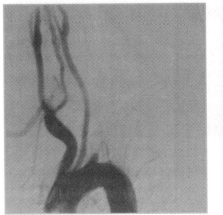

Fig 6.9a

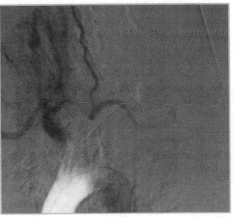

Fig 6.9b

1. What do you see on the first image?
2. What is demonstrated in the second image?
3. What is the diagnosis?
4. What are the causes? What syndrome does a disease in this vessel cause?
5. What are the clinical features?
6. What are the radiological features?
7. What are the complications?
8. What is the treatment?

Answers on pages 451–474

Chest Questions

A 45-year-old woman presented with uncontrollable hypertension. On examination, her BP was 210/118 mm Hg and there was a bruit in the abdomen.

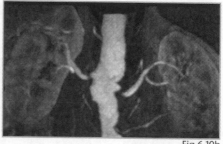

Fig 6.10b

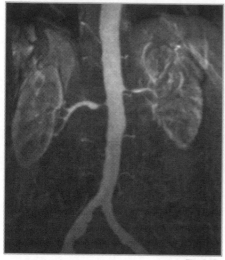

Fig 6.10a

1. What is this investigation and what do you observe?
2. What is the diagnosis?
3. What are the causes of this disease?
4. What are the haemodynamically significant lesions?
5. Who needs screening?
6. What are the radiological features?
7. What are the complications?
8. What is the management?

Answers *on pages 451–474*

Case 6.11

A 47-year-old man presented with chest pain and hypertension. On examination there were asymmetrical pulses and blood pressure in the arms.

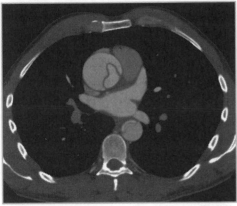

Fig 6.11a

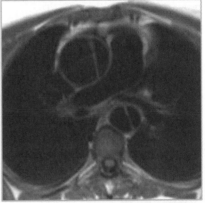

Fig 6.11b

1. What do you find on the CT and MR scans?
2. What is the diagnosis?
3. What are the causes of this disease?
4. What are the locations?
5. What are the types?
6. What are the radiological features?
7. What are the complications?
8. What is the management?

Answers on pages 451–474

Case 6.12

A 61-year-old man, with a history of medically controlled hypertension, presents with severe abdominal pain. On examination, he has a palpable, tender mass in the umbilical region, which is tender, and the patient is hypotensive.

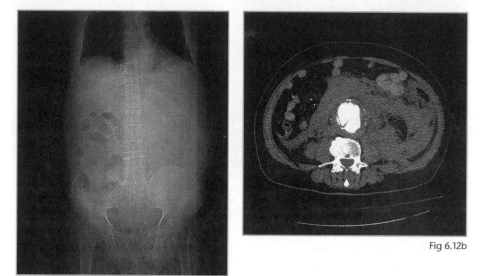

Fig 6.12b

Fig 6.12a

1. What do you find on the abdominal X-ray and CT scan?
2. What is the diagnosis?
3. What are the causes of this disease?
4. What are the associations?
5. What are the types?
6. What are the complications?
7. What are the radiological features?
8. What is the management?

Answers on pages 451–474

Case 6.13

A 56-year-old woman presents with right-sided chest and bilateral leg pain after recent travel. On examination, she has tenderness in both legs. Doppler ultrasonography showed bilateral thrombi.

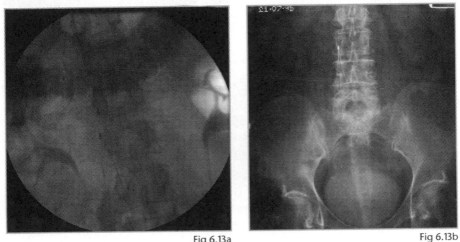

Fig 6.13a   Fig 6.13b

1. What procedure is being done on the first film?

2. What do you note on the second film?

3. What is the indication for this?

4. What are the types?

5. How is it inserted?

6. What are the precautions?

7. What are the contraindications?

Answers on pages 451–474

A 33-year-old man presents with infertility and testicular pain. He was investigated thoroughly for infertility. A scrotal ultrasound was performed, which was followed by a definitive procedure for treatment of infertility.

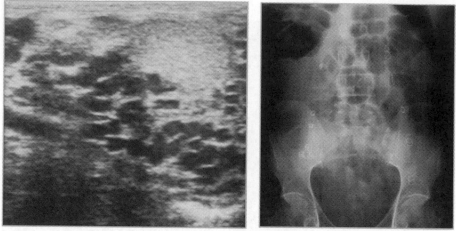

Fig 6.14a   Fig 6.14b

1. What do you see on ultrasonography?
2. What do you observe on the second film? What procedure has been done?
3. What is the diagnosis?
4. What is the aetiology of this condition?
5. What is the anatomy?
6. What are the clinical features and the complications?
7. What are the radiological findings?
8. What are the treatment options?

Answers *on pages 451–474*

Case 6.15

A 38-year-old woman presented with irregular uterine bleeding.
Clinical examination revealed multiple, irregular masses in the uterus.
Ultrasonography also showed multiple benign tumours. The patient was
referred to radiology for treatment.

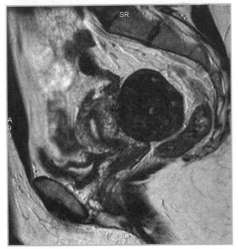

Fig 6.15a

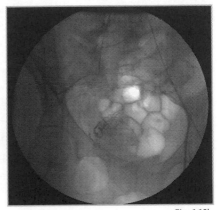

Fig 6.15b

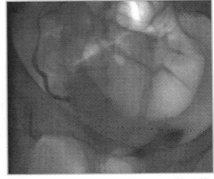

Fig 6.15c

Chest Questions

1. What do you observe on MRI of this patient?
2. What is the diagnosis?
3. What is the procedure being performed on the second picture?
4. What are the clinical features of this disease?
5. What are the radiological features?
6. What are the treatment options and the indications of the procedure shown above?
7. What are the results of this procedure?
8. What are the complications?

Answers on pages 451–474

A 52-year-old woman presents with a lump behind the left knee. On clinical examination, the lump is pulsatile. The patient was sent for further investigations.

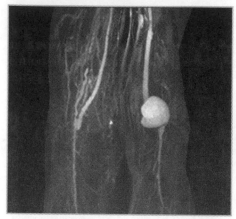

Fig 6.16a

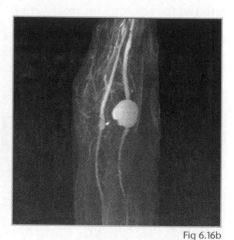

Fig 6.16b

1. What do you see on MRA?
2. What is the diagnosis?
3. What are the causes?
4. What are the radiological and clinical features?
5. What are the complications?
6. What are the differential diagnoses?
7. What is the treatment?

Answers on pages 451–474

A 65-year-old patient presents with intermittent episodes of weakness in his right arm. He is hypertensive and diabetic.

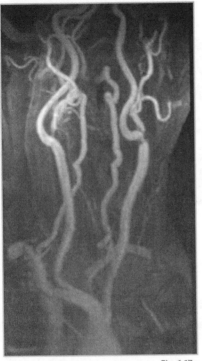

Fig 6.17a

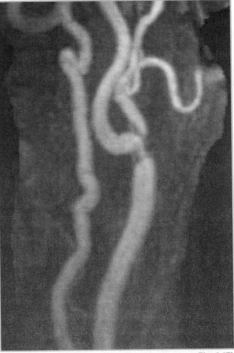

Fig 6.17b

1. What are the findings on MRA?
2. What is the diagnosis?
3. What are the causes of this disease?
4. What are the common locations?
5. What are the indications for carotid ultrasonography?
6. What are the appearances on ultrasonography and angiography?
7. What are the risks and treatment?

Answers on pages 451–474

A 57-year-old man presents with multiple episodes of haemoptysis and coughing. He has a 20-year history of smoking. On examination, there are crackles and bronchial breathing in the right lung.

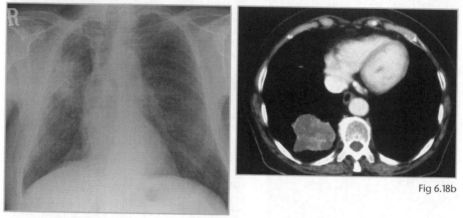

Fig 6.18b

Fig 6.18a

1. What do you observe on the chest X-ray and CT scan?
2. What are the predisposing factors and clinical features?
3. What are the different types of this disease?
4. What are the clinical features?
5. What are the radiological features?
6. How is the diagnosis confirmed and what further investigations are required?
7. What is the differential diagnosis?

Answers on pages 451–474

A 58-year-old man, who is an intravenous drug abuser, presents with pain and swelling in his left groin. On examination, there is a tender, red, pulsatile mass in the left inguinal region. Doppler ultrasound of the left groin and CT scan of pelvis were performed.

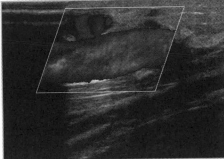

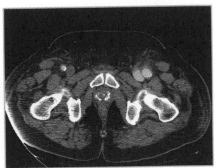

For colour version , see *Colour Images* section from page 475.

Fig 6.19a

Fig 6.19b

1. What do you see on Doppler ultrasonography and on the CT scan?
2. What is the diagnosis?
3. What are the causes?
4. What are the clinical and radiological features?
5. What are the complications?
6. What is the differential diagnosis?
7. What is the role of radiology in treatment?

Answers *on pages 451–474*

Chest Questions

Case 6.1: Answers

1. The heart is enlarged and there are prominent pulmonary vessels. There are also bilateral, perihilar, fluffy, alveolar shadowing, consistent with pulmonary oedema. There are small, bilateral pleural effusions.

2. Congestive cardiac failure.

3. Causes of cardiac failure:

    Underlying cause: structural abnormalities that affect coronary or peripheral arterial circulation, myocardium, pericardium, valves

    Fundamental causes: biochemical or physiological mechanisms that increase haemodynamic burden

    Precipitating cause: arrhythmia, infection, PE, exertion, drugs, high-output states.

4. X-rays show an enlarged heart (heart is not enlarged in acute heat failure):

    Normal left atrial pressure 5–10 mmHg.

    Cephalisation 10–15 mm – prominent upper lobe vessels.

    Kerley B lines 15–20 mm – horizontal lines at base near costophrenic angle.

    Interstitial oedema 20–25 mm – fine reticular opacities in bases.

    Alveolar oedema > 25 mm – confluent, perihilar fluffy opacities.

    Cephalisation: when pressure > 10 mmHg, the fluid leaks into the interstitium and compresses the lower lobes first. This recruits the resting upper lobe vessels to carry more blood. Other features are peribronchial cuffing (interstitial fluid around bronchi), loss of definition of vessels, thickened fissures and pleural effusions. Laminar effusions are seen beneath visceral pleura in the loose connective tissue between the pleura and lung. Pseudotumours can be seen resulting from loculated collections in the fissures.

    Kerley B lines: distended interlobular septa, 1–2 cm long at bases, horizontal, perpendicular to pleural surface.

    Kerley A lines: connective tissue near bronchoarterial bundle, near hilum, oblique, longer.

    Kerley C lines: reticular network of lines.

    There is a 12-hour radiological lag from onset of symptoms. Radiological findings persist for several days despite clinical recovery.

5. A batwing/butterfly shape is caused by an increased accumulation of oedematous fluid in the parahilar region. There are various theories for this appearance. The autoregulation is poorer in the central than in the peripheral region; lymphatics are not efficient in the central region, probably secondary to reduced ventilation in the centre. Lower lung zones are more affected than upper zones. Usually it clears in 2–3 days from the periphery to the centre.

6. Cardiac failure results in clinical symptoms such as dyspnoea, orthopnoea, paroxysmal nocturnal dyspnoea, fatigue, weakness, nocturia and syncope.

7. Differential diagnoses for alveolar opacities: infection, haemorrhage, aspiration, lymphoma, pulmonary alveolar proteinosis. Causes of pulmonary oedema can be cardiac, renal or ARDS: in **cardiac**, even distribution in 90%; in **renal**, central distribution in 70%; in **ARDS**, peripheral in 45% and even in 35%. Air bronchograms are more common in ARDS and pleural effusions more common in cardiac than renal. Radiologically, it is difficult to differentiate oedema, infection, haemorrhage and ARDS.

Case 6.2: Answers

1. The X-ray shows a faint line in the right hemithorax, which separates a collapsed lung and a lucent lateral collection of air without any underlying lung vascular markings.

2. Spontaneous pneumothorax.

3. Pneumothorax can be:

Closed: when the chest wall is intact

Open: when there is a chest wound, producing communication between the pleura and the exterior

Tension: check valve mechanism where air enters the pleural space, but cannot leave it

Hydropneumothorax: air and fluid.

4. Spontaneous, trauma, iatrogenic, airway disease (asthma, histiocytosis, tuberous sclerosis, cystic fibrosis), infections (lung abscess, necrotising pneumonia, bacterial, *Pneumocystis jiroveci* [*carinii*] pneumonia, TB), sarcoidosis, berylliosis, lung cancer, metastasis (osteosarcoma), connective tissue disorder (scleroderma, Marfan syndrome, Ehlers–Danlos syndrome, rheumatoid), pneumonconiosis (silicosis, berylliosis), infarction, catamenial (during menstruation, endometriosis of diaphragm) and complications of honeycomb lung are the different causes of this condition.

5. Spontaneous pneumothorax is caused by rupture of subpleural bulla in the apical region. It is common in tall young men who present with chest pain and dyspnoea. Recurrence is common in 30%, on the same or opposite side.

6. In pneumothorax, there is a lucent collection of air in the pleural space, with a visceral pleural line demarcating it from the collapsed lung. A small pneumothorax requires meticulous inspection to identify it, and it is best demonstrated by a PA chest film taken on expiration. The most important diagnosis that should not be missed is a tension pneumothorax. In tension pneumothorax, there is a large pneumothorax, with inversion of the diaphragm, collapse of the lung, displacement of the trachea and heart to the opposite side. Deep sulcus sign is seen due to large costodiaphragmatic recess. Air–fluid level is seen in hydropneumothorax. If the pneumothorax is localised in the anteromedial location, there is outline of the medial diaphragm under cardiac shadow, with sharp delineation of medial diaphragmatic contour. When there is subpulmonic pneumothorax, there is a hyperlucent upper abdomen, with deep lateral costophrenic sulcus and visualisation of the inferior surface of the liver. In postomedial pneumothorax, a lucent triangle is seen with vertex at the hilum, and a V-shaped base delineating costovertebral sulcus.

7. Treatment of primary spontaneous pneumothorax includes observation, simple aspiration and chest tube placement. Secondary spontaneous and traumatic pneumothoraces require chest tube placement. An iatrogenic pneumothorax is treated with observation or simple aspiration. A tension pneumothorax is a medical emergency and requires immediate needle decompression and chest tube placement, with aspiration of tube drainage in severe cases. Observation is appropriate when a pneumothorax is < 15% chest volume. Pneumothorax > 35% volume requires a chest tube. O_2 administration at 3–10 l/min increases the rate of pleural air absorption. A pneumothorax is reabsorbed at the rate of 1.25%/day. A recurrent pneumothorax is managed with pleurodesis.

Case 6.3: Answers

1. This is CT pulmonary angiography; 150 ml iodinated contrast is injected at the rate of 4–5 ml/s into the antecubital vein and images are taken throughout the chest during peak enhancement in the pulmonary arteries.

2. There is a hypodense lesion within the right pulmonary artery, which is occluding the lumen. The main pulmonary artery and left pulmonary artery are normal.

3. Pulmonary embolism.

4. In a patient with suspected PE, a chest X-ray is performed. If the chest X-ray is normal, a ventilation perfusion lung scintigraphy is performed. Ventilation scan is done by inhalation of radioactive tracer gas such as Krypton. Areas of lung that receive too much air are seen as hot spots and areas not receiving enough air are seen as cold spots. On a perfusion scan, radioactive tracer, such as albumin macroaggregates, is injected intravenously. Areas of the lungs not receiving enough blood, will be seen as defects. In PE, the ventilation scans will be normal and perfusion scans will be abnormal, giving the characteristic mismatched ventilation and perfusion defects. If chest X-ray is abnormal or the ventilation perfusion scan is indeterminate, a CT pulmonary angiography is performed. With the modern 64-slice multidetector CT scanners, embolus can be detected even in tiny peripheral pulmonary arterial branches. The overall negative predictive value of CT angiography for pulmonary embolism is greater than 99%. CT scan also find features of right-heart strain, such as a big pulmonary artery and bowing of the interventricular septum, which are bad prognostic indicators. PE can also be diagnosed indirectly, by demonstrating deep venous thrombus by colour Doppler ultrasound of the extremities.

5. Hypercoagulable states, DVT, recent surgery, pregnancy, immobilisation and underlying malignancy are predisposing features.

6. Chest pain, back pain, shoulder pain, dyspnoea, haemoptysis, wheeze, syncope and cardiac arrhythmia are clinical features. Low PO_2, raised D-dimer and raised WBC count are lab findings.

7. Myocardial infarction, angina, pneumonia and oesophageal reflux are differential diagnoses.

8. Oxygen, fluids, anticoagulants and fibrinolytics are used for treating pulmonary embolism. Fibrinolytic therapy is the standard of care for PE, unless there is a contraindication to fibrinolysis. Heparin is used to slow or prevent clot progression and reduce the risk of further embolism. Occasionally, embolectomy may be necessary. IVC filters are used for recurrent PE. Sudden death, cardiac arrest, pulmonary hypertension and cor pulmonale are the complications.

Case 6.4: Answers

1. The X-ray shows a tortuous, enlarged descending thoracic aorta, causing superior mediastinal widening. The CT scan with contrast shows a normal ascending aorta, but there is a massively enlarged descending thoracic aorta, which has thrombus within it. The coronal CT scan shows the complete extent of the aneurysm filled with thrombus.

2. Descending thoracic aortic aneurysm.

3. Atherosclerosis, cystic medial necrosis, Marfan syndrome, Ehler–Danlos syndrome, infection, arteritis and trauma are recognised causes. In the past, syphilis was a major cause of thoracic aortic aneurysm.

4. Crawford classification:

   Type I involves the descending thoracic aorta from the left subclavian artery down to the abdominal aorta above the renal arteries.

   Type II extends from the left subclavian artery to the renal arteries and may continue distally to the aortic bifurcation.

   Type III begins at the mid-to-distal descending thoracic aorta and involves most of the abdominal aorta as far distal as the aortic bifurcation.

   Type IV extends from the upper abdominal aorta and all or most of the infrarenal aorta.

5. Usually they are asymptomatic and incidentally discovered on imaging studies. They can present with pain and hypertension. On X-rays aneurysms cause mediastinal widening. Transoesophageal echocardiography is good for assessment of aortic valve, ascending/proximal descending aorta, but limited for arch and distal descending aorta. Transoesophageal echocardiography can differentiate aneurysm

and dissection. Contrast-enhanced CT is the main investigation used in diagnosis of aortic aneurysms. It evaluates the aorta rapidly. The location, extent and size of the aneurysm, the relationship of the aneurysm to branch vessels and surrounding structures, and the size, dissection, thrombus, intramural haematoma and rupture are all evaluated. Multiplanar reconstructions are obtained. A CT scan is done before stent graft insertion to determine the adequacy of the proximal landing zone, patency of vertebral arteries and whether the left subclavian artery should be covered by a stent graft. MRI and MRA can also determine the location, extent, size, and relationship to branch vessels and surrounding organs.

6. Complications include rupture and compression of adjacent structures. Tracheal compression produces dyspnoea, stridor and wheezing. SVC compression produces dilated veins and ecchymosi. Compression of the oesophagus causes dysphagia and haematemesis. Compression of the spine produces back pain and paralysis. Distal thromboemboli and aortic insufficiency may be encountered.

7. Surgical repair is indicated in all symptomatic patients. Elective repair is indicated in ascending aortic aneuryms > 5.5 cm and descending aortic aneuryms > 6.5 cm (> 5 and 6 cm respectively in Marfan syndrome) and any aneurysm that grows more than 1 cm/year. Symptoms, dissection and rupture are indications for emergency repair. Descending thoracic aneurysms may be repaired with open surgery or endovascular stent grafting techniques.

8. Arch aneuryms have the highest morbidity and mortality as a result of associated neurological complications.

Case 6.5: Answers

1. The chest X-ray shows a large pleural effusion on the right side, without a mediastinal shift. The CT scan shows a large pleural effusion with lobulated soft-tissue masses arising from the pleural surface over the chest wall.

2. Malignant mesothelioma.

3. Malignant mesothelioma is a malignant tumour of serosal lining of the pleura, usually involving the parietal pleura and to a lesser extent the visceral pleura. Predisposing factors are asbestos exposure, TB, empyema and radiation. In asbestos exposure, crocidolite fibres are the most common and 10% of workers exposed to asbestos develop malignant mesothelioma. Smoking is not a risk factor.

4. Latent period is 20–45 years. It is seen in men aged 50–70 years. Histological types are epithelioid, sarcomatoid and biphasic.

5. Mesothelioma is associated with hypertrophic pulmonary osteoarthropathy, peritoneal mesothelioma and the changes noted with asbestos exposure in lungs.

6. Clinical features are cough, chest pain, coughing up of asbestos bodies, weakness, fever and dyspnoea. Spread can be contiguous to the lung, chest wall, mediastinum, pericardium, diaphragm and peritoneum. Lymphatic spread is to the hila, mediastinum, and supraclavicular, axillary and cervical nodes. Haematogenous metastasis occurs in the liver, lungs and bones.

7. An X-ray shows a large pleural effusion and a pleurally based, lobulated opacity with no contralateral mediastinal shift as a result of tumour fixing the mediastinum. Rib destruction can be seen. A CT scan shows pleural effusion. The volume of the lung is reduced with fixed mediastinum or ipsilateral mediastinal shift, narrowed intercostal spaces and elevated diaphragm. The fissures are thickened as a result of tumour infiltration. There is a large, lobulated, pleural mass, with destruction of the ribs. The tumour might spread to abdominal peritoneum, causing ascites. Calcified pleural plaques and underlying asbestosis can be seen. Features of asbestos exposure, such as pleural thickening and calcified diaphragmatic/mediastinal pleural plaques, are also seen.

8. Metastatic adenocarcinoma, benign mesothelioma, pleural fibrosis, fibrothorax and empyema are the differential diagnoses. Metastatic adenocarcinoma is commonly seen in breast carcinoma and the appearances are similar, but there are no telltale signs of asbestos exposure, such as pleural thickening and plaques.

1. The first picture shows atherosclerotic changes of sacculations and stenosis of the left common iliac artery. Significant stenosis is also noted in the external iliac arteries on both sides.

2. The second film shows normal flow in the previously narrowed left common and external iliac arteries. The previously stenosed segment of the right external iliac artery also appears dilated.

3. Percutaneous transluminal balloon angioplasty (PTA) of both the iliac arteries has been performed. (See catheters within the arterial lumens as lucent lines.)

4. Atherosclerosis, thromboangiitis obliterans and diabetes are the common causes of arterial narrowing.

5. PTA fractures the vascular intima and the plaques, and stretches the media, improving the luminal diameter of the stenosed segments. Healing is by intimal hyperplasia.

6. Claudication, non-healing wound, tissue loss and inflow for distal bypass graft are the indications for balloon angioplasty. For the femoral artery, an ipsilateral approach is preferred and for iliac arteries, a contralateral approach is used. The lesion is crossed by a guidewire. If there is significant pressure gradient across the stenosis, a balloon catheter is passed, with optimal diameter, and inflated. The wire remains across the lesion. After angioplasty, the pressure measurements and angiogram are repeated to assess the result.

7. In the femoral artery, there is a 90% initial success with 70% 5-year patency. Good prognostic indicators are large vessel, proximal lesions, stenosis rather than occlusion, short stenosis, isolated disease, good inflow and outflow. Poor prognosis is seen in diabetes, limb salvage interventions and in patients who continue to smoke.

8. Complications are thrombosis, dissection, perforation, occlusion, recurrent stenosis and groin haematoma and puncture site pseudoaneurysm.

Case 6.7: Answers

1. The angiogram of the left leg shows occlusion of the proximal left superficial femoral artery, which is reconstituted distally by collaterals from the profunda femoris artery.

2. The second picture shows a metallic stent deployed in the occluded femoral artery. The third picture obtained after stent deployment shows normal flow through the stent and the artery is now patent.

3. Vascular stenting involves the placement of a small wire mesh tube called a stent into the newly opened artery. Occluded arteries are first opened with balloon angioplasty. Stenting may be necessary after some angioplasty procedures if the artery is considerably narrowed or completely blocked. The stent is a permanent device that is left in the artery and may be needed to help the artery heal in an open position after the angioplasty. Stents are used when angioplasty is unsuccessful and stenosis recurrent in all venous obstructions and TIPSS. Stents are useful in long segment stenosis, total occlusion, or ineffective or unsuccessful PTA with residual stenosis/pressure gradient, recurrent stenosis after PTA, ulcerated plaque and renal ostial lesions.

4. A stent can be a bare metal stent, a covered stent/stent graft or a drug-eluting stent. A stent graft is a tubular device that is composed of a special fabric supported by a rigid structure, usually metal. The rigid structure is the stent. An average stent on its own has no covering and is usually just a metal mesh. Stent grafts are used in endovascular surgery, including in the repair of an abdominal aortic aneurysm. Once inside the aorta, the stent graft acts as false lumen for blood to pass through, rather than the aneurysm sack. There are two major types of metallic stent: the balloon expandable stent and the self-expandable stent. Balloon expandable stents are made of Nitinol, and are less flexible and distended with balloon. Self-expandable stents, such as the Wallstent, are made of stainless steel; placement is less precise, but they can be used in tortuous vessels.

5. Vascular stenting is used in peripheral vascular disease, renal vascular disease, coronary artery disease, carotid stenosis, for haemodialysis access and in strictures and occlusion of veins.

6. Complications of stent placement are haemorrhage, dissection, thrombosis, embolus, maldeployment, stent migration, rupture and sudden closure of a vessel.

Case 6.8: Answers

1. A venogram shows multiple, small, filling defects in the popliteal vein, extending to the femoral vein. Doppler ultrasonography shows colour flow within the femoral artery, but no colour flow within the femoral vein, which is filled with echogenic material.

2. DVT in the left leg.

3. DVT is caused in hypercoagulability states, stasis, intimal injury or platelet aggregation. The predisposing factors are surgery, trauma, prolonged immobilisation, obesity, malignancy, diabetes, pregnancy, oral contraceptive pills, cardiac failure, myocardial infarction, old age, varicose veins, previous DVT, polycythaemia and smoking.

4. The most common location is the dorsal veins of the calf. Other locations are the iliofemoral veins. It is rare in an internal iliac vein, ovarian vein and ascending lumbar vein. It is more common in the left side as a result of compression of the left common iliac vein by the left common iliac artery, which leads to chronic endothelial injury. Patients present with swelling, pain, warmth, tenderness and calf pain, exacerbated by dorsiflexion of the foot.

5. Doppler ultrasonography shows expansion of the veins. Thrombus is hypo- or isoechoic. Normal veins can be compressed with the ultrasound probe, but this is not possible with a thrombosed vein. There is no cyclical variation in flow with respiration and there is no augmentation on distal compression. Soft-tissue oedema can be seen. Doppler ultrasonography is efficient in detection of DVT of calf veins.

6. Venography shows a filling defect in deep veins, but it does not demonstrate satisfactorily the calf veins, common femoral vein or iliac veins. ^{125}I-labelled fibrinogen localises to the clot. Venous occlusion plethysmography shows delay in venous outflow.

7. Complications are PE (77% risk from iliac veins, 35–70% for femoropopliteal veins, 0–50% for calf veins), post-phlebitic syndrome and phlegmasia cerulea/alba dolens with gangrene.

8. Tibial/peroneal venous thrombi resolve in 40%. Treatment is with intravenous heparin, systemic anticoagulation with warfarin for > 3 months. An IVC filter is placed in patients with contraindications/complications from anticoagulent treatment and recurrent DVT.

Case 6.9: Answers

1. This is an angiogram of the aortic arch, which shows occlusion of the left subclavian artery close to its origin from the aortic arch.

2. The second image taken with delay of a few seconds, shows retrograde flow through the left vertebral artery filling the left subclavian artery, distal to the stenosis.

3. Subclavian stenosis, with subclavian steal syndrome.

4. Subclavian stenosis is most commonly caused by atherosclerosis. Subclavian steal syndrome is a subclavian artery occlusive disease proximal to the origin of the vertebral artery, which is associated with flow reversal in the vertebral artery. When the subclavian artery is occluded or stenosed, the decreased blood pressure in the arm distally causes vertebral artery flow alteration. Subsequently, there is no flow through the vertebral artery. A compensatory collateral circulation is established from the circle of Willis, which reverses flow into the vertebral artery; this then flows into the distal subclavian artery. There are four types: vertebro-vertebral, carotid basilar, external carotid–vertebral and carotid–subclavian.

5. The patient may be asymptomatic or present with arm pain, claudication, dizziness, vertigo, unsteadiness and visual changes. Symptoms are provoked by an increased blood flow requirement to the compromised arm such as an arm exercise, arm cuff inflation or during neck movements, which restricts compensatory flow.

Chest Answers

6. Angiography is the modality of choice. An angiogram shows occlusion or stenosis of the subclavian artery proximal to the vertebral artery. Delayed films show retrograde filling of the vertebral artery. Alternatively, the normal carotid circulation can be catheterised and there will be retrograde flow into the affected vertebral artery. MRI or CT angiography can be done instead of the invasive conventional angiography. Doppler ultrasonography shows subclavian artery stenosis and reversal of vertebral artery flow.

7. Complications are arm ischaemia and stroke.

8. Treatment is with angioplasty and stenting, failing which surgical revascularisation is performed.

Case 6.10: Answers

1. This is MRA (MR Angiography) of the abdominal aorta and renal arteries. There is bilateral, high-grade narrowing of both renal arteries.

2. Bilateral renal arterial stenosis.

3. Causes of renal arterial stenosis are: atherosclerosis 60–90% (ostia and proximal 2 cm), fibromuscular dysplasia, dissection, thromboembolism, aneurysm, AV fistula, vasculitis, polyarteritis nodosa, radiation, neurofibromatosis and retroperitoneal fibrosis.

4. Due to stenosis, there is decreased flow, which leads to decreased perfusion pressure of glomeruli, which in turn produces renin in the juxtaglomerular apparatus. Renin converts angiotensinogen to angiotensin I converted by ACE (angiotensin-converting enzyme) in the vascular endothelium to angiotensin II, which releases aldosterone; this increases salt and water retention and vasoconstriction. Haemodynamically significant lesions are: renin ratio between affected side and normal side >1.5:1; collateral vessels; >70% stenosis; trans-stenotic pressure gradient >40 mmHg; and decrease in renal size. Patients present with abdominal pain, flank pain, haematuria, hypertension, oliguria/anuria and low urine sodium.

5. Screening is indicated for those with hypertension and bruit, accelerated/malignant hypertension, severe hypertension, onset <25 years or >50 years, unilateral small kidney, diastolic pressure >105 mmHg, sudden worsening, refractory and impaired renal function after ACE inhibitors.

6. Investigations used for diagnosis are IVU, Doppler ultrasonography of the abdomen, CT/MRA and captopril scintigraphy. IVU shows delayed appearance of contrast with increased density and delayed washout and notching of the ureter as a result of collaterals. Doppler ultrasonography may visualise the stenotic areas but it is technically challenging as a result of bowel gas, presence of collaterals and multiple renal arteries. Peak systolic velocity in renal artery is > 150 cm/s, ratio of peak renal artery velocity:peak aortic centre stream velocity > 35, post-stenotic spectral broadening, absent flow during diastole. CT and MRA show good visualisation of renal arteries and preclude the need for conventional angiography unless intervention is contemplated.

7. Complications are renal failure, hypertension, cardiac failure and stroke.

8. Antihypertensive therapy is started for mild cases. Renal angioplasty is indicated for high-grade stenosis with stent placement. There is high success rate for non-osteal lesions (80%). Surgical revascularisation should be considered if angioplasty fails. However the result of surgery for controlling renal hypertension in the older age group is poor.

Case 6.11: Answers

1. The CT scan shows a curvilinear flap within the lumen of the thoracic aorta. The flap is seen in the proximal ascending aorta (which is dilated) as well as the descending thoracic aorta. Similar findings are seen in the MRI scan, where the blood is seen as black and the flap is seen within the dark lumen.

2. Aortic dissection, type A

3. Dissection is separation of the aortic intima and adventitia by blood accessing the media of aorta, splitting it into two. It is caused by a combination of medial degeneration that decreases cohesiveness, within the aortic wall, and the hydrodynamic forces of systemic hypertension.

No intimal tear is identified in 5%. Common causes of dissection are hypertension, Marfan syndrome, Ehlers–Danlos syndrome, coarctation, bicuspid aortic valve, prosthetic valve, trauma, aortic stenosis, relapsing polychondritis, Turner syndrome, pregnancy, SLE and cocaine. Syphilis does not cause dissection.

4. The most common site is the anterior and right lateral wall of the ascending aorta, just distal to the valve. Other sites are the superior and posterior wall of the transverse aortic arch, and the posterior left lateral wall of the upper descending aorta distal to the left subclavian artery.

5. There are two classification systems.

    Stanford's: type A affects ascending aorta; type B – ascending aorta not involved.

    Debakey's: I – entire aorta; II – ascending aorta only; III – descending aorta.

6. A chest X-ray is normal or shows displacement of calcification in a patient with known disease, by 4–10 mm from the outer aortic contour. The contour of the aorta is irregular and the superior mediastinum widened (> 8 cm). Left pleural effusion and left basal atelectasis are seen. CT with contrast is the investigation of choice. Non-contrast CT may show high-density clot within a false lumen. A contrast scan shows intimal flap separating the true and false lumina. The flap displaces calcification internally. MRI shows similar appearances and may also show cobwebs, marking the false lumen. Differential diagnosis is a penetrating ulcer of the thoracic aorta.

7. Complications are aortic insufficiency, coronary artery occlusion, pericardial effusion, pleural effusion, rupture into right ventricle/left atrium/SVC/pulmonary artery, producing left-to-right shunt and occlusion of branch vessels as a result of flap entering the branch vessel origin or covering it like a curtain. Organs can receive a blood supply from a true lumen, a false lumen or both. An aneurysm can originate from the lumina.

8. Type A dissections require immediate surgical graft reinforcement of the aortic wall to prevent rupture and aortic insufficiency. Type B dissections require antihypertensives. There is a 10–35% mortality rate from surgery.

Case 6.12: Answers

1. The abdominal X-ray shows a large soft tissue mass in the lower part of the abdomen, which obliterates the left psoas outline and displaces the bowel loops. CT scan of the abdomen shows a large calcified abdominal aorta. The contrast-filled lumen appears irregular due to intraluminal thrombosis. There is extensive retroperitoneal infiltrate in the periaortic region, extending to both flanks. The mixed density of the infiltrate represents a retroperitoneal leak of blood.

2. Ruptured abdominal aortic aneurysm (AAA).

3. Causes of an AAA: atherosclerosis, syphilis, mycotic, trauma, cystic medial necrosis, arteritis (Takayasu's arteritis, giant cell arteritis, rheumatic arteritis, ankylosing spondylitis, Reiter syndrome, SLE, ulcerative colitis, scleroderma, Behçet's disease), hypertension and aortic regurgitation.

4. An AAA can be associated with aneurysm of the visceral arteries, renal arteries, iliac artery, femoral artery aneurysm, stenosis/occlusion of SMA/ coeliac trunk/renal artery/inferior mesenteric artery/lumbar arteries.

5. An AAA is dilatation of an abdominal aorta. A measurement of 3 cm is used to diagnose an aneurysm. It is common in men, especially aged > 60 years. The aneurysm can be true (all layers of wall present) or false (focal perforation with all layers disrupted, contained by adventitia). Based on the shape it can be fusiform or saccular.

6. Rupture, thrombosis, embolism, infection and occlusion are complications of abdominal aortic aneurysm. Rupture usually occurs into retroperitoneum on the left side, into the GI tract, or into the IVC.

7. Abdominal aortic aneurysms are often discovered incidentally in ultrasound or CT. In ultrasound the aorta is enlarged, with patent lumen, often with intraluminal thrombosis. On contrast enhanced CT, the aorta is enlarged, with eccentric thrombus and small, but patent lumen. CT scan is very useful for treatment planning, since it gives the dimensions and distance from renal arteries and iliac arteries, which are important factors for placing an endograft. Similar information can be obtained by MRI and MR angiography. When the aneurysm ruptures, it is seen as soft tissue opacity in the plain X-ray, with loss of psoas outline. When the

rupture is contained, there is hyperdense clot in the thrombus. Crescent sign indicates high-density crescent in the aneurysm, signifying impending rupture. When there is frank rupture, the CT shows a large retroperitoneal haematoma in the non-contrast scan. Contrast extravasation is seen and there is anterior displacement of the kidney. Fluid collection/haematoma is seen in posterior pararenal space/perirenal space/psoas, with free intraperitoneal fluid. There is perinephric stranding. When the rupture is contained, there is extraluminal haematoma surrounding the aorta.

8. In asymptomatic individuals, abdominal aneurysm can be followed by annual ultrasonography. A CT scan is used for surgical and endoprosthesis planning. The factors assessed are location, type, infra-/suprarenal, proximal extent, neck, sac, distance from bifurcation and iliac artery involvement. Enlarging aneurysms > 5 cm undergo repair. Ruptured aneurysms require emergency surgery. The mortality rate is 30–80% for ruptured aneurysms.

Case 6.13: Answers

1. The first picture shows a catheter in the IVC. A metallic device is being deployed in the distal aspect of the catheter.

2. The second film shows a metallic stent in the optimal portion in the IVC.

3. Indications for IVC filter are:

    DVT or PE in a patient with a contraindication to anticoagulation

    DVT/PE in a patient with complications from anticoagulation

    Failure of anticoagulation therapy

    Free floating iliofemoral or caval thrombosis

    Prophylaxis to prevent PE in high-risk patients (surgery, chronic pulmonary hypertension, caner, trauma).

4. IVC filters are either temporary and retrievable or permanent. There are many different types of IVC filter, including the Mobin–Uddin umbrella filter, titanium Greenfield filter, etc. The filter should trap most of the thrombi, be non-thrombogenic, biocompatible, structurally strong, should not migrate, should not cause perforation, should be non-ferromagnetic and retrievable when required.

5. Filters are placed under fluoroscopic guidance. Most are placed in the infrarenal IVC. A suprarenal filter is placed when there has been renal vein thrombosis, IVC thrombosis extending above the level of the renal veins, thrombus in the infrarenal IVC, recurrent PE despite infrarenal filter, PE after ovarian vein thrombosis and pregnancy. One of the femoral veins is punctured. A guidewire is passed into the femoral vein and the filter system passed over the guidewire. Then the filter is deployed at the infrarenal portion.

6. Before the procedure, DVT/PE is confirmed. The coagulation profile is tested and, if the patient is already on anticoagulants, it is discontinued before the procedure. The IVC should be assessed for size, configuration, anatomical variation and thrombosis. This can be done by Doppler ultrasonography, cavography, CT or MRI.

7. Contraindications are thrombus between venous access site and deployment site, and therapeutic anticoagulation.

Case 6.14: Answers

1. This is Doppler ultrasonography of the scrotum. There are very prominent venous structures in the scrotum in the spermatic cord and testis.

2. The second film is a plain X-ray, which shows small coils on both sides of the abdomen and groin, along the distribution of the testicular vein.

3. Varicocele, with coil embolisation.

4. A varicocele is dilatation and tortuosity of pampiniform plexus secondary to retrograde flow into the internal spermatic vein (ISV). It is caused by an incompetent or absent valve at the level of the left renal vein/IVC on the right side or compression of the left renal vein by tumour or thrombosis, or an aberrant renal artery.

5. Pampiniform plexus consists of the ISV draining the testis, veins of vas deferens draining the epididymis and the cremasteric vein draining the scrotal wall.

6. Of varicoceles 80% are seen on the left side. Clinically varicoceles are graded:

1: palpable only during Valsalva's manoeuvre

2: palpable without Valsalva's manoeuvre

3: visually detectable.

Scrotal pain, scrotal swelling, altered sperm count, impaired motility and immature sperm are features. Infertility is seen in varicoceles because of increased local temperature, reflux of toxic substances from the adrenal gland, alteration of Leydig cell function and hypoxia of germinal tissue, as a result of venous reflux causing venous hypertension and stasis.

7. Ultrasound with Doppler is the diagnostic procedure of choice. There are two types of varicocele, the **shunt** and the **stop** type. In the **shunt** type, there are insufficient valves in the ISV, which allows continuous and spontaneous reflux into the cremasteric and vas deferens veins. These varicoceles are large and show continuous reflux during Valsalva manoeuvre and are associated with a low sperm count. In the **stop** type, the valves are intact and there is only a brief period of reflux into the other veins during the Valsalva manoeuvre. If the varicoceles are subclinical or small, with a short phase of retrograde flow during Valsalva, sperm quantity is normal. Ultrasound is used to grade varicoceles. In normal patients, the dominant vein in the inguinal canal measures 2.2 mm in the upright position and 2.7 mm during the Valsalva manoeuvre. Small varicoceles are 2.5–4 mm; moderate varicoceles are 4–5 mm; large varicoceles are >5 mm. Venous reflux is graded as static (grade I), intermittent (grade II), or continuous (grade III). Venography can demonstrate reflux in subclinical varicoceles.

8. Varicoceles can be treated by surgery, where the testicular veins are ligated above the inguinal ligament, but recurrence is high due to the presence of collateral channels. Varicoceles can also be treated by embolisation of the left internal spermatic vein, with interruption of retrograde venous flow. Indications are: large varicoceles, varicoceles associated with infertility, pain or atrophy, and recurrent varicoceles. A preliminary diagnostic venogram is obtained. The internal spermatic vein is occluded with detachable balloons, stainless steel or platinum spring-like coils, or various sclerosing agents such as sodium tetradecyl sulphate.

Case 6.15: Answers

1. MRI shows a large, encapsulated lesion of low intensity arising from the posterior wall of the uterus and extending into the whole thickness of the posterior wall of the uterus.

2. Large uterine leiomyoma (fibroid).

3. Uterine artery embolisation with occlusion of the arterial supply to the uterine fibroid.

4. Leiomyomas are benign tumours of the uterus that arise from the overgrowth of smooth muscle and connective tissue in the uterus. Leiomyomas occur most commonly in women > 30 years, but they can occur in females of any age. Most fibroids are intramural (95%), although some could be subserosal or submucosal. Most women with fibroids are asymptomatic. Only 10–20% of patients require treatment. Menorrhagia, abdominal cramps, urinary frequency, urgency, incontinence and infertility are the clinical features. The complications are degeneration, infertility and malignant degeneration (1%). Fibroids in pregnancy cause complications including preterm labour and obstruction of the birth canal.

5. On ultrasonography, the fibroids appear as hypoechoic masses and are more heterogeneous when there is degeneration. On the CT scan they are hypodense and show patchy enhancement. On MRI, they are of low signal intensity on T1- and T2-weighted images as a result of the fibrous content and they show contrast enhancement.

6. Treatment options for fibroids vary and include conservative management, myomectomy and hysterectomy. Uterine artery embolisation is a non-invasive alternative. On a diagnostic angiogram before embolisation, there is distortion and enlargement of the uterine arteries supplying the normal myometrium and fibroids. The flow in the fibroid is substantially increased and perifibroid arteries are larger, although the tumour itself is hypovascular and small centripetal arteries originating in perifibroid arterial plexus supply the interior. Embolisation of these arteries results in a decrease in size and symptoms of the fibroid. Imaging is very important in planning for uterine fibroid embolisation. The factors to be assessed are the size, number, location and degree of vascularisation of the fibroids. Complete occlusion of the uterine arteries with stasis of contrast material is the usual angiographic endpoint when embolisation is performed with a non-spherical polyvinyl alcohol particle.

7. After embolisation, a 35–60% reduction in uterine volume and a 40–80% reduction in fibroid volume have been observed at 3–6 months. Recurrence is observed when the fibroids are not infarcted after unilateral uterine artery embolisation because of either additional supply from other sources or associated adenomyosis.

8. Major complications include passage of fibroid following necrosis, infections, DVT, PE, inadvertent embolisation of a malignant leiomyosarcoma, ovarian dysfunction, regrowth, uterine necrosis and even death. Minor complications include haematoma, UTI, retention of urine, transient pain, and vessel or nerve injury at the puncture site.

Case 6.16: Answers

1. MRA shows a saccular protrusion from the popliteal artery. A patent sapheno-popliteal artery bypass graft is noted on the right side.

2. Popliteal artery aneurysm.

3. Popliteal artery aneurysms are the most common peripheral artery aneurysms; 90% are atherosclerotic. Theories of formation are: turbulence distal to relative stenosis of tendinous hiatus of adductor magnus, and repeated flexion at knee. Most of these aneurysms are fusiform and they are bilateral in 25–70%. They are associated with abdominal aortic aneurysm in 40% of cases, and 1–2% of abdominal aortic aneurysms are associated with popliteal artery aneurysms. Most popliteal artery aneurysms measure 3–4 cm.

4. Doppler ultrasound is the initial investigation. It shows the aneurysm, flow within the lumen, and thrombus when present. It also differentiates aneurysm from Baker's cyst. Angiography is done for evaluation of inflow and outflow. MR angiography is a non-invasive method of assessing the popliteal artery. CT angiography is also very efficient, but involves a high dose of radiation. Clinical presentation is with a palpable pulsatile mass, lower extremity ischaemia, or compression of adjacent structures.

5. Complications are thrombus, embolus, compression of adjacent structures, rupture and limb-threatening ischaemia.

6. The differential diagnosis is Baker's cyst, which is non-pulsatile and shows communication with the joint cavity.

7. Symptomatic aneurysms require repair irrespective of size, because the main complication is thromboembolism, not rupture. Other indications are asymptomatic aneurysms > 2 cm and any aneurysm with thrombus. The aneurysm is ligated and bypassed with a graft. Endoaneurysmorrhapy can be performed with the graft through the aneurysm. Another alternative is resection of the aneurysm and bypass. An endoprosthesis can be placed.

Case 6.17: Answers

1. This is MRA of the carotid vessels, which shows a severe narrowing of the bifurcation of the left common carotid artery (left CCA).

2. Left carotid artery stenosis at its bifurcation. This is a small segment stenosis (<2 cm), with considerable luminal narrowing (>70%).

3. Carotid stenosis is caused by hardening of the arterial wall, which could be a result of diffuse intimal thickening, atherosclerosis, Monckberg's medial sclerosis or hypertensive arteriosclerosis. Reduction of blood flow occurs at 50–60% narrowing. When the narrowing is 75%, it is haemodynamically significant and associated with a 16% incidence of stroke. Plaque ulceration, necrosis and haemorrhage can cause embolic stroke.

4. The most common location of stenosis originates in the right internal carotid artery (ICA). Other locations originate in the left ICA, right vertebral artery and left vertebral artery; 68% of stenoses are stable and 25% have progressive stenosis to > 50% diameter reduction.

5. Carotid Doppler ultrasonography is done to screen for a suspected carotid disease, neurological symptoms, transient ischaemic accident (TIA), stroke, carotid bruit, retinal embolus, preoperative evaluation before major surgery and intraoperative monitoring during endarterectomy.

6. Doppler ultrasound of the neck is a very reliable technique for identifying and grading stenosis. In a normal patient, normal colour flow is seen. When there is stenosis, there is narrowing or complete occlusion and colour flow is not seen. Doppler analysis of the waveform is useful for quantifying the stenosis. Normally the peak systolic velocity is <125 cm/second with a clear window under systole without spectral broadening and no evidence of plaque. In the haemodynamically significant stenosis >70%, the peak systolic velocity is >230 cm/sec, end-diastole is >100 cm/sec, peak velocity ratio of ICA/CCA is >4.0, peak systolic velocity ICA + end diastolic velocity CCA is >15. When the vessel is occluded, there is no flow in ICA, there is absence of diastolic flow in CCA and diastolic flow reversal in CCA. With ultrasound, the plaques may be of the following types – **hypoechoic**: fibrofatty/haemorrhage; **isoechoic**: smooth muscle proliferation; **hyperechoic**: fibrous, calcified; **homogeneous**: fatty and fibrous, no haemorrhage or necrosis; **heterogeneous**: unstable plaque, 27% risk of neurological deficit. Ultrasound is not good for characterising plaque surface. CT and MR angiography are also accurate methods of diagnosing and grading carotid stenosis/occlusion.

7. Significant carotid artery stenosis increases risk for TIA, stroke, occlusion, embolism. Carotid endarterectomy is done if there is haemodynamically significant stenosis. There is 17% reduction of stroke at 2 years for those who undergo surgery. The surgery carries a mortality of 1%.

Case 6.18: Answers

1. The chest X-ray shows a spiculated mass in the right midzone. The CT scan shows a heterogeneous, necrotic mass in the posterior aspect of the right lung.

2. Bronchogenic carcinoma.

3. Lung cancers are broadly divided into small cell cancers and non-small cell cancers (NSCLCs), which include adenocarcinoma, squamous cell carcinoma, bronchoalveolar carcinoma and large cell carcinoma.

4. Lung cancer is the most common fatal malignant neoplasm in men. Predisposing factors are smoking, asbestos, arsenic, chromium, chloromethyl ether, mustard gas and genetic factors. Idiopathic pulmonary fibrosis, systemic sclerosis and TB increase the risk of adenocarcinomas. Patients with central tumours present with wheezing, haemoptysis, cough, infection, laryngeal nerve palsy, pleural or chest wall pain, SVC obstruction

and paraneoplastic syndromes (clubbing, hypertrophic osteoarthropathy, osteomalacia, Cushing syndrome, hyponatraemia, neuromuscular dysfunction, myopathy, neuropathy, cerebellar degeneration and encephalomyelopathy).

5. Chest X-ray is the first investigation with which the tumour is first identified. A CT scan is used for diagnosis and staging. The CT appearances depend on the type of tumour. Adenocarcinomas and bronchoalveolar carcinomas are peripheral and can present as a solitary pulmonary nodule, multifocal disease or a rapidly progressing pneumonic form. Squamous cell carcinomas are usually central, large and often cavitatory. Large cell carcinoma is seen as an ill-defined, large, peripheral mass. Small cell carcinomas are central and present as a hilar mass with obstructive collapse/pneumonia and early metastasis. A CT scan should include the adrenals, because it is a common organ of spread in lung cancers.

6. Diagnosis is confirmed by a biopsy. Central tumours are biopsied through bronchoscopy and peripheral tumours are accessed percutaneously under CT guidance. Bone spread can be assessed by a bone scan. A PET scan assesses systemic metastasis. Brain MRI is indicated if neurological symptoms are present. Chest MRI is useful for assessing chest wall or brachial plexus invasion. Staging is done using the TNM system.

7. Differential diagnoses for lung mass: tuberculoma, histoplasmosis, abscess, atypical pneumonia, lymphoma, metastasis, progressive massive fibrosis, pleural tumours and other nodular lesions of the lungs.

Case 6.19: Answers

1. Doppler ultrasound demonstrates a saccular structure arising from the left femoral artery, which shows swirling flow within it. CT scan in the same patient shows a saccular, contrast-enhancing structure arising from the medial aspect of the proximal common femoral artery.

2. Femoral artery pseudoaneurysm.

3. Pseudoaneurysm is formed as a result of disruption in arterial wall continuity by trauma, inflammation, iatrogenic causes such as surgery, arterial puncture for angiography, biopsy and drainage. The incidence of pseudoaneurysm with angiography is high as 7% with the use of large-bore sheaths, periprocedural anticoagulation and antiplatelet therapy.

4. Clinical features are a mass with a palpable thrill, an audible bruit, a pulsatile mass and secondary effect on adjacent structures. Necrosis of skin and subcutaneous tissue is seen as a result of pressure. Ultrasonography shows a hypoechoic cystic structure adjacent to the femoral artery, demonstrating the size, connection of the sac to the artery, lobes in sac, and the length and width of the neck. Doppler ultrasonography shows a swirling motion called the yin–yang sign. The main finding on Doppler ultrasonography is demonstration of a communicating channel or neck between the sac and feeding artery with a to-and-fro waveform on duplex Doppler ultrasonography. The 'to' component is blood entering the pseudoaneurysm in systole and the 'fro' component is blood exiting it during diastole. CT angiography and MRA are also diagnostic

5. Rupture is the major complication. Haemorrhage and thrombus are other complications.

6. The most important differential diagnosis is an abscess, especially in someone who is an intravenous drug abuser. Abscess is hypoechoic and shows no flow within it. Hernia, enlarged lymph node and soft tissue mass are other lesions which are included in the differential diagnosis. Doppler sonography can be used to differentiate these, as flow is not seen in any of these lesions.

7. Small asymptomatic pseudoaneuryms are just observed, but symptomatic pseudoaneurysms are treated. Pseudoaneurysms are usually treated under radiological guidance The options are US-guided compression, ultrasound-guided percutaneous thrombin injection and endovascular management with embolisation/stent graft placement. Pressure is applied to the pseudoaneurysm neck for 10–30 minutes. Compression eliminates flow to the aneurysm, which then clots, but flow to the extremity continues. Thrombin can be injected into the pseudoaneurysm, which converts inactive fibrinogen into fibrin leading to thrombus formation. Thrombin is injected slowly (0.5–1.0 mL), until the flow of blood ceases within the pseudoaneurysm.

COLOUR IMAGES

Case 2.25

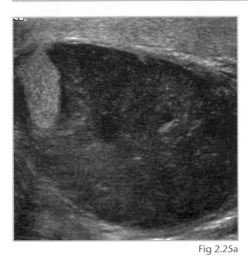

Fig 2.25a

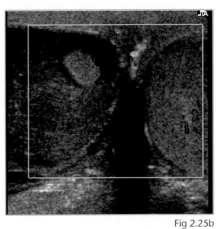

Fig 2.25b

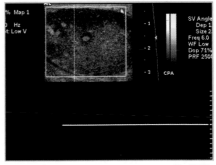

Fig 2.25c

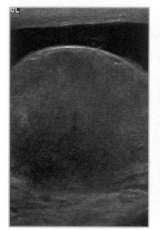

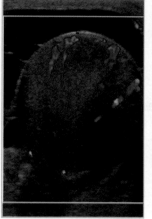

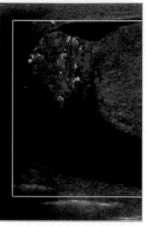

Fig 2.26a   Fig 2.26b   Fig 2.26c

Case 6.8

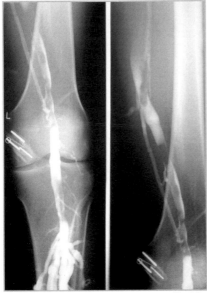

Fig 6.8a

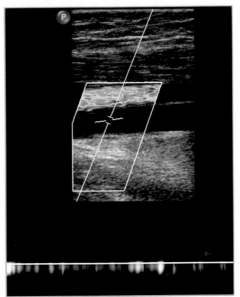

Fig 6.8b

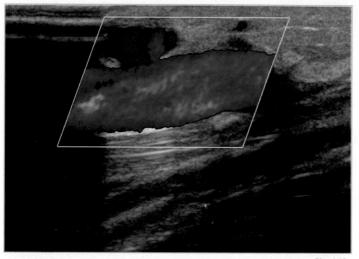

Fig 6.19a

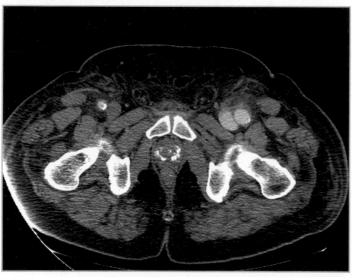

Fig 6.19b

INDEX